T0375365

# CARDIAC FIBRILLATION-DEFIBRILLATION

## Clinical and Engineering Aspects

# SERIES ON BIOENGINEERING AND BIOMEDICAL ENGINEERING

**Series Editor**: John K-J Li *(Department of Biomedical Engineering, Rutgers University, USA)*

Series on Bioengineering & Biomedical Engineering – Vol. 6

# CARDIAC FIBRILLATION-DEFIBRILLATION
## Clinical and Engineering Aspects

### Max E Valentinuzzi
University of Buenos Aires, Argentina &
University of Tucumán, Argentina

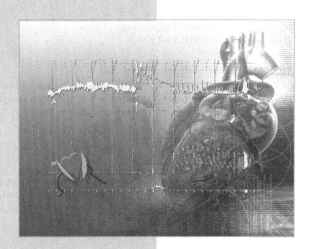

**World Scientific**

NEW JERSEY · LONDON · SINGAPORE · BEIJING · SHANGHAI · HONG KONG · TAIPEI · CHENNAI

*Published by*

World Scientific Publishing Co. Pte. Ltd.

5 Toh Tuck Link, Singapore 596224

*USA office:* 27 Warren Street, Suite 401-402, Hackensack, NJ 07601

*UK office:* 57 Shelton Street, Covent Garden, London WC2H 9HE

**British Library Cataloguing-in-Publication Data**
A catalogue record for this book is available from the British Library.

**Series on Bioengineering and Biomedical Engineering — Vol. 6**
**CARDIAC FIBRILLATION-DEFIBRILLATION**
**Clinical and Engineering Aspects**

ISBN-13 978-981-4293-63-1
ISBN-10 981-4293-63-6

Typeset by Stallion Press
Email: enquiries@stallionpress.com

Printed in Singapore.

To Nilda,
my lifelong love.
For she was there,
during laughs and tears, health and sickness, joy and grief,
ups and downs.
Through storms and sunny days, behind weaknesses
and by strengths,
when darkness came over and when the light was back on.
Near, very near, even if physically distant.
Yes, she was always there... unyieldingly and stubbornly there...

And, by the way...
do you know how many dogs docilely gave their lives
in the experimental laboratory to
improve our knowledge of cardiac arrhythmias?
Only the Great Engineer has the right and exact number,
but whatever it is, it is for sure
large, large, large... and those lives were given
to and for us, human beings.
Thus, as someone said, if Heaven is not the place where dogs go
after death, wherever that
place is, I want to go to that same place when my time come.

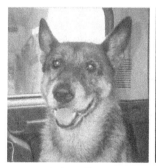 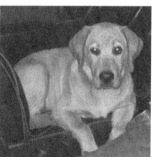 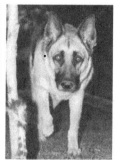

**Apollo** **Tropi** **Huanki**
**(1993–2005)** **(2007–)** **(1993–2005)**

A memento also to
Leslie Alexander Geddes
(May 24, 1921–October 25, 2009)

He taught me that the objective of a project must always start
with a verb in infinitive, to mean action;
He showed me the failing meanders of a fibrillating heart
and amazed me when that huge machine delivered impressive
high shocks in its vain attempt to recover the equine ventricles;
He put me in front of an open-chest dog to massage its rapid waving
cardiac fibers as if "milking a cow in reverse";
He was my teacher, made me feel his collaborator, and gently
pushed me in this long fascinating bumpy road.

May the Great Engineer find, up there, a good lab for you!


Max E. Valentinuzzi
Yerba Buena, Tucumán, Argentina
February 7, 2010

# CONTENTS

# PREFACE

After a number of years at Baylor College of Medicine, in Houston, Texas, under the mentorship of Drs. Hebbel E. Hoff and Leslie A. Geddes, my family and I returned to our native country, Argentina, in 1972, about one year after the return of Dr. René G. Favaloro, who also had been in the USA for considerable time, at the Cleveland Clinic, Ohio, where he developed the coronary by-pass surgery. Hebbel and Les deeply influenced my academic life and introduced me to cardiac fibrillation–defibrillation. Vivid in my memory still are the many experiments carried out over the years...and I brought the subject over to Tucumán, well kept in my portfolio of plans and dreams. Those were not easy years in Argentina, plagued with upheaval, social unrest, and increasing violence. The country was taken over by a cruel military dictatorship, which fortunately ended in 1983, when democracy came back after the disastrous and insane Malvinas' Islands War of 1982. How many sad, dramatic stories we could tell!

In 1981, while struggling to hold and put things together in a rather indifferent and even hostile environment, I was lucky enough to meet René in Buenos Aires through a common old friend, Dr. Ricardo H. Pichel, now President of the Favaloro University. That was the beginning of scientific collaboration between his group and ours, both in their early stages yet, that lasted for several productive years working on the intra-ventricular pressure–volume loop concept, as a tool to better grasp cardiac performance. His ideas and ideals as well as mine, so many times discussed in private informal chats, either over the phone or facing a cup of tea, matched perfectly, we were meant for each other. He had a clear understanding of what academic life, scientific research, technical development, bioengineering, medical practice and human sympathy and empathy are about. His influence was also profound, and I will never stop mourning his undeserved abrupt departure (Pichel and Valentinuzzi, 2001).

Mainly based on a first period of research and development at the Laboratory of Bioengineering of the *Universidad Nacional de Tucumán*, roughly between 1974 and 1984, always signed by shortage of funds, meager overall support and recognition, a small book was published in Spanish in 1986, I dare say in spite of the streams against. A small group of young and enthusiastic collaborators plus a few dedicated believers, all hard workers, were no doubt an essential driving force. René, kindly, wrote a nice presenting prologue reminiscing some of his own experiences (Valentinuzzi *et al.*, 1986). That book (Geddes, 1987), well received by the medical and bioengineering audiences at that time (its publisher, -INTERMEDICA-, kindly authorized the reproduction of several of its figures) was the seed, indeed, of the present new one, now fully updated and revamped, for many advances and changes took place in the elapsed 25 years or more. Our laboratory added also some results because we continued to be active in the area for a few more years after the book was out in the market.

Hence, the product is here and a brief overall introductory description appears convenient so that the potential reader/user has a picture of what the book is about. Let us start with its sources, which are recognized as four,

— Personal experience in the subject as active researcher for many years;
— The regular literature published in main stream journals and books;
— The World Wide Web (often downloading pieces clearly indicating their origin); and
— Personal contacts with a few authors.

All these are carefully referenced as the text develops. Such bibliography is not exhaustive because this book, I emphasize, does not intend to be a review. Moreover, by now after more than 100 years of laboratory and clinical research and technological development of so many people in so many places, the amount of material found in the specialized literature is so huge that I think it defies the would-be intention of any serious author who might dare into such project. As a consequence, we apologize for those and to those whose contributions are not discussed, quoted, or referred to herein, either by sheer ignorance or for not having considered them as necessary.

INTERNET has played a fundamental role in the process of globalization and its impact on scientific literature is impressive and in growing process, even though sometimes not always is fully reliable. Through it, several databases are available, too, some with open access abstracts or full texts or with some restrictions (PubMed, MEDLINE, SCOPE). WIKIPEDIA is another nice and easy source, widely accessed by students, which quickly orients the searcher where to proceed (but do not take as granted everything it says). Papers and books nowadays

make use of specific websites as references and this book is no exception
to that tendency. Recall that a great amount of information is freely and
generously offered, as the true scientific spirit is (contrasting with the patent
spirit, which tends to hide in the expectation of future potential profits).
These words intend to neutralize possible and probable criticisms when
readers discover that this or that paragraph is similar to one found in
INTERNET ... well, yes, it is true, and no shame about it, no plagiarism
at all, full credit is given and full recognition is made to the many often
unknown authors. To them all, and deeply, thanks a lot! And if something or
someone was unwillingly or inadvertently skipped, please, let me know, and
accept my sincere apologies. However, even though gratuity of such publicly
available information is granted, in all cases the Website address is given
and many times the scientific and technical papers' references too, where
full details are to be found. Where copyright was needed and required,
proper permission was requested to either the authors or the editors or
publishers.

Given the characteristics of the subject at large, almost all chapters
show a certain degree of repetition, sometimes in more detail or in other
places rather superficially, and such repetition is good and acceptable from
a didactic point of view. It is, for example, unavoidable to refer to time
as one of the fibrillation variables and to come back to it when dealing
with cardiopulmonary resuscitation, or to speak of the impedance seen
by the defibrillating paddles and to return to it when defining the load
presented to the machine or when insisting on the different components
of that load. Besides, the book is *interdisciplinary*, *multidisciplinary*, and
*transdisciplinary*, as any bioengineering product should be, and recognizing
the relatively minor etymological and linguistic differences in the meanings
of these words; the suffixes *inter-*, *multi-* and *trans-*, respectively, indicate
crossing from one discipline into other, participation of more than one
discipline, and the latter a form of knowledge integration.

Historically, the advances in fibrillation–defibrillation knowledge may
be divided into three intermixed aspects:

1. Recognition of fibrillation as a unique life threatening cardiac
   arrhythmia;
2. Discovery of the electric discharge in its double role of culprit and
   savior; and
3. Technological and steadily improved contributions, from very crude and
   rudimentary equipment, to the automatic external pieces, to the recent

very small and "clever" implanted combined models of defibrillator–
pacemakers. The word "clever" above is shyly and respectfully employed
after reading a little and difficult book by a group of highly recognized
neuroscientists and philosophers (Bennet *et al.*, 2007), for its many
implications could greatly complicate the scenery. Thus, since no other
better word seems available, "clever" is simply used as technological
qualification.

The last two broad types, external and internal defibrillators, will
continue to be produced, used, and improved for they have very specific
applications: the former are intended for the open-chest surgery room and
the domestic or industrial or public cardiac emergency, while the latter is
specific to the ambulatory risk cardiac patient.

Injuries due to defibrillating shocks will be only marginally mentioned,
for two reasons: First, the subject has been discussed at large by several
authors (Tacker and Geddes, 1980; Valentinuzzi *et al.*, 1986; Wilson *et al.*,
1989), and second, advances in electrodes, leads and technology, especially
with the implanted type, have considerably reduced the applied energy
levels, so that now the problem has relatively taken a backward step.
Nonetheless, post-defibrillation cardiac damage continuous to be a risk,
even at the low intensities so far achieved. Selection of waveforms may help
but there is not yet a definite fully preventive prescription.

The book is composed of an INTRODUCTION and eight CHAPTERS.
The INTRODUCTION sets up the subject, especially within the overall
context of the Framingham Study. The first CHAPTER deals with
fibrillation, including its definition, mechanisms, causes, types, clinical
significance, variables, and thresholds. Chapter 2 takes care of defibrillation,
as an intervention. Definition and early developments, chemical and
electrical defibrillation, variables, thresholds, and the concept of dose
are introduced, proceeding thereafter with cardiopulmonary resuscitation
(CPR) and cardioversion or atrial defibrillation. Finally, ablation is also
touched.

Defibrillators are the well-controlled generators to deliver the reversing
discharge; they are described in Chap. 3, which is divided into five sections:
types of defibrillators, external defibrillators, internal defibrillators,
implantable defibrillators and, finally, the defibrillator's cousins, the
pacemakers. However, do not expect to find the latest model in it. This
book is NOT a prescription; besides, technologies constantly evolve.

Chapter 4 deals with the touchy detection of fibrillation. It is coauthored with a young and able researcher, specialist in cardiac signal processing, Dr. Eric Laciar, currently a Professor and Investigator at the Engineering School of the *Universidad Nacional de San Juan*, Argentina. The criteria for detection, parameter evaluation, and several algorithms are presented, closing with the possible defibrillation pain that may occur when the shock is applied too soon.

Interfaces are often, if not always, a bottleneck, so that ELECTRODES and PASTES constitute the subject matter of Chap. 5, where the electrode–tissue impedance is considered along with the type of electrodes and the electrolytic material needed to reduce electric current hindrance during transchest shocks, for the direct procedure, being intrinsically wet, does not require any.

A Clinical Engineering concern regarding medical equipment lies on how efficacious and safe the procedure is, and no wonder, since the subject is strongly linked to legal liabilities. Hence, Chap. 6 defines and discusses safety levels (patient, operator, and equipment), the concept of isolation, electromagnetic interference, and possible incompatibility with other devices. Standards are briefly touched ending with any possible pain (here we find a repetition, as mentioned before). A former student of mine, Juan M. Olivera, EE, MSc, currently Assistant Professor at the Department of Bioengineering of the *Universidad Nacional de Tucumán*, lent me a kind hand, especially in those aspects dealing with standards.

Not every reader will be attracted to or interested in or even may not be prepared for Chap. 7 because it handles theoretical models. Such reader can skip the chapter without losing touch with the overall subject. It is coauthored with Drs. Diego Gonzalez and Simone Giannerini, longstanding investigators at the University of Bologna, in Italy.

The final Chap. 8 attempts to lump everything in few essential concepts trying also to show new avenues for research, development, and possible applications. A definite and not yet resolved area is a good theoretical background which might lead to better predictions. So far, the area is rather empirical.

Interspersed in the text, subjects are also seen from their historical side for often, beyond mere curiosity, such view helps understanding and setting them up. Moreover, each chapter is preceded by an abstract and finished with conclusions and a set of simple review questions.

This book is addressed to undergraduate and graduate biomedical engineering students, physicians going into cardiology, clinical engineers and clinical engineering technicians, nurses, paramedics, and emergency medical personnel. Those who are interested only in the practical aspects, may skip Chaps. 4 (detection) and 7 (theoretical models), which are more demanding in terms of previous knowledge. Full requirements call for algebra, differential and integral calculus, basic circuit theory, cardiovascular physiology, electrophysiology, and elementary physics, but with the exception of the two mentioned chapters, any nurse or physician or technician or undergraduate student of any level can delve into the rest without problem. The book stands on the well-known philosophy of Education Based on Problems (or EBP), that is, take fibrillation as a medical daily problem and search for that knowledge, technique or principle, no matter where it comes from, that solves it, either partially or fully, and most of the time the advance is in small partial steps. In simple words, you must be an active reader and, if possible, an actor!

Max E. Valentinuzzi
Yerba Buena (at the foothill of the *Cerros*),
Tucumán, Argentina
January 7, 2010
maxvalentinuzzi@arnet.com.ar
maxvalentinuzzi@hotmail.com
maxvalentinuzzi@gmail.com
maxvalentinuzzi@ieee.org

# ACKNOWLEDGMENTS

This book took a long time and hard effort. Recognition must be given to several persons who, one way or another, made the project crystallize.

First of all, I must recall the personnel of the Laboratory of Bioengineering, at the *Universidad Nacional de Tucumán* (UNT), who during my active research years produced many papers on the subject. Grants in that period came from the *Secretaría de Ciencia y Técnica* (SECYT), *Consejo Nacional de Investigaciones Científicas y Técnicas* (CONICET), and *Consejo de Investigaciones de la Universidad Nacional de Tucumán* (CIUNT), all in Argentina.

The publisher, WSP, where Dr. John K. Li and Ms. Yubin Zhai were key persons, for their confidence and support. To Mr. Steven Patt, editor, constantly giving me practical details to proceed. To the unknown reviewers of the initial proposal, for comments and suggestions.

Dr. Eric Laciar Leber, from the *Universidad Nacional de San Juan*, Argentina, and Drs. Diego González and Simone Giannerini, from the *Università di Bologna*, Italy, for the co-authorship, respectively, of Chaps. 4 and 7.

To Prof. Juan M. Olivera, from the Department of Bioengineering, UNT, for reviewing Chap. 6.

To Leslie A. Geddes, one of my teachers, long and heavy contributor to the subject, and to his memory; he reviewed the outline of this book and gave me some advices, among them, for example, are the simple questions at the end of each chapter.

# INTRODUCTION

*If the heart trembles,*
*it has little power and sinks,*
*the disease is advancing and death is near.*
*Ebers Papyrus ~3500 BC*

As the translated words quoted above would indicate, the phenomenon is as old as our heart and, thus, it should not surprise us if now, many centuries away, cardiovascular disease (CVD) is considered the leading cause of death and serious illness, not only in the United States, but also all over the world, with relatively minor numerical variations from site to site. Early in time, not many people reached an age old enough to develop heart disease (they died rather young mostly of other causes), thus, its significant incidence started to show up when life expectancy grew to the levels we encounter nowadays in the more advanced societies. The Center for Health Statistics, Department of Health, USA (http://www.cdc.gov/NCHS/data/ nvsr/nvsr57/nvsr57_14.pdf) gives, for the years 2003–2006, the rank of deaths due to heart disease by age group: deaths under 14 years of age fell well below and were not ranked; at age between 14 and 24 ranked 5; at age 25–44 ranked 4; at age 45–64 ranked 2; and only over 65 the number of deaths due to heart disease took the first place (see *National Vital Statistics Reports*, vol 57, number 14, April 17, 2009). Good figures are needed for world deaths due to malnutrition and car accidents, the latter in younger groups far exceed cardiac origin.

In 1948, the Framingham Heart Study, under the direction of the National Heart Institute (now known as the National Heart, Lung, and Blood Institute; NHLBI), embarked on an ambitious project in health research. At the time, little was known about the general causes of heart disease and stroke, but the death rates for CVD had been increasing steadily since the beginning of the century and had become an American epidemic. Since 1971, the Framingham Heart Study has been conducted in collaboration with Boston University.

**The town of Framingham** ($\cong$70,000 people) is located in eastern Massachusetts, near Boston. In 1948, it was selected by the U.S. Public Health Service as a cardiovascular study site, and 5,209 healthy residents between 30 and 60 years of age, both men and women, were enrolled as the first cohort. It was the first major cardiovascular study to recruit women participants, so beginning the first round of extensive physical examinations and lifestyle interviews that they would later analyze. Since that date, the subjects have continued to return to the study every two years for a detailed medical history, physical examination, and laboratory tests. In its first year, the study responsibilities were assumed by the National Heart Institute, now the National Heart, Lung, and Blood Institute. Through a contract with the NHLBI, researchers from the Boston University School of Medicine (BUSM) have played an important role in the Framingham Heart Study. Both NHLBI and BUSM scientists have added to our knowledge about reducing disability and death from heart disease. In 1971, the study recruited 5,124 children (and their spouses) of the original cohort for a second study, the "Offspring Study." With two generations of data, the Framingham Project acquired an unmatched amount of information. These studies have become regarded as overestimating risk, but they are generally accepted as outstanding and useful.

The objective of the Framingham Heart Study was to identify the common factors or characteristics that contribute to CVD by following its development over a long period of time in a large group of participants who had not yet developed overt symptoms. Among the already well-established facts, the following should be listed as beyond discussion or without any hint of doubt: In 1960, cigarette smoking found to increase the risk of heart disease; in 1961, cholesterol level, blood pressure, and electrocardiogram abnormalities found to increase the risk of heart disease; in 1967, physical activity found to reduce the risk of heart disease and obesity to increase the risk of heart disease; in 1970, high blood pressure found to increase the risk of stroke; in 1976, menopause found to increase the risk of heart disease; in 1978, psychosocial factors found to affect heart disease; in 1988, high levels of high-density lipoproteins (HDL) found to reduce risk of death; in 1994, enlarged left ventricle shown to increase the risk of stroke; and in 1996, progression from hypertension to heart failure was described.

A similar longitudinal study has been carried out in a high proportion of the residents of Busselton, a town in Western Australia, over a period of many years; however, Framingham is more widely cited. Other references regarding risk factors include an editorial of the *British Medical Journal* (2003) and contributions as that of Levy and Brink (2005), to mention only a few. Available material for research is indeed abundant.

Fibrillation is a specific subject encompassed within the overall framework of cardiac pathologies. Moss (2003), for example, offered an account on the history of atrial fibrillation, while Wang *et al.* (2003) proposed a risk score for predicting stroke or death for individuals with atrial fibrillation. This book deals specifically with both types of fibrillation, atrial and ventricular, the former compatible with life and the latter fully incompatible, stressing that many of the frequently referred to as *he/she died of a heart attack* in the daily common language is nothing else than ventricular fibrillation. Since the previous condition of the patient and the circumstances surrounding the event may strongly influence the outcome (survival or death), it is appropriate here to cite a joint position paper authored by the American College of Sports Medicine and the American Heart Association (freely available in the WEB). It was published concurrently, in 2002, in *Medicine & Science in Sports & Exercise* and in *Circulation*, written by a group of experts (Gary J. Balady, Bernard Chaitman, Carl Foster, Erika Froelicher, Neil Gordon, and Steven Van Camp) under the title "Automated external defibrillators (AED) in health-fitness facilities". And why in health-fitness facilities? To answer the question, the report clearly says:

"Obviously, the risk of a cardiovascular event is greater among individuals with cardiovascular disease than among presumably healthy people. As the demographics of the more than 30 million individuals who exercise at health-fitness facilities demonstrate a steady increase in the number of members older than 35 yr (approximately 55% of current membership), it is reasonable to presume that the number of members with cardiovascular disease is rising as well. Although there are no data regarding the incidence of cardiac arrest at health-fitness facilities, two recent surveys provide some important insight. A large database consisting of more than 2.9 million members of a large commercial health-fitness facility chain demonstrates 71 deaths (mean age 52-13 yr; 61 men, 10 women) occurring over a 2-year period, yielding a rate of **1 death/100,000 members/year**. The death rate was highest among those members who exercised less frequently, such that nearly half of exercise-related deaths were in those who exercised less than once/week. A recent survey of 65 randomly chosen health-fitness facilities in Ohio reports the occurrence of sudden cardiac arrest or heart attack in 17% of facilities during a 5-year period. Notably, only 3% of facilities had an AED on site. Thus, it is prudent to conclude that health-fitness facilities should be considered among the sites in which Public Access Defibrillation (PAD) programs should be established." Well, all the subjects barely anticipated above are covered in the following chapters, hopefully with enough detail and depth.

Quite interesting, but not surprising, patients with heart attacks and other forms of chest pain were found as three to five times more likely to experience serious complications after hospital admission when treated in a crowded emergency department (ED), according to Pines *et al.*'s (2009) report.

Life expectancy has significantly increased, daily habits along with quality of life have also changed, and large city technological facilities have improved making us envision deeper changes . . . at least in First World Countries . . . in the rest, the so-called Third World, things show a different picture, darker and less promising (Valentinuzzi, 2004). An overt and dear wish, as author well rooted in this beautiful and at the same time painful Latin America (part of that Third World, although politicians often try to sell a brighter picture), is that this book reach also the working desk of the many professionals, at all levels, working in hospitals and laboratories, health dispensaries and small industries, medical, engineering and technical schools, carrying not only information in this particular cardiology subject to contribute to its understanding and to assist in saving lives, but a message urging to,

LEARN ALL YOU ARE ABLE TO, BECAUSE YOU HAVE BRAIN;
MAKE THE DECISION, BECAUSE YOU KNOW;
DO IT, BECAUSE YOU CAN.

And finally, always remember and honor your teachers (even those that were not so good), simultaneously respecting and honoring your disciples, too (Valentinuzzi, 2008).

# Chapter 1

# FIBRILLATION

*Like a handful of worms...*

The arrhythmia called fibrillation is introduced as a generalized disordered activity of the cardiac fibers with no actual output of blood from the chambers. Its mechanisms of maintenance are tentatively explained by the reentry, the multiple ectopic foci, or the rotor theories, which are supported only partially by experimental and/or theoretical evidence. By and large, a disturbance starts up the arrhythmia, often in a sensitized heart, but not necessarily always so. Thus, the *setting* of the phenomenon and the *type of disturbance* become relevant, leading to the so-called *clinical fibrillation* (due to disease), *industrial* or *domestic fibrillation* (due to electric accidental shock), and *surgical fibrillation* (due probably to handling). Since the mammalian heart is structurally and electrophysiologically inhomogeneous, a disturbance can be viewed as some added extra-inhomogeneity, which increases the probability of triggering the phenomenon. Thus, electrical, mechanical, chemical, and thermal energies are the different disturbances to add inhomogeneity. Cardiac fibrillation can be classified on the basis of its *etiology* (primary or secondary), *localization* (atrial or ventricular), or *characteristics* (strong or weak). Its clinical and surgical significance is underlined while the fibrillation variables, divided into electrophysiologic and metabolic, are discussed. Since the arrhythmia is a group phenomenon, the concept of minimal mass appears as a pertinent quantity yet to be numerically determined. The minimum magnitude (amplitude in adequate units, of whatever kind) required to trigger fibrillation is called *fibrillation threshold*. When electrically induced, it is called electrical fibrillation threshold (EFT), as a parameter to evaluate and test the sensitivity of the myocardium to the arrhythmia. Single rectangular pulses or train of pulses, either synchronized or not with the QRS complex, can be used as testing signal, wherefrom a time window of weakness called vulnerable period is found, which roughly coincides with the duration of the T-wave. Some numerical illustrative values taken from the literatures are offered.

## 1.1. Definition

Cardiac electrical activity triggers the mechanical activity of the heart — its contraction — both in the atria and in the ventricles. Mechanical contraction absolutely cannot occur without the former while cases of the

1

opposite situation may be found, that is, existence of electrical activity and no contraction whatsoever. In normal conditions, there is a time sequence of events: First, atrial electrical activity (the P-wave) followed by atrial contraction and, thereafter, ventricular electrical activity (the QRS complex) followed by ventricular contraction and its important physiological consequence, ejection of blood, via the aorta from the left ventricle and pulmonary artery from the right side, to the peripheral and to the lung circulations, respectively. The nomenclature P and QRS belongs to the traditional wave identification in the electrocardiogram (ECG), as established by its founder, Wilhelm Einthoven (1903).

The electrical activity, first in the atria and second in the ventricles, after rapid conduction and distribution throughout the whole myocardial mass takes place in synchronism, thus giving a degree of simultaneity, to the atria first and to the ventricles thereafter — i.e. there is overall depolarization of the fibers — essential for an effective systolic action. Under certain circumstances, however, such synchronism is lost and the atria or the ventricles fall in the state known as *fibrillation*. Therefore, *cardiac fibrillation can be defined as the phenomenon of asynchronic or uncoordinated or chaotic activity either of the atrial or of the ventricular fibers*.

Overall asynchronism is electrical and mechanical, and effective ejection disappears. Figures 1.1 and 1.2 illustrate, respectively, records of atrial and ventricular fibrillation (VF), both recorded from experimental dogs. The electrical activity shows a chaotic nature, with no clear rhythmicity even though frequencies in the order of 300–600 cycles per minute can be detected if the Fourier spectrum is calculated (Clayton *et al.*, 1994); there are, however, reports of somewhat higher values. In fibrillation, the atria do not eject blood any more to the ventricles although ventricular filling is still accomplished due to passive pressure gradient; in the second case, VF, aortic and pulmonary artery pressures, instead, fall rapidly to essentially zero. When the myocardium is looked at, it resembles a handful of moving worms, for which reason sometimes the phenomenon has been described as *worm-like activity*.

In order to illustrate with an analogy (Fig. 1.3), let us consider a team of rowers when competing with their boat in a race. The helmsman, usually a smaller and light guy, steers the boat and acts as pacemaker by rhythmically shouting so that the rowers move their oars in synchronism. If for some reason a disturbance takes place, as for example a bee stings one of the rowers and he slaps it, he may break the synchronism bringing very likely

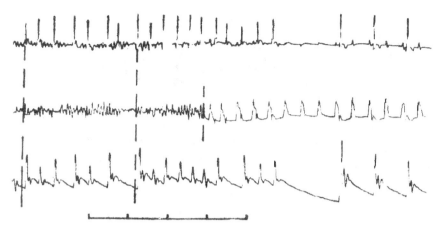

Fig. 1.1.   Induced atrial fibrillation in the dog. Top: Surface ECG. Middle: Jugular lead into the right atrium. Bottom: Carotid blood pressure. Time marks below one sec apart. Observe the pulse deficit within the time interval between the two vertical dashed bars on the left when comparing the top and the bottom channels. Spontaneous defibrillation at the third vertical dashed bar followed by AV block. Records obtained by the author at the Laboratory of Bioengineering; reproduced from Valentinuzzi *et al.*, 1986, with kind permission of the publisher.

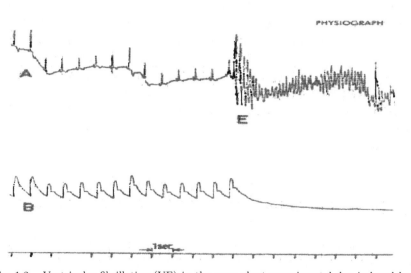

Fig. 1.2.   Ventricular fibrillation (VF) in the open chest experimental dog induced by an electric stimulus (E) applied to the myocardium. Channel A is the surface ECG (lead II). Blood pressure, in Channel B, fell rapidly to almost zero level. Obtained by the author at the Laboratory of Bioengineering, UNT, Tucumán. Valentinuzzi *et al.*, 1986, with kind permission of its publisher.

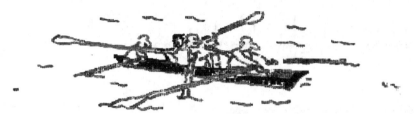

Fig. 1.3.   Analogy: A team of rowers needs to row in synchronism if they are to win the race. Here the rowers are shown fully out of phase, that is, they would hardly advance. In similar way, cardiac fibers tend to act on their own when in fibrillation, both electrically and mechanically.

the rest of the team into disorganized movements. Each tends to act on his own, as the fibers of a fibrillating heart with mixed action potentials result in different not coordinated fiber lengths.

## 1.2. Mechanisms

There are two basic and rather simple theories that traditionally try to explain the phenomenon of cardiac fibrillation. The first one was proposed early in the 1900s, independently and within less than one year span, by Mines (1913, 1914) and Garrey (1914). It is known as the **Theory of Circus Motion** or **Reentry**. The second is called the **Multiple Ectopic Foci Theory**. Even a third position claims the arrhythmia to be a consequence of a combined effect of the previous two events. Also Lewis (1925), McKenzie's disciple, in his classical treatise, described these mechanisms. More recent insights, however, say since the 1980s, based on some experimental evidence and mathematical and computer models, have proposed the more complex and still unsettled **Rotor or Vortex Theory** (Rogers and Ideker, 2000; Jalife and Berenfeld, 2004; Massé *et al.*, 2007).

### 1.2.1. *Reentry*

Figure 1.4 describes a model of this mechanism. On the left, a ring of excitable homogeneous tissue is represented as a circle. At point A, an electrical stimulus is applied triggering the appearance of an action potential that propagates both to the right and to the left. The two excitation waves, one running clockwise and the other counter-clockwise, collide about halfway in their attempt to return to the starting site A and the whole process ends. On the right side of the figure, the same piece of

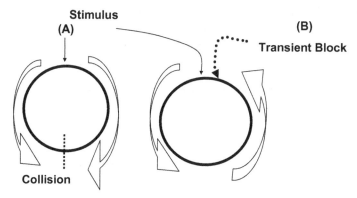

Fig. 1.4. Re-entry mechanism. Left: A ring of excitable homogeneous tissue (circle) is stimulated at point A triggering the appearance of an action potential that propagates both to the right and to the left. Right: The same tissue, but a transient block appears at B at the stimulation moment. Thus, the action potential can only propagate to the left, running the whole circuit to get back to the starting place A.

tissue is depicted but a transient block has appeared at B, at the stimulation moment. In such case, the triggered action potential can only propagate to the left and run the whole circuit to get back to the starting place A. Two possibilities then may occur: the block continues to exist or the block has vanished. If the former happens, the excitation wave dies out; if the latter takes place, the wave re-stimulates site A and a second turn begins so that excitation can keep going on indefinitely establishing a re-entry circuit. Precisely, Mines and Garrey performed experiments with rings of excitable tissue of variable size and they were able to demonstrate the phenomenon. It is, indeed, a beautiful and clear plausible concept. An Old Italian motto says, *se non e vero, è ben trovato* (even if not true, the explanation is nice).

Several aspects need discussion in the previous model to further clarify it. What variables play a role to actually lead to a circus motion?

(1) The velocity of propagation $V_p$ of the action potential is a first element; if it is too high, the excitatory wave will get back to the starting point when the block still persists and will not be able to continue. On the other hand, if such velocity is low enough, the action potential will find point A fully recovered and re-excitation will be possible.

(2) A second element is the refractory period $\tau$ of the action potential; if short enough, the possibility of reactivation of the site is clear. However, if it is too long, reentry could not happen for the excitatory wave would find the site unresponsive.

(3) The third element is the length $(L)$ of the circuit, which relates to the heart size (and to the possible wavelength): the longer, the higher the probability of re-stimulation, while the opposite occurs in the case of short pathways.

Thus, after the above-mentioned settings, we may write down the following relationship,

$$V_\mathrm{p} = L/\tau \tag{1.1}$$

or, better as inequality, because the pathway must at least be equal to or longer than the solved for product,

$$L \geq V_\mathrm{p}\tau \tag{1.1a}$$

as the necessary condition for the establishment of a continuously running action potential, a circus motion or a reentry in a ring-like piece of excitable tissue. Each factor in Eq. (1.1), using the international system of units SI, should be measured in meters (m), meters/second (m/s), and seconds (s), respectively. Expressed in words, **a low propagation velocity, short refractory period, and/or long pathway certainly favor the establishment of a reentrant wave front**. Any action, exogenous or endogenous (as drug injection, cooling, blood flow change, metabolic alteration or the like), affecting any of these three parameters will have an influence, too, on the probability of reentry and, thus, appears as corollary of the latter statement.

How can the appearance of transient blocks be explained? Inhomogeneities may be a first cause, because they tend to hinder normal conduction of the electrical impulse, and cardiac tissue, especially in the mammalian heart, is far from being homogeneous, both histologically and electrophysiologically.

Study of the fibers composing the atria and ventricles clearly shows the existence of different types: contractile, conductive, tendinous, pacemaker-like, of the atrioventricular node, of the sinus node, Purkinje fibers, atrial fibers. They are organized as a *syncytium*, which has a wavy complex structure and is biologically defined as a multi-nucleated mass of cytoplasm not fully separated into individual cells. A unique feature of the heart is the existence of intercalated discs that act as specialized cell junctions, which offer little resistance to the passage of an action potential. Their resistance is very low, so much that ions move freely through the junction allowing the entire atrial or ventricular mass to function as one huge cell. For this reason, cardiac muscle is frequently referred to as a *functional syncytium*, or a single functional unit. It has been found that abnormal intercellular coupling in the heart, resulting from defects in the expression of *connexin* 43, the major constituent of cardiac gap junctions, plays a key role in the initiation and maintenance of sustained arrhythmias (Cancelas *et al.*, 2000; Gutstein *et al.*, 2005). Gap junctions provide for a unique system of intercellular communication allowing rapid transport of small molecules from cell-to-cell. Such junctions are formed by a large family of proteins named *connexins*. From a cardiovascular viewpoint, cell-to-cell communication, under normal conditions, is essential in cardiac embryogenesis, electrical impulse transmission, synchronization of cardiac contractile activity, transmission of vascular reflex signals, and other biological functions. Under pathological conditions, either by inherited or acquired genetic mutation, intercellular communications participate in the development of congenital cardiopathies, arrhythmogenesis and electrical remodeling, atherosclerosis and myocardial ischemia, arterial hypertension and myocardial remodeling (Suárez and Bravo, 2006). Another important fact refers to the direction the electric impulse moves: conduction velocity along myocardial fibers was found to be usually several times larger than that vertical to them. In pathological conditions, the phenomenon seems to be more marked (Toyomi *et al.*, 1959). In short, structural inhomogeneity and pathways associated with it are facts that may become decisive in triggering fibrillation.

Microelectrode records of cardiac action potentials have demonstrated long time back substantial morphological differences when comparing several fiber types (Hoffman and Cranefield, 1960). Figure 1.5 is a traditional didactic set of intracellular signals based on a long row of careful experiments first published by the previously mentioned authors and, thereafter, reproduced over and over in the literature. They are quite illustrative; the delay between them is clearly discernible. Time marks (shown at the bottom) are 100 ms apart. Not all fibers over the myocardial mass find themselves at one given instant at the same electrophysiological state, due either to temporal shift or to differences in the recovery time. Such differences are more marked during repolarization, which, when looked at from the position of a standard surface ECG, correspond approximately to the location of the T-wave. In short, there is lack of temporal electrophysiological homogeneity and that may favor also the establishment of reentry pathways.

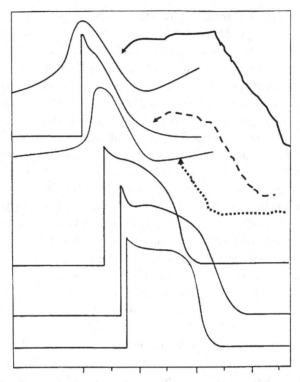

Fig. 1.5. Six cardiac action potentials recorded with microelectrodes from six types of cardiac fibers. They have similar characteristics, but they also show significant differences. Upper one: Produced by one myocyte of the sinoatrial node. The second came from an atrial fiber and the third from a cell located at the atrioventricular node. The lower three action potentials came from the left ventricle: bundle of HIS, distal Purkinje fiber, and a contractile fiber, respectively. Time marks: 100 ms apart (As shown in Hoffman and Cranefield, 1960, and in many textbooks).

### 1.2.2. *Multiple Ectopic Foci*

A single cardiac electrical impulse out of its anatomical normal site is, by definition, an ectopic beat (from Greek, *ektopos*, out of place, formed by *ex* out + *topos* place). It may show up at any myocardial spot and it may trigger or not a consequent contraction. It usually falls also out of the regular expected time, eventually before time (as premature beat) or sometimes rather late in the cycle. Isolated ectopics do not have physiological significance. Young people may have them and, as they grow older, such cardiac manifestations disappear. Their shape is characteristic and depends on the origin; by and large, the depolarization wave (QRS complex) is opposite in polarity to the recovery wave (T-wave).

A sensitized myocardium (say, ischemic) may produce one or more trains of ectopics; the longer the strip and the more frequent, the more worrying the cardiac condition of the subject because they indicate perhaps tissue injury. If the morphology of the beats making up the tachyarrhythmic episodes changes, it means there are several foci that tend to act as quasi-pacemakers and, at a given time, may easily involve enough muscle mass to turn into fibrillation. Whether such event is the result of just several foci, as some sort of electrical overall bombardment, or a combination of them with reentrant circuits elicited in some other way, becomes a speculative matter of perhaps not much relevance. Figure 1.6 illustrates a basal ectopic beat, Fig. 1.7 points out different places in the myocardium where the unwanted activity might arise and Fig. 1.8 shows a dangerous run of ectopics, also-called extra-systoles or extrasystolia.

### 1.2.3. *Rotor Theory*

An old idea, put forward by Thomas Lewis in 1925, on the mechanism of fibrillation has re-emerged from theoretical and experimental studies; it says that wave propagation during VF is not totally random. The postulate is that *rotors* or *vortices* (Webster Dictionary says it is *a part that revolves*

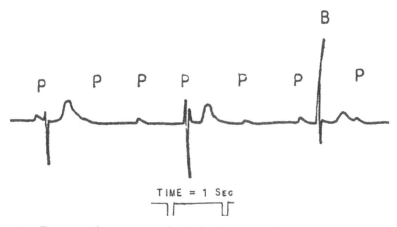

Fig. 1.6.    Two ectopic beats originated at the basal region of the ventricles. QRS complexes opposite to T-waves. There is total A-V dissociation. The third beat B is supraventricular and looks very similar to a normal one, but is not. Obtained from an experimental dog at the Department of Physiology, Baylor College of Medicine, Houston, TX.

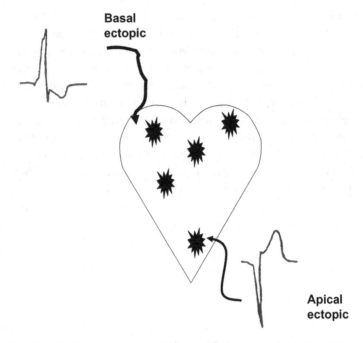

Fig. 1.7.  Multiple ectopic foci. Records obtained from experimental dogs.

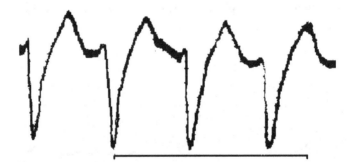

Fig. 1.8.  Sequence of apical extra-systoles. It may become a precursor of ventricular fibrillation. Also called extrasystolia. Horizontal bar corresponds to 1 sec. Courtesy of Sofia Berman, MD, Tucuman, Argentina.

*in a stationary part*) are the major organizing centers of fibrillation and that certain specific molecular properties of the cardiac muscle at the ion channel level contribute to the establishment of such rotors and to the overall complexity of the arrhythmia. There is emerging evidence of spatiotemporal organization during early VF. The mechanism is, so far, unknown in myopathic hearts. The model is based on the theoretical and experimental findings that the heart could maintain electrical waves that rotate about *functional*, rather than *anatomical*, obstacles. These so-called *rotors* were taken as the primary "organizing centers" for fibrillation, and refractory period heterogeneity was considered a secondary factor, possibly modulating and masking the activity of rotors, but not driving the rhythm. Transient unstable rotors might explain VF in terms of how rotors break up to form the turbulent state seen in epicardial maps, that is, there would be "mother rotors" breaking up into "daughter rotors," which in turn break up in a continual chain of succession (Jalife, 2000; Rogers and Ideker, 2000; Jalife and Berenfeld, 2004; Chorro *et al.*, 2007). Even though somewhat repeating the concept, it deserves quoting the nice description given by the first investigator (Jalife, 2000), from the Department of Pharmacology, SUNY Health Science Center, Syracuse, New York, who says that "traditionally, VF has been defined as turbulent cardiac electrical activity, which implies a large amount of irregularity in the electrical waves that underlie ventricular excitation. During VF, the heart rate is too high (>550 excitations/min) to allow adequate pumping of blood. In the electrocardiogram (ECG), ventricular complexes that are ever-changing in frequency, contour, and amplitude characterize VF. Recent experiments and computer simulations suggest that VF may be explained in terms of highly periodic three-dimensional rotors that activate the ventricles at exceedingly high frequency. Such rotors may show at least two different behaviors:

(a) At one extreme, they may drift throughout the heart at high speeds producing beat-to-beat changes in the activation sequence.
(b) At the other extreme, rotors may be relatively stationary, activating the ventricles at such high frequencies that the wave fronts emanating from them break up at varying distances, resulting in complex spatiotemporal patterns of fibrillatory conduction.

In either case, the recorded ECG patterns are indistinguishable from VF"".

The same group called attention to possible dynamic differences in the case of heart failure remodeling, because there is a decrease in VF rate. Besides, acute stretch partially may reverse such effect by a mechanism that is independent of remodeling (Moreno *et al.*, 2005).

Several authors have contributed to the theory. For example, Massé *et al.* (2007) reported that "rotors were present in myopathic hearts studied during VF and cumulatively lasted a mean of $(3.2 \pm 2.0)$ s of the $(7.0 \pm 4.0)$ s of the VF segments analyzed. For each surface mapped, $(3.6 \pm 2.9)$ rotors were identified for the duration mapped. The average number of cycles completed by these rotors was $(4.9 \pm 4.9)$. The longest rotor took $(10.2 \pm 6.2)$ rotations and lasted $(2.0 \pm 1.2)$ s. The rotors on the endocardium had a cycle length of $(192 \pm 33)$ ms compared with $(220 \pm 15)$ ms on the epicardium". They found centrifugal activation of electrical activity from these rotors, frequently localized at border regions of the myocardium. The subject, however, remains yet unsettled and calls for further and deeper research; no doubt, it is greatly attractive. It might be asked whether a reentry circuit can be considered as a rotor (or is a rotor) and, if not, what the difference between the two phenomena is. The indication seems to be a vortex-like activity moving or shifting along a reentry circuit.

## 1.3. Causes

By and large, a disturbance starts up the arrhythmia, often in a sensitized heart, but not necessarily so. Thus, classification criteria depend on the *setting* the phenomenon takes place and on the *type of disturbance*.

### 1.3.1. *Setting*

(a) *Clinical fibrillation*, which etiologically stems mainly in myocardial ischemia or infarct. This is definitely the case of a sensitized myocardium, which speaks precisely of the high-risk patients, candidates to be confined in a coronary unit. Previous clinical studies have diagnosed in them, for example, ventricular hypertrophy or dilatation, hypokinesia, weakened contractility, insufficiency along with very low ejection fraction. Perhaps, they also show hypercholesterolemia and atherosclerosis and a history of hypertension, diabetes, angioplasty, *stents*,[a] smoking habits, and even hereditary factors. It is difficult to determine what the perturbation triggered the arrhythmia, but endogenous catecholamine release due to stress, either physical or psychological, may well be the initial stimulus, or perhaps a minor local metabolic alteration. This fibrillation may not be easy to revert.

---

[a] *Stent*, a short narrow metal or plastic tube often in the form of a mesh that is inserted into the lumen of vessels, as an artery or a bile duct, especially to keep a previously blocked passageway open, apparently introduced by Charles Thomas *Stent*, died 1885, English dentist (Webster Dictionary).

(b) *Industrial or domestic fibrillation*, which mainly happens at home or in the industrial environment. It is the accidental macroshock (see Chap. 6), due to faulty equipment or installations or improper handling, which most of the time catches a young and healthy heart (because it belongs probably to a worker). Thus, it is not an easy organ to surrender and, if fibrillation is triggered, its probability to be reverted is high. The disturbance in this case clearly is an electrical stimulus.

(c) *Surgical fibrillation*, which takes place in the operating room, most often during cardiac interventions. The disturbance probably is mechanical handling of a sensitized myocardium, or it may be related to the level and kind of anesthesia. It is simply detected by visual inspection and counter-measures can be applied right on.

## 1.3.2. Type of Disturbance

As described above, the mammalian heart is structurally and electrophysiologically inhomogeneous, which means it is relatively prone to fall into a fibrillary chaotic activity. If, in the form of a perturbation, some extra-inhomogeneity is added, the probability of triggering the phenomenon increases. The question, hence, settles on what kind of disturbance appears as more appropriate. Here is where energy comes up as a handy concept since the cardiac mass during normal and pathological conditions develops metabolic activity involving electrical, mechanical, chemical, and thermal energies. Therefore, these are the different disturbances to add inhomogeneity:

(a) *Electric energy*, either as a pulse or as a train of pulses, definitely can initiate the phenomenon. In experimental conditions, it represents obviously the best method because it is easy to control, be it in terms of voltage or current.

(b) *Mechanical energy*, as a thump or several thumps produced with a tool or just with the naked fingers. The resulting minor back and forth compression perhaps produces a redistribution of the membrane electrical charges. Cardiac surgeons are quite familiar with this kind of event.

(c) *Chemical energy*, as the addition of certain amount of an electrolytic solution containing, for example, potassium ions, or some other exogenous or endogenous agent changing electrophysiological properties. Alcohol feeding is one of the many possible examples (Khedun *et al.*, 1991). Type and amount of anesthesia is another.

(d) *Thermal energy*, as the addition of certain amount of either warm or cold physiological solution (see Sec. 1.4.2). Gradients of temperature tend to increase the degree of local inhomogeneity by modifying, for example, conductive characteristics of the tissue (Todd, 1983).

There is ample empirical and controlled experimental evidence that any of the above-mentioned perturbations to the heart may lead it into fibrillation.

## 1.4. Types of Fibrillation

Cardiac fibrillation can be classified on the basis of its *etiology, localization,* or *characteristics*. Perhaps, these criteria deserve a deeper insight and revision, but they are still useful and have didactic value.

### 1.4.1. *Etiology*

The word *etiology* refers to the causes of a disease or disorder; thus, we must search for the origin of the specific fibrillation we are faced to. When the origin lies within the heart itself, as ischemia or infarct, it is denominated *primary fibrillation*. Fibrillation triggered by accidental electrocution is usually included in this class.

*Secondary fibrillation* stems, instead, in other non-cardiac pathologies, as for example in electrolytic imbalance due to renal failure. Diabetes, hormonal disorders, genetic factors, sympathetic over-discharge, or anesthesia may be the underlying causes. Let us illustrate with a few examples:

Resuscitation from cardiac arrest caused by volatile substance abuse is rarely successful. Large doses of catecholamines given during resuscitation, in the presence of butane, may cause recurrent VF. Edwards and Wenstone (2000) reported a case of prolonged resuscitation in a young man, who had inhaled butane. Cardiac output was restored 10 min after the administration of intravenous amiodarone. They suggest that antiarrhythmic agents should be used early during resuscitation to prevent recurrent arrhythmias.

An interesting example is described by Munhoz Da Fontoura Tavares *et al.* (2004), from Brazil: a patient with recurrent VF secondary to an aortic tumor. These tumors can obstruct the coronary arteries, secondarily causing ischemia and VF. Such a mechanism must be considered in the differential diagnosis of sudden death.

Upile *et al.* (2006) reported a rare case of atrial fibrillation (AF) secondary to a mega-esophagus occurring in an old woman. Achalasia (from *a* + Greek *chalasis*, slackening, herein interpreted as, failure of a ring of muscle, as the anal sphincter or one of the esophagus to relax) is associated with a degeneration of ganglion cells of the *Auerbach plexus* resulting in the absence of esophageal peristalsis and failure of lower esophageal sphincter relaxation. This leads to esophageal dilatation (mega-esophagus). There is a correlation between achalasia and cardiac arrhythmia. Patients with this disorder tend to perform a Valsalva maneuver to aid the transit of food over the stenotic esophageal segment. Besides, recall the anatomical proximity of the esophagus to the left atrium and the possibility of mechanical pressure. More than that, abnormalities of heart rate responses to the Valsalva maneuver (Valentinuzzi *et al.*, 1974), deep breathing, and standing were noted in patients with autonomic defects. This is consistent with the hypothesis that abnormal vagal discharge may contribute to the pathogenesis of achalasia. Vagal firing through acetylcholine release reduces atrial electrical refractory period (the classic negative *bathmotropic* effect), which potentiates AF (Valentinuzzi *et al.*, 1973).

Anyhow, the literature abounds and, unfortunately, often it is not clear enough in its definitions and criteria regarding this matter, pointing out perhaps to a pending subject for revision.

### 1.4.2. *Localization*

Since the heart is composed of two atria and two ventricles, the phenomenon may take place in any of them or in both simultaneously. In lower species, as herptiles (frogs, lizards, snakes, or turtles) it may occur also in the *sinus venosus* (SV), which is their first cardiac chamber, where the pacemaker is located. While the overall sequence of normal events is well documented, the arrhythmia at the SV, however, is extremely difficult to demonstrate and only in very rare circumstances and for very short periods it can be recorded (Valentinuzzi and Hoff, 1970, 1972; Valentinuzzi *et al.*, 1986; Savino and Valentinuzzi, 1988). Figure 1.9 shows rare VF records obtained from an experimental open chest turtle (*Pseudemys floridana*). The four channels, A, B, C, and D, correspond to ventricular myograms, i.e., the heart was hooked from the ventricular apex and attached by a thin thread at an almost 90 degrees angle to a photoelectric transducer. On the left of A, five normal beats are clearly seen with a rate of about 28/min. Just at the occurrence of the sixth beat (vertical arrow), a brief train of rectangular pulses (10 V,

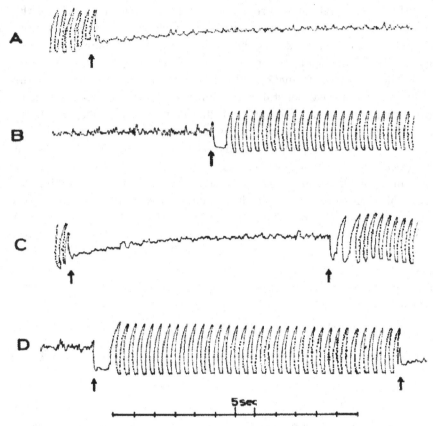

Fig. 1.9.   Ventricular fibrillation in an experimental turtle (*Pseudemys floridana*). Time marks below are 5 s apart. See text for details. Obtained by the author at the Department of Physiology, Baylor College of Medicine, Houston, TX, USA, back in the 1960s, during his graduate student years. Also appearing in Valentinuzzi *et al.*, 1986, with the publisher's permission.

2 ms, 25 pps) was directly applied to the ventricles by means of a pair of electrodes triggering the arrhythmia, manifested by the small amplitude grass-like shivering. The second channel B, a continuation of the former above, after 2 min 30 s of fibrillation, displays on the right spontaneous defibrillation (vertical arrow): normal regular beating was resumed. The third channel C, always on the same animal, depicts another episode of fibrillation similar to the first one above, which this time lasted slightly over 1 min and was terminated by the sudden application of cold saline solution. Finally, the lower trace D shows a spontaneous defibrillation on the left (first arrow) followed by another fibrillation triggered with electrical

stimulation. This particular turtle was relatively big, 3 kg of body weight, a fact that could have favored the phenomenon. However, this behavior is far from frequent and no rules can be offered to repeat the experiment.

*AF* is one of the classical cardiac disorders. It was studied for the first time by James Mackenzie, who is to be considered as the first cardiologist (Hoff *et al.*, 1966). It is a clinical disorder, compatible with life that requires care and medical follow-up because of its persistency and common cause of arrhythmia-related hospitalizations. In addition, it is a major contributor to stroke. Figure 1.1 displays a set of three simultaneous records (surface ECG, semidirect atrial electrogram and arterial blood pressure). Its typical characteristics are clearly seen,

(1) The ECG does not show the typical P-waves preceding each QRS complex; instead, they have been replaced by a grass-like hum usually termed the $f$-waves.
(2) Ventricular frequency is high (tachycardia) and irregular. There is tachycardia because of rapid stimulation from the atria to the ventricles via the AV node and it is irregular because not all stimuli can traverse successfully the node, by nature with relatively poor conductive properties.
(3) There is pulse deficit, that is, when considering an arbitrary time period (say, 30 or 60 s), the number of QRS is larger than the number of arterial pulses. In the figure, compare eight beats in channel 1 vs seven in channel 3, when the records between the two vertical bars are inspected. Besides, the pulse amplitude is irregular because some ejections are weak to open the aortic valve (remember Starling's law of the heart); they are too premature and do not allow for an adequate ventricular filling. Clinically, the physician can detect these features by simple peripheral pulse palpation (irregular tachycardia and irregular pulse strength).
(4) Atrial effective contraction does not exist, meaning that ventricular filling misses the last part. In normal conditions, however, atrial contribution amounts to not more than 20–25% of ventricular filling, hence, and as stated above, the disorder is compatible with life.

AF may persist during many years (10, 20, or more), it needs treatment, and it leads to atrial hypertrophy and rarely, if ever, at least in man, reverts spontaneously to normal rhythm. It is considered serious. In the dog, probably due to heart size, most of the time does not last longer than a few minutes.

In an editorial article, Efimov and Fedorov (2005) discussed quite clearly four traditional and still challenging questions: (1) Is AF myogenic or neurogenic in nature?; (2) Is AF maintained by reentry or by focal activity?; (3) Is AF maintained by a single source, or are multiple sources required?; and (4) Is there a critical mass of myocardium required to maintain AF? They suggest possible avenues of research as well as requirements that might be needed to reach full answers. One important outcome is that AF appears as not fully similar to VF.

An even more recent review article highlights groundbreaking work in AF genetics that has provided with a better understanding of the origins of this dysrhythmia (Damani and Topol, 2009). Historically, many studies have identified the familial predisposition for AF, however, up to 30% of patients are affected without any known familial association and the absence of any other risk factors, such as hypertension or diabetes. Other studies found mutations associated with the disease, but it was not until recent work using sequencing technology, that the 4q25 locus was recognized as a susceptibility factor for AF. The gene *PITX2*, which is known to have a role in embryonic cardiac development, has also been identified as the causal variant within the 4q25 susceptibility locus. Translation of these findings will lead to improved screening, prognosis, and treatment, as well as the future possibility of a personalized approach for the treatment of AF.

*Atrial flutter* can be considered a variant of the former arrhythmia, even though it shows lower frequency components and appears as more regular, its hemodynamic effects, however, are similar to those of AF. It is a common tachycardia that can be caused by scarring in the heart resulting from prior cardiac disease or heart surgery, but it can also occur in some patients with no other identifiable heart problems. During atrial flutter, instead of the electrical activity starting in the sinus node, electrical activity begins in that chamber. The rapid beating of the atria can in turn cause the ventricles to beat rapidly. It typically originates from the right atrium and most often involves a large circuit that travels around the area of the tricuspid valve that is between the right atrium and the right ventricle. This type of flutter is referred to as *typical atrial flutter*. Less commonly, atrial flutter can result from circuits in other areas of the atria. Flutter that results from these less common types of circuits is referred to as *atypical atrial flutter* (Boyer and Koplan, 2005). Figure 1.10 illustrates a clinical example.

*VF* spreads throughout the ventricular mass (Fig. 1.2). It was observed in 1543 by Andrea Vesalius, author of the first modern anatomy treatise.

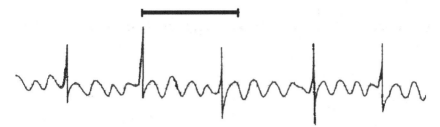

Fig. 1.10. Atrial flutter. The horizontal bar above corresponds to 1 second. QRS complexes are clearly shown while the atrial P-waves have been replaced by a rather regular high rhythm in the order of 300 per minute. Courtesy of Gabriela Feldman, MD, Tucumán City, Argentina.

Hoffa and Ludwig triggered it electrically in 1850 in the experimental animal searching for "tetanic contraction of the heart", which is now well-known that it cannot take place due to its long refractory period. In 1874, Edmé Félix Alfred Vulpian (1826–1887, French neurologist) coined the term *mouvement fibrillaire* and John A. MacWilliam, a physiologist trained under Karl Ludwig, gave an accurate description in 1887. Clearly, this arrhythmic arrhythmia is incompatible with life posing a serious emergency to be attended to within no longer than a few minutes. Most of the commonly named "heart attack" or "heart collapse" falls in this category. It is the typical emergency of the cardiac surgeon, of the coronary unit, of the street collapse, of the domestic, or industrial accidental electrocution.

### 1.4.3. *Characteristics*

Once the ECG is disrupted into the fibrillatory waves, its characteristics change suddenly and sharply, from the periodic three-component polymorphic form to the irregular already described pattern. By and large, the first 2–3 min of fibrillation appear as composed of high frequencies with relatively high amplitudes. If the heart is visible, the uncoordinated movements impress as strong and vigorous; this is referred to as *Fibrillation Type* 1, with good possibilities for reversion. As time goes by, the fibrillary contractions weaken as does the probability of reversion. The electrical signal loses amplitude, too, and lower frequency components prevail. It is called *Fibrillation Type* 2. Emergency personnel well know by experience the importance of the fastest possible intervention for the defibrillating procedure to succeed. Animal experimentation has led to the same

*Cardiac Fibrillation-Defibrillation*

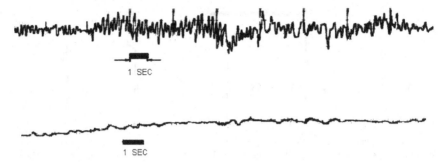

Fig. 1.11.   Type 1 (upper trace) and Type 2 (lower trace) Ventricular Fibrillation in the dog. Observe the higher frequencies and amplitudes in the former as compared to the latter, which seems to be fading off. Obtained by the author in the Laboratory of Bioengineering, Universidad Nacional de Tucumán, Argentina.

conclusion. Figure 1.11 depicts both types recorded from an experimental dog. Up to here, the above description is purely qualitative.

A good number of reports fill the literature determining quantitatively the fibrillation frequency components under different conditions. Not all coincide fully; however, ranges are not too far off. It has been found, for example, that during cardiopulmonary by-pass and after inducing VF at a core body temperature of 34°C (normothermia) or at a core body temperature of 29.8°C (hypothermia), by using fast Fourier transform of the ECG signal, median fibrillation frequencies were 5.4 Hz and 3.6 Hz, respectively (Strohmenger *et al.*, 1997).

A team from Austria and Norway (Strohmenger *et al.*, 2001) evaluated VF frequency and amplitude variables in 89 patients with out-of-hospital cardiac arrest. ECG recordings of 594 countershock attempts were collected and analyzed. By using fast Fourier transformation analysis of the VF ECG signal — and quoting from that paper — median frequency, dominant frequency, spectral edge frequency, and amplitude were as follows: 4.4 (2.4–7.5) Hz, 4.0 (0.7–7.0) Hz, 7.7 (3.7–13.7) Hz, and 0.94 (0.24–1.95) mV, respectively, before successful countershock ($n = 59$). These values were 3.8 (0.8–7.7) Hz, 3.0 (0.3–9.7) Hz, 7.3 (2.0–14.0) Hz, and 0.53 (0.03–3.03) mV, respectively, before unsuccessful countershock (number of cases, $n = 535$). In patients in whom bystander CPR was performed ($n = 51$), VF frequency and amplitude before the first defibrillation attempt were higher than in patients without bystander CPR ($n = 38$) (median frequency, 4.4 (2.4–7.5) vs 3.7 (1.8–5.3) Hz, dominant frequency, 3.8 (0.9–7.7) vs 2.6 (0.8–5.9) Hz; spectral edge frequency, 8.4 (4.8–12.9) vs 7.2 (3.9–12.1) Hz; amplitude, 0.79

(0.06–4.72) vs 0.67 (0.16–2.29) mV. Clearly, the unsuccessful interventions were dealing with fibrillations of the second type.


## 1.5. Clinical and Surgical Significance

Sudden cardiac death (SCD) stems in primary cardiac causes, often without previous symptoms. In the USA, about 325,000 people (about 0.2% of the population) a year die of coronary heart disease without being hospitalized or admitted to an emergency room. Most of these are deaths caused by cardiac arrest and are due to ventricular tachycardia or VF or both. Some cardiac arrests, however, are due to extreme slowing of the heart or *bradycardia*. The figures herein cited are approximately the same for the Western countries, all perhaps strained and stressed by similar socio-economic and labor problems. Economic crises, unemployment, and crime increase in big cities are combined factors that have built up a sensation of lack of security. Globalization seems to impose a toll on humankind, giving quite a piece of material not only for the medical sciences but also for psychologists and social workers alike. Politicians should take a look, too, and be concerned at least.

The incidence of SCD parallels the incidence of coronary artery disease (CAD), with the peak of SCD occurring in people aged 45–75 years. The incidence increases with age in men, women, whites, and non-whites. However, the proportion of deaths that are sudden from CAD decreases with age. In the Framingham study (http://www.nhlbi.nih.gov/about/framingham/), the proportion of CAD deaths that were sudden was 62% in men aged 45–54 years, but this fell to 58% in men aged 55–64 years and to 42% in men aged 65–74 years (www.americanheart.org/presenter.jhtml; www.emedicine.com/med/topic276.htm).

Fibrillation, either atrial or ventricular, is no doubt a cardiologic clinical problem of current standings. If we recall what is presented in the previous paragraphs above, it is also a potential surgery event; occasionally, it may be deliberately triggered to quiet down the contracting heart, which, during an intervention under the control of a heart–lung machine, acts as a disturbance. However, it is a controversial issue and some authors favor hypothermia or cardioplegic solutions as stabilizing methods during cardiac surgery. By definition, **cardioplegia** is the intentional and temporary cessation of cardiac activity. Most frequently, it is obtained by injection of a cold crystalloid because it protects the myocardium from damage. Sometimes, the patient is first exposed to hypothermia and, thereafter, iced solution of dextrose and potassium chloride is introduced into the heart (http://en.wikipedia.org/wiki/Cardioplegia).

All this points out to a whole battery of associated laboratory and imaging studies to complement and back up a therapeutic decision: ECG to help identify ischemic or pro-arrhythmic conditions, serum electrolyte levels (including calcium and magnesium), cardiac enzymes to identify myocardial injury, complete blood count (CBC) to detect possible anemia, arterial blood gases to assess the degree of acidosis or hypoxemia, and even the determination of eventual toxic substances. Images include the traditional X-rays or any of the more sophisticated single photon emission computed tomography (SPECT), positron emission tomography (PET), nuclear magnetic resonance (NMR), and/or Doppler echocardiography to identify hypokinesia, aspiration pneumonia, pulmonary edema, cardiomegaly, or injury, as secondary to cardiopulmonary resuscitation CPR.

## 1.6. Fibrillation Variables

The fibrillating arrhythmia can happen either in the atria or in the ventricles or simultaneously in both. Qualitative description is usually the case (as up to here in this text, interspersed with a few quantitative parameters), but no absolute quantification has so far been developed, as with other physiological variables (for example, blood pressure, blood flow, or concentration of substances). We cannot offer a statement like "this fibrillation is very serious because it measures so many units or because it is of grade 3 or 4"; at most, Types 1 and 2 are feebly distinguished, as described before. The only true statement refers to just a normally beating heart or to a fibrillating heart, as states. Besides, some stimuli (see above) may induce the passage from one state to the other, either way, and there are factors or variables that favor the transition. Finally, once the transition takes place (from normal beating to fibrillation or vice versa), the stimulus does not have to be maintained, for either spreading of fibrillation to the whole mass or reversion to the regular beat, act by themselves, as self-sustained events.

### 1.6.1. *Electrophysiological Variables*

Everything related to the movement of charges *in* and *out* of or *along* the cardiac fibers belongs to this group. Hence, diastolic potential, action potential amplitude, action potential duration (APD) (refractory period), propagation velocity, diastolic depolarization, and depolarization rate, are to be taken into account. Membrane permeabilities to sodium, potassium, and calcium ions are also members of the set. In short, all that encompasses the electrophysiological behavior of the myocardium.

### 1.6.2. *Metabolic Variables*

Cardiac tissue consumes energy and delivers work. All the complex processes involved in such actions include availability, synthesis, processing, and breaking down of a variety of substances such as oxygen, carbon dioxide, adenosine triphosphate (ATP), enzymes, chemical and hormonal mediators, and the like. They influence the above-mentioned variables, sometimes very deeply, as hypoxia would do. Over 30 years ago, attention was called over some of these factors including hypothalamic influence, too (Verrier *et al.*, 1975; Obeid *et al.*, 1978).

All variables influencing the probability of triggering fibrillation are no doubt inter-related and not precisely in a simple form. The best we can do is trying to qualitatively anticipate how high that probability is in a particular individual given a number of previously measured variables and cardiac history. This is the way to classify a patient as of "high or medium cardiac risk".

### 1.6.3. *Myocardial Mass*

Garrey (1914) proposed the concept of *critical mass* as essential in the establishment of the fibrillatory waves and estimated a value not in weight but in square units, suggesting $400\,mm^2$ as possible figure. In fact, MacWilliam long before, in 1887, advanced the same idea. The size of the heart is obviously related to the possible length of the reentry circuits and it is easily visualized that a longer pathway tends to facilitate the phenomenon. Small hearts would not fibrillate easily or would not at all. The opposite should hold true. Homogeneous hearts (that are small, too), as those of lower animals, would not either; however, there are reports of uncontrolled cases in which the phenomenon was sporadically seen (Valentinuzzi *et al.*, 1986; Savino and Valentinuzzi, 1988; see also Fig. 1.9).

A few investigators have tried to numerically estimate that *minimum fibrillating mass*. Moe and Abildskov (1959), for example, claimed it is in the order of 1 g; much later, Ruiz and Valentinuzzi (1994) considered a *minimal defibrillating mass* (perhaps around 11–12 g), that is — and anticipating the concept to be discussed in the chapter on defibrillation — the smallest mass (in essence, number of fibers) to depolarize in order to revert the phenomenon; such mass is conceptually similar but not necessarily numerically the same as the former.

Nolasco and Dahlen (1968) reported that if the relation of the APD and its preceding diastolic interval (the so-called *restitution relation*) is equal or larger than 1, electrical alternans may show up, while the latter phenomenon does not take place when such relation is smaller than 1. Recall that alternans may well become a preliminary event to fibrillation; recall also that if a heart is driven by slowly increasing the stimulation frequency, the diastolic interval gets shorter and, as the process continues, repolarization of one pulse touches at some instant the depolarization phase of the following pulse so signaling in all probability the beginning of fibrillation. In such case, the electrical diastolic interval $T_D$ tends to zero or becomes zero and $APD/T_D$ tends to a large value. Years later, and following Nolasco and Dahlen's lead, Wu *et al.* (1999) studied how the restitution characteristics might influence the *fibrillation critical mass*, since the latter might be influenced by the former. The goal of these authors was to evaluate the relationship between repolarization characteristics and critical mass for VF in diseased human cardiac tissues. Hearts from transplant recipients were used. After a rather sophisticated methodology, it was found that at baseline, VF did not occur either spontaneously or during rewarming, and it could not be induced by electrical stimulation. Reproducing now almost verbatim from their paper: "The mean APD at 90% depolarization at a cycle length of 600 msec was $(227 \pm 49)$ msec, and the mean slope of the APD restitution curve was $0.22\pm0.08$. The weight of these samples averaged $(111\pm23)$ g (range 85 to 138). However, after cromakalim infusion, sustained VF ($>30$ min in duration) was consistently induced. As compared with the baseline in the same tissues, cromakalim shortened the APD at 90% from $(243 \pm 32)$ msec to $(55 \pm 18)$ msec and increased the maximum slope of the restitution curve from $0.24 \pm 0.11$ to $1.43 \pm 0.10$. They concluded that at baseline, the critical mass for VF in diseased human hearts *in vitro* is $>111$ g. However, the critical mass for VF can vary, as it can be reduced by shortening APD and increasing the slope of the APD restitution curve". Observe that this value is more than 100 times higher than that estimated by Moe and Abildskov 40 years ago, although it admits different figures, presumably lower, if the APD shortens.

Winfree (1994) predicted 100–200 mm$^2$, i.e., one-fourth to one-half smaller than Garrey's value, basing his assumption on the vortex-like reentry; he also advanced 12 cm$^3$ or 12 g, as possible value for the critical mass. He expressed the idea in a different way, too: a minimum size of six times the rotor diameter, which would lead to a volume of about 12 g, although it is not clear how the latter figure was actually obtained. Vaidya *et al.* (1999), in a beautifully presented article, reflectively state that sustained fibrillation should not be possible in the mouse heart with ventricular areas of some 100 mm$^2$ and masses around 200 mg. They wanted to determine whether arrhythmias are possible in the adult mouse ventricle and, after careful experimental design, they found that such Langendorff perfused heart can, indeed, sustain rotors and VF. The result is surprising because the wavelength (10–30 mm), as the authors themselves assert, is larger than the available length, which may mean that wavelength is not a good fibrillation predictor, at least in the mouse. The paper offers several previous references that suggested reentry in small pieces of cardiac tissue and concludes that an area just larger than that required for reentry could support fibrillation. The latter sounds quite sensible.

In a not too clear paper, Fatema *et al.* (2008) sought to compare the predictive power and reproducibility between minimum and maximum left atrial (LA) volume for the development of first AF or flutter. It was a prospective study in 574 adults (mean age 74 ± 6 years), in sinus arrhythmia, with no history of prior atrial arrhythmias. After a mean follow-up period of (1.9 ± 1.2) year, 30 of them (that is, 5.2%) developed either AF or flutter. Without giving actual volume values or explaining how such parameter was determined (apparently, echocardiography was used), these authors concluded that "*minimal LA volume was an independent predictor of first AF/flutter*". Is this contribution related to the concept of minimal fibrillating mass? The answer tends to the affirmative, but from the information made available it becomes rather difficult to assess. A large volume does not necessarily mean a large mass for it may be due to blood overload of the cavity.

Panfilov (2006) put forward the concept of *effective size*, which takes into account the wavelength of reentry, as determining factor. The paper deserves a more detailed consideration because its ideas are attractive, indeed. From Eq. (1.1) above, such wavelength $L$ in a physical pathway is given by the refractory period $\tau$ multiplied by the velocity $V_p$ (or $L = \tau \, V_p$). However, cardiac reentry is usually characterized by a spiral shape, with a specific geometry, so that wavelength $L$ is defined in a slightly different way, as this author clearly says. For isotropic tissue far from the spiral wave core, such shape can be approximated in polar coordinates $(r, \varphi)$ as $r \cong \lambda\varphi2\pi$; in the latter, the wavelength $\lambda = V_p(T)T$, where $T$ stands for the period of spiral wave rotation and $V_p(T)$ represents the wave propagation velocity at that particular period $T$. Hence, the spiral wave depends only on $\lambda$, which in turn means that the number of spiral turns is a function of the tissue size $S$ relative to $\lambda$, so that Panfilov (2006) defines the *effective size* $S_e$ as $S/\lambda$. However, tissue size (or heart size) is a rather undetermined parameter because of the complex shapes involved that calls for further elaboration if a quantitative value is searched for. Panfilov, then, very ingeniously proceeds assuming that the shapes of two different ventricles or atria have the same ratios relative to their respective anisotropic properties. In such situation, relative sizes can be estimated from the cubic roots of their masses (Winfree, 1994). Heart weight can be measured or approximated as 0.6% of the body weight, while the spiral wavelength is the period of the tachycardia or fibrillation (easily obtained from the ECG). Unfortunately, data regarding the propagation velocity *at the arrhythmia frequency* are rarely, if ever, available, meaning that an exact computation of the wavelength is not possible. Panfilow, again quite slyly, states that arrhythmia wavelengths can be compared by comparing their periods under the approximate assumption that conduction velocities are the same, and so defines for a particular species the relative effective size of the heart $S_{re}$ as,

$$S_{re} = \frac{\sqrt[3]{(HW)}}{T}. \tag{1.2}$$

The above expression is a rough approximation, as he clearly recognizes, but gives the possibility of comparing VF of different animals, including man. With Eq. (1.2), Panfilov (2006) estimated effective sizes for rabbit, dog, pig, and human hearts during VF reporting the following $S_{re}$ values:

Rabbit,   $33.2 \pm 12.9$, estimated heart weights,   $(18$ to $30)\,\text{g}$

Dog,   $53.1 \pm 15.3$, estimated heart weight,   $(150 \pm 40)\,\text{g}$

Pig,   $59.4 \pm 12.7$, estimated heart weight,   $(210 \pm 40)\,\text{g}$

Human,   $37.4 \pm 9.3$, estimated heart weight,   $(420 \pm 60)\,\text{g}$

Observe how the relative effective size grows to a maximum falling back to almost the initial value as the heart weight increases (Fig. 1.12). The maximum corresponds to approximately $250\,\text{g}$ and, while the range of mass is rather wide, between 25 and $500\,\text{g}$, the range of the effective fibrillating size appears as considerably narrower, only from 30 to 60, the former being about 16 times larger than the latter. Anyhow, speculating on this interesting proposal would not lead anywhere. It must be underlined, too, that in Eq. (1.1), there are two overlapping concepts: one is $L$, the

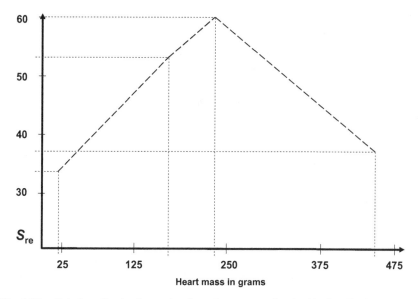

Fig. 1.12. Relative effective heart size $S_{re}$ vs heart mass. Inspired in Panfilov's Figure 1b (2006) and using his average data. With the latter author's kind permission.

physical available length over the tissue; and $\lambda$, the wavelength of the electrical circulating signal, that at first sight ought to fit into the former path, even though, as reported above by some authors, is not always so.

Closing this section, we underline that whatever the actual value of the critical mass, it is clear that fibrillation is a *group concept*, in the sense that for one fiber the phenomenon does not have meaning, even for just a few fibers it would be questionable. Obviously, it calls for more and quite attractive research, both experimentally and theoretically. Besides, heart and body weights are related and it has been known for a long time that obese people tend to have larger hearts, which are easier to fibrillate and more difficult to defibrillate (DeSilva and Lown, 1978).

## 1.7. Electrical Fibrillation Thresholds (EFTs)

### 1.7.1. *Definition*

The minimum magnitude (amplitude in adequate units, of whatever kind) required to trigger fibrillation is called *fibrillation threshold*. A small increment assures fibrillation, while the same decrement will never produce the event. It is like walking on the borderline of a step ladder: a bit to the flat side, and we are safer; a bit to the cliff side, and we fall off. Perhaps a better definition should state: *That amplitude with 50% probability of triggering the phenomenon is the fibrillation threshold.* It is interesting to note that as early as 1940, Wiggers and Wegria proposed the fibrillation threshold concept as a parameter to quantitatively evaluate myocardial susceptibility or sensitivity to the arrhythmia, which no doubt continues as valid practical piece of information; an ischemic ventricle, for example, requires less current than a healthy heart to fall into the uncoordinated activity.

To deepen into the concept two aspects need further discussion: *Methods of Stimulation* and the so-called *Ventricular Vulnerable Period*.

### 1.7.2. *Methods of Stimulation*

Cardiac stimulation is frequently used in experimental physiology and in clinical studies as a method to evaluate the effects of drugs or the responses in a given pathology. The outstanding saga of electrophysiologists, among a wealth of superb contributions, has led to the now fully recognized rectangular waveform as the best controllable electrical stimulus.

As a *single pulse*, the stimulus is characterized primarily by its duration and amplitude and, secondarily, by the rising and falling times, usually defined as the times elapsed between the 10% and 90% levels of the maximum amplitude. The two latter time parameters are more than met by the current electronic technology, i.e., they are short enough and negligible in comparison with the durations found in cardiac electrophysiology, which at most covers a range of 10–500 ms. In other words, the pulse behaves as if it were a perfect rectangle.

As a *train of rectangular pulses*, the stimulus needs two other characteristics to be specified: the *repetition frequency* and the *on–off ratio*. The former is measured in number of pulses per second or pulses per minute (p/s or ppm) and the latter as a number between 0 and 1, which describes the ratio of the time current (or voltage) is applied to the repetition period; thus, a 0.5 or a 50% ratio would mean pulses that apply current during one-half of the total cycle. Sometimes, it is also-called the *stimulation duty ratio* or *duty cycle*. Besides, the train has always an *overall duration*, from start to end, which includes a definite total number of pulses.

### 1.7.3. *Vulnerable Period*

A single electrical pulse can trigger fibrillation, however, to study the conditions for this to happen requires the exploration of the cardiac cycle, from QRS to QRS complex; say, from beat $N$ to beat $(N+1)$. A pair of electrodes picks up the ECG and this signal is connected to the stimulator trigger input. Besides, the output from the stimulator is connected via adequate electrodes to the myocardial mass. When the stimulator is manually turned on, it does not yet deliver the stimulus but it waits a predetermined time — an *adjustable delay* — being triggered by the next and immediately oncoming R-wave. In this way, all the cycle is explored, from zero delay, i.e., applying a stimulus to the heart in coincidence with the R-wave, up to the following (R + 1)-wave. For each cycle location, the stimulating single pulse is raised from zero amplitude up to the value that actually triggers fibrillation or to a maximum value in the case fibrillation is not met. A given pulse width must be selected (say, 1, 2, or 5 ms or longer, if necessary) and either voltage (in Volts) or current (in mA) should be chosen as the electrical parameter to apply. Plotting those pulse amplitudes vs the cycle location would produce the threshold curve for fibrillation (Fig. 1.13); those values on the upper region should always lead to fibrillation while values below never will. Values at the far left or at the far right will never trigger fibrillation because the ventricles are in the refractory period. However, there is a clear region where the curve falls off rather sharply showing a definite minimum, precisely in coincidence with the T-wave of the ECG. In other words, with one single pulse, either of voltage or of current, at a given pulse width, a definite duration in the order of 30 ms (roughly the duration of the T-wave) is found over each beat where fibrillation is more likely to occur. Like a window letting bad air

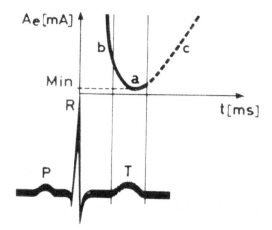

Fig. 1.13.   Ventricular Vulnerable Period. The T-wave duration of each cardiac beat is more sensitive to a single electrical stimulus. Amplitudes above display a clear minimum at *a*. Vertical axis can be expressed either in mA or in volts as well.

in, that is the *vulnerable period* of the heart. Thus, the *electrical fibrillation threshold (EFT) to single pulse stimulation is that minimum amplitude with a 50% probability of triggering the phenomenon when directly applied to the myocardium during the vulnerable period.*

A train of pulses can also be synchronized with the QRS complex (Fig. 1.14, lower panel) or can be applied at any random instant. Depending on its overall length, the train may fully cross the T-wave region or it may fall short. Most of the time, however, pulses bombard all through the vulnerable period greatly favoring the discharge of the arrhythmia. A fibrillation threshold is also defined for this situation and, as expected, this second value is always considerably lower than to single pulses. In other words, a burst of electrical pulses is more likely to produce cardiac fibrillation than an isolated pulse; this conclusion has relevance when electrical safety is considered (alternate current is more dangerous than direct current). With single pulse, the probability of hitting the vulnerable period is low, about $D_T/T_C$, where the numerator stands for the ECG T-wave duration and the denominator represents the cardiac period, roughly 10% at the most.

Hence, EFTs depend on many factors, patho-physiological, pharmacological, technological, and procedural (Ruiz *et al.*, 1987); numerical values are only illustrative, as orienting references, and should not be taken as absolute. Comparisons are acceptable exclusively when similar conditions are met. Let us offer examples reported in the literature. Some papers published before 1986 dealing with this specific subject are referred to in Valentinuzzi *et al.* (1986).

Aupetit *et al.* (1993) found a beneficial effect of calcium antagonists when studying the vulnerability to fibrillation. The threshold intensity for fibrillation electrically induced with impulses of 100 ms and 180 ppm (3 Hz) was measured during the course of ischemias obtained by total occlusion of the left anterior descending coronary artery near its origin in open-chest pigs. The variations of EFT with ischemia duration (30, 60, 120, 180, 240, 360) s were compared under control conditions and after diltiazem. EFT was not influenced by diltiazem before, but raised during ischemia, particularly from the 60th second, from 1.7 to 4.0 mA. In six pigs out of eight, fibrillation was even avoided in the longest of the ischemic periods considered (360 s). These experimental results obtained with diltiazem are consistent with the clinical effectiveness of calcium antagonists recently observed in the prevention of post-infarction sudden death, provided that myocardial contractility is not too much adversely affected.

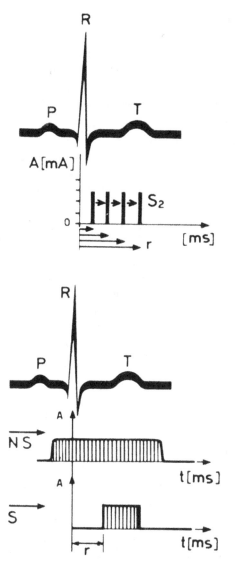

Fig. 1.14.   Upper part: Synchronized single stimulus with adjustable delay. See also the preceding Fig. 1.13. Lower part: Non-synchronized (NS) and synchronized (S) trains of pulses; the latter with adjustable delay.

Ruiz and Valentinuzzi (1994) determined in a group of 17 dogs an average EFT of $(14.1 \pm 4.3)$ mA applying with spoon electrodes ($664\,\text{mm}^2$, i.e. a current density of $0.21\,\text{mA/mm}^2$) directly to the ventricles non-synchronized train of pulses of 2 ms width, 50 Hz repetition rate and overall duration of 1 s (meaning that 50 pulses were delivered). In a group of 33 animals, instead, the average EFT was $(0.91 \pm 0.44)$ mA with the same type of stimulus but using hook electrodes inserted on the myocardium ($11 \, mm^2$, i.e. a current density of $0.08 \, mA/mm^2$). On the other hand, with synchronized single pulses of 5 ms duration using hook electrodes, the average value over the same group of 33 dogs was $(16.8 \pm 7.4) \, mA/mm^2$, or a density of $1.53 \, mA/mm^2$. Obviously, a single pulse was less effective than a train to trigger fibrillation; besides, hook electrodes were more effective than large electrodes applying trains because the former concentrate the stimulus on a small spot creating a focalized inhomogeneity. In the previous report, the threshold for each animal was obtained from the threshold band concept (Valentinuzzi *et al.*, 1984), that is, the applied current attempting fibrillation was plotted as a function of time. A band can be bounded between the maximum value that did not trigger fibrillation and the minimum that did produce the arrhythmia. The mid-range value of such band was taken as the ventricular EFT for that particular animal. The width of the band can well be considered as an estimator of intra-animal repeatability. Numerical data collected from dogs, sloths, and cats yielded that the mid-range value does not differ significantly from the average value within the band. This "fibrillation band" contains values that may or may not trigger the phenomenon with a 50% probability of success. Thus, this definition would take account of the random variations intrinsic to the threshold concept.

Opposite to diltiazem, as described above, myocardial ischemia sensitizes the cardiotoxic effects of bupivacaine, especially the propensity to VF. In anesthetized, open chest pigs, determination of EFT was performed with impulses of 100 ms duration at the rate of 180 bpm, in the absence of ischemia and at the end of increasing periods of ischemia (30, 60, 120, 180) s obtained by complete occlusion of the left anterior descending coronary artery, that is, similar conditions as described by the same group (Aupetit *et al.*, 1993). Bupivacaine significantly increased the fibrillation threshold before coronary occlusion from approximately 7.0 to 9.5 mA. In contrast, during ischemia, the fibrillation threshold was shifted to the left and down, with a hastening of spontaneous fibrillation. Recording of monophasic action potentials in the ischemic area revealed that conduction time was prolonged by more than 100% under the combined influence of ischemia and bupivacaine, whereas the major enhancement of excitability due to ischemia was not attenuated by bupivacaine. Therefore, bupivacaine should be used with caution in the condition of ischemia, especially if heart rate is rapid. Besides, tachycardia may be another factor in the enhancement of bupivacaine effects on conduction (Freysz *et al.*, 1995).

Left ventricular hypertrophy (LVH) is associated with an increased risk of death, susceptibility to ventricular arrhythmia, and multiple electrophysiological abnormalities. Do such susceptibility and electrical abnormalities persist after regression of hypertrophy? Rials *et al.* (1995) placed constricting bands on the ascending aorta of cats or performed sham operations. Serial cardiac echocardiography was performed to measure left ventricular wall thickness. After LVH had developed in the banded animals, the constricting bands were removed and serial echocardiograms were used to monitor for regression of hypertrophy. Cats with persistent LVH had a higher incidence of ventricular tachycardia compared with those that regressed or with sham and had lower VF thresholds $(9 \pm 2)$ mA against $(17 \pm 4)$ mA or $(16 \pm 3)$ mA. Persistent LVH was associated with prolongation of epicardial monophasic action potential duration (MAPD). Dispersion of refractoriness was greater in the group with no regression vs the other two groups. The authors concluded that LVH produces multiple electrophysiological abnormalities and increased vulnerability to inducible polymorphic ventricular arrhythmia.

The latter same group (Rials *et al.*, 1997) addressed the possible regression of ventricular hypertrophy using captopril, including its vulnerability to fibrillation. They used rabbits which had undergone unilateral renal artery banding and contralateral nephrectomy to induce LVH or were placed in the control group. Their description states: "Both groups were studied 3 months later by *in vivo* and *in vitro* electrophysiological techniques. Banded rabbits had increased mean arterial pressure, increased left ventricular weight and wall thickness, increased dispersion of refractoriness, and lower ventricular fibrillation thresholds than control rabbits. Action potential duration and cell capacitance were also greater in the banded group. Additional rabbits were treated beginning 3 months after banding with either captopril or vehicle added to their diet for an additional 3 months. These rabbits and age-matched controls were then studied by *in vivo* and *in vitro* electrophysiological techniques. In banded rabbits that received vehicle and were studied 6 months after banding, increased dispersion of refractoriness, a lower ventricular fibrillation threshold, and action potential prolongation persisted and were unchanged from animals studied 3 months after banding. Captopril, started 3 months after banding, caused regression of hypertrophy and normalization of the *in vivo* and *in vitro* electrophysiological abnormalities.

Addition of captopril to the tissue bath during *in vitro* electrophysiological study showed no effect on cells from control or banded rabbits. That is, pharmacological regression of LVH with captopril normalized the *in vivo* and *in vitro* electrophysiological abnormalities of ventricular hypertrophy and reduced the vulnerability to ventricular fibrillation".

## 1.8. Conclusions and Review Questions

The fibrillation process is a complex and still not well understood phenomenon, even though at least three theories have been so far proposed: re-entrant and persistent excitatory waves, appearance of many pacemaker sites, and formation of relatively organized vortices that tend to generate other vortices as they wander. Perhaps, the latter are a different and more sophisticated way of looking at the circular motions. Several causes have been identified that can be placed either in the clinical, industrial (or domestic), or surgical setting; in the end they amount to the concept of disturbance or to added inhomogeneity to a tissue which is by nature highly inhomogeneous. The latter leads to the traditional four kinds of applicable energies: electric, mechanic, chemical, or thermal. Primary and secondary fibrillations are also distinguished as according to its anatomical localization, that is, atrial or ventricular, the former compatible with life and considered as clinical, and the latter classified as an urgent emergency. The so-called fibrillation variables were introduced along with the not yet well-documented idea of critical fibrillatory mass. Finally, EFT, which can be widely changed by a number of parameters and by methods of stimulation, was presented; it is linked to the extremely important concept of vulnerable window.

*Review questions* (T = True; F = False)

1. Mechanical contraction of the ventricles means the presence of previous electrical activity.                                        T          F
2. During normal cardiac activity the sequence of events is: *sinus node-atrial/atrial contraction/AV node-ventricular conduction system-ventricular mass/ ventricular contraction.*                                        T          F
3. Cardiac fibrillation is the phenomenon of asynchronic or incoordinated or chaotic activity either of the atrial or of the ventricular fibers.                                        T          F

4. Atrial fibrillation is not compatible with life while ventricular fibrillation is.                                     T          F

5. The circus motion theory of fibrillation says essentially that many hyper-excitable points all over the myocardial mass tend to take over the control of cardiac action.                                                        T          F

6. Cold may slow down the propagation of action potentials along the myocardial fibers, while acetylcholine may hinder conduction across the AV node.                                                                  T          F

7. Mammalian myocardial tissue is inherently homogeneous, very much like in a lower heart.                  T          F

8. A vigorous fibrillation, that is, with high frequency components and good amplitude, has better probability of being reverted.                                      T          F

9. A single cardiac fiber may enter into fibrillation.        T          F

10. An electrical stimulus with amplitude having 50% probability of triggering fibrillation is called electrical fibrillation threshold or EFT.                                T          F

11. A sudden accidental human body connection to a direct current power generator...

    (A) will very likely trigger cardiac fibrillation.
    (B) will never trigger cardiac fibrillation.
    (C) may trigger cardiac fibrillation.
        Finish the above statement with either (A), (B), or (C), as the most appropriate form to express the concept.

12. The ventricles of a mammalian heart are electrophysiologically more unstable during the duration of the T-wave.                                          T          F

13. A short action potential...

    (A) does not have any effect on the probability of fibrillation.
    (B) tends to favor the arrhythmia.
    (C) does not favor the arrhythmia.
        Finish the sentence above with the most plausible option.

14. Abnormal intercellular coupling in the heart, resulting
    say from defects in the expression of *connexin* 43, plays
    a key role in the initiation and maintenance of sustained
    arrhythmias.                                              T     F

15. Electrical waves rotating around functional obstacles
    act as primary organizing centers for fibrillation.

    ABSOLUTELY TRUE     PERHAPS TRUE
    ABSOLUTELY NO

16. Ventricular hypertrophy or dilatation, hypokinesia,
    weakened contractility, insufficiency, low ejection
    fraction, atherosclerosis do not favor the probability of
    fibrillation.                                             T     F

17. The type of anesthesia may favor ventricular fibrillation.   T     F

18. Mark at least three possible etiologic factors
    favoring cardiac fibrillation:

    CATECHOLAMINES     BRONCHITIS
        VAGAL FIRING       DEPRESSION
    AORTIC TUMOR

19. Lower animals fibrillate very easily.                     T     F

20. Fibrillation of the second type is characterized by . . .

    (A) high frequency components.
    (B) a wide spectrum.
    (C) low frequency components.
        Select the best answer.

21. Fibrillation is a group phenomenon, that is, one single
    fiber cannot fibrillate.                                  T     F

22. A minimum mass of cardiac tissue is needed for
    fibrillation to take place.                               T     F

23. An electrical amplitude with 50% probability of
    triggering the phenomenon is called the electrical
    fibrillation threshold.                                   T     F

24. The electrocardiographic T-wave marks a period of...

   (A) no susceptibility to electrical pulses.

   (B) high susceptibility to electrical pulses.

25. Is cardiac fibrillation a fully understood arrhythmia?        YES     NO

# Chapter 2

# DEFIBRILLATION

*A sharp and loud shout from the teacher brought back to silence the lecture room full of noisy children...*

This chapter is devoted to the process of arresting the incoordinate and hemodynamically useless cardiac fibrillary movements and, by so doing, offer them the chance to return to the normal beat. In case of ventricular fibrillation, it means a resuscitatory act. The historical development is reviewed, since its inception back in the middle 1700s until the twentieth century pioneers, as example of knowledge acquisition. Thereafter, and even though there are many drawbacks and controversial aspects, chemical defibrillation is also described since it might become the ultimate procedure when the arrhythmia is refractory to the electric shock. Most of this chapter deals with electrical defibrillation, which, so far, is the only available life-saving procedure, either in its direct or indirect forms, depending on the emergency circumstances. The core of this chapter appears in the section dealing with the variables affecting defibrillation, threshold definition, and the concept of dose. For convenience, variables are divided in two groups: *physiopathological* and *technological*. The former includes the *critical defibrillatory mass, heart size*, $K^+$, $Ca^{++}$, $H^+$, *oxygen concentrations*, and *temperature*, all influential variables in the probability of a successful defibrillation. When *myocardial injury* is present and/or *pharmacological agents* have been administered, the situation changes radically, bringing into the forefront the so-called *risk patient*. The last added factor is *fibrillation time*: the longer, the lower the probability of getting out, because damage to the tissues increases. The technological electrical variables constitute determinant factors in the success of a defibrillating discharge. The manufacturer, the physician, the biomedical engineer, and the intervening paramedics must have a clear understanding of them and of the estimated values to apply. Hence, *voltage* V, *current* I, *resistance* R, *power* P, and energy E are briefly reviewed, particularly underlining the resistive hindrance imposed either by the myocardium or the thorax, which usually is referred to as *cardiac* or *thoracic impedance*. Thereafter, the concepts of defibrillation threshold and dose are defined, emphasizing that current, in amperes, should be the parameter to be used because it directly relates to membrane behavior and, if possible, it should be scaled to body weight. For this matter, old basic laws, such as Weiss' and Lapicque's, are recalled. The conceptual and numerical distinctions between defibrillatory threshold and electric dose for defibrillation are underlined. The former is defined as the minimum value (either expressed as current or energy) needed to defibrillate or, in other words, the electric value with a 50% probability of success. The latter, instead, corresponds to the value necessary to defibrillate with at least 90% probability of success and minimum or no damage to the myocardium. Threshold is a reference value while dose is a working quantity related to the previous one by a safety factor. To end, the reader will find cardiopulmonary resuscitation (CPR), cardioversion, and electrical ablation of re-entrant circuits as other techniques to deal with the lethal or very serious arrhthymic arrhythmias.

## 2.1. Definition and Early Developments

Once ventricular fibrillation (VF) is triggered, it must be stopped within a very short time (usually not longer than 3 min, as recommended) because, otherwise, the risk of death ensues due to lack of perfusion to the essential organs (brain, myocardium itself, kidneys). Cardiac fibers, at least most of them if not all, have to be depolarized in order to give them a chance to resume their natural self-sustained normal rhythm. This emergency medical act is called *defibrillation* and frequently is associated with artificial respiration, too, the whole procedure encompassed under the term *cardiopulmonary resuscitation* (CPR).

One definition we can find in the WEB says that "defibrillation is the application of a controlled electrical shock to terminate ventricular fibrillation (VF) or pulseless ventricular tachycardia (VT). The shock is delivered through the chest wall or directly to the heart in an attempt to completely depolarize the myocardium and provide an opportunity for the SA (sino-atrial) node to take over. The longer the myocardium is in VF or VT, the more damage, and the lesser the chance of survival. In other simpler words, the probability of successful defibrillation diminishes rapidly over time."

The origins of defibrillation appear somewhat mixed with charlatanism and rather confusing evidences. In the course of the 1700s and 1800s, numerous trials intended to revive animals and human beings by means of electrical shocks (Schechter, 1971; Geddes, 1984). Perhaps, the first documented electro-resuscitation took place in 1774 and was documented in the *Registers of the Royal Humane Society* of London, when a man named Mr. Squires, from Soho (district of central London, in Westminster), brought back to life a girl, Sofia Greenhill, who had fallen off a window from a second floor. He used a device that was no other than a charged Leyden bottle (that is, a capacitor) applied through electrodes to the girl's thorax. Was it a defibrillation? Perhaps not, but the procedure was truly sound and actual. By a similar token, Luigi Galvani's nephew, Prof. Giovanni Aldini

(1762–1834), of Bologna — a physicist walking the borders of quackery — described resuscitation of the dead or half-dead by electrical shocks delivered from an Alessandro Volta's pile. He traveled all over Europe publicly electrifying human and animal bodies, with performances that were theatrical spectacles, applying it to the bodies of various criminals after execution and heads of animals, too. These experiments were described in a book he published in London in 1803 (*An account of the late improvements in galvanism, with a series of curious and interesting experiments performed before the commissioners of the French National Institute, and repeated lately in the anatomical theaters of London*). Parenthetically and interestingly enough, a description is given in this book of the magnetization of steel needles through connection to one of these voltaic cells (see http://www.corrosion-doctors.org/Biographies/AldiniBio.htm).

The first true and documented defibrillation of the canine heart was demonstrated by the Swiss researchers Prevost and Batelli (1899a, 1989b, 1989c, 1989d; 1900) bringing into light an apparent paradox: an electric current could led the cardiac chambers into fibrillation and another similar, but much higher one, was able to stop it. The studies by these authors were carried out under contract with the power company of those days in Switzerland due to accidental deaths, especially of workers, bringing the matter of electric risk under the spot.

The development of knowledge regarding defibrillation spans well over one hundred years (see http://efimov.wustl.edu/defibrillation/history/defibrillation_history.htm, a site authored by Igor R. Efimov, from Washington University) and it is full of stories, misunderstandings, setbacks, and true advances. Even capital punishment was involved when the decision was taken to use alternating current (ac) for the installation of the first two electric chairs, one in New York and the other in San Francisco, after Edison counsel prevailed; he said (rightly, but probably biased, too) that ac was better suited to kill (see Chap. 1). George Westinghouse (1846–1914) reacted by forbidding his factory to supply the generators (Bernstein, 1973). However, the subject remained controversial for many years including medical, ethical, and moral issues from the very beginning (MacDonald, 1892; Hillman, 1983).

William Kouwenhouven, an electrical engineer, Claude S. Beck, a surgeon, and Paul M. Zoll, a cardiologist, the former in Baltimore, Maryland, the second in Cleveland, Ohio, and the latter in Harvard, Massachusetts, carried out pioneering work leading to clinical and open-chest defibrillation (Kouwenhoven and Hooker, 1933; Beck *et al.*, 1947;

Zoll *et al.*, 1956; Kouwenhoven *et al.*, 1957). Thus, over a period of about 25 years, the procedure advanced enough to be established in medical emergency practice, both in the surgery room and in the general hospital wards, and nowadays even in public spaces. Kouwenhoven, who died in 1975, devoted his entire life to the subject at Johns Hopkins University. He received prizes and distinctions, including the American Medical Association's, the Lasker Award for Clinical and Medical Research and the *Honoris Causa* Medical Doctor Degree from Johns Hopkins, the latter, in 1969, being an honor which very rarely, if ever, is awarded to a person without the medical degree. There is, however, an almost forgotten and not well-recognized previous contribution by Robinovitch (1907, 1909), a Jewish physician of Russian origin, who suffered considerable double discrimination, by genre and by race. Robinovitch elaborated on the idea that bradycardia could be treated by periodic pulses of direct current (dc) in a course of experiments performed in the early 1900s on the resuscitation of victims of electrocution, drowning and excessive anesthesia. It might be speculated that she was aware of Prevost and Batelli's contributions, which is perfectly acceptable and even expected in the advancement of scientific and technical knowledge, without detracting from her at all. She apparently applied pulses for the first time. She also did pioneering research in electro-anesthesia during the 1900–1920s and cardiac physiology. In New York City, she brought wide attention of the press, too.

Defibrillation has been reviewed extensively by several authors (Geddes, 1976; Kerber and Sarnat, 1979; Crampton, 1980; Tacker and Geddes, 1980). This author and his group (Valentinuzzi *et al.*, 1986) published also a critical small book, in Spanish, mostly based on animal experimentation and this present account, in a sense, is its updated continuation. Very recently, Efimov *et al.* (2008), as editors, produced an impressively comprehensive work that goes beyond the mere defibrillation process, coauthored by a team of highly recognized and experienced experts. The most advanced ideas are collected and put forward in it. Besides, several websites, full of practical details, can be easily found by the interested reader, including references to encyclopedias, one of the most reliable is that of the American Heart Association, which periodically updates its contents.

## 2.2. Chemical Defibrillation

The resting membrane potential is mainly dominated by the high ionic potassium concentration within the intracellular fluid while outside its concentration remains much lower. If potassium is added to the extracellular fluid, the transmembrane potential can be significantly reduced by depolarization (i.e. the external side of the excitable membrane becomes less positive with respect to the internal part); thus, a sudden injection of a potassium-rich solution into, say, the coronary circulation, thereafter followed by a wash-out solution, massively depolarizes cardiac cells giving them the chance to resume their natural rhythm.

Hooker (1930) experimented chemical defibrillation in dogs by means of KCl (0.5%) followed by $CaCl_2$ (0.023%), both in NaCl (at 0.5% and 0.9%, respectively). These oxygen saturated solutions, at body temperature, were sequentially injected into the carotid artery at a pressure of 150 mmHg, the second calcium one acting as wash-out, which has also positive inotropic properties. The technique, however, is not easy to implement because the injected doses must be well measured and balanced; excess of $K^+$ would easily bring the ventricles hypodynamic, while excess of $Ca^{++}$ leads to hyperexcitability and, thus, would favor refibrillation.

Due to the above-mentioned reasons, chemical defibrillation was abandoned, nonetheless, there were some come backs. Robicsek (1984), for example, in North Carolina, after a few procedural changes, advocated it, especially during open-chest interventions. Cammili *et al.* (1991), from the Cardiac Pacing Center, Firenze, Italy, proposed an implantable pharmacological defibrillator. As the predecessors did, it consists of replacing the electric shock with a "chemical" shock, i.e. a bolus retroperfused in the coronary sinus (CS) immediately after VF arises. Preliminary investigations were performed in rabbits, sheep, and swine. The perfused drugs were lidocaine and bretylium tosylate, the former with 86% success and the latter with 14% success. These figures refer to the total number of animals irrespective of the species. Lidocaine immediately terminated VF in 100% of the rabbits followed by sinus rhythm restoration, while in the other two species results were less conclusive. New compounds, such as bethanidine, clofilium, tricyclic antidepressants and phenotiazine derivatives, were suggested by these authors as defibrillating agents in dogs, sheep and swine, and also in humans during routine electropharmacological studies.

There are other reports offering support to chemical defibrillation. Theoretical and computer studies, as well as experimental evidence, have suggested that fibrillation is created and sustained by the property of restitution of the cardiac action potential duration, that is, its dependence on the previous diastolic interval (DI). Somewhat repeating what was said in the previous chapter, the **restitution hypothesis states that steeply sloped restitution curves create unstable wave propagation that results in wave break,** i.e. the cardiac action potential duration (APD) and its conduction velocity (CV) both depend on the previous DI, which is the rest period between repolarization and the next excitation. A critical prediction says that a **drug that reduces the slope of the curve should have potent antifibrillatory effects.** In particular, the action of bretylium would appear as a prototype for the future development of effective antifibrillatory agents because it flattens such curve. It even converts existing fibrillation, either to a periodic state (ventricular tachycardia (VT), which is much more easily controlled) or to quiescent healthy tissue (Garfinkel *et al.*, 2000). In slightly different wording: recalling the multiple vortex-like of reentrant waves described in Chap. 1, electrical excitation meanders erratically through the ventricular muscle. It usually begins with a more orderly stage (sometimes named Wiggers' stage I), consisting of just one or a pair of spiral waves, which then break down into the multi-spiral disordered state that is the actual VF. Heterogeneity, either histological or electrophysiological, is probably a cause (Chap. 1), while several theorists suggested that dynamic heterogeneity arising from restitution properties may be more critical.

Even though there are many drawbacks, doubts, and controversial aspects, perhaps chemical action could become the ultimate procedure when fibrillation is refractory to the electrical shock. It should be considered an area still open to basic research. Just the whole restitution hypothesis (a term that to the author of this book sounds as more confusing than truly descriptive) appears somewhat aside and, in itself, as lying in its investigative stage.

## 2.3. Electrical Defibrillation

### 2.3.1. *Transventricular or Direct*

In spite of the claims already described above, the electrical counter-shock is so far the established, accepted, and rather reliable method to revert VF. Successful defibrillation depends strongly on a cross-lateral transventricular current density large enough to depolarize a myocardial mass equal to or bigger than the *critical defibrillatory mass* (which is different and not related to the *critical fibrillatory mass*). Cardiac surgeons, who often face the arrhythmia, use the method by embracing with spoon electrodes

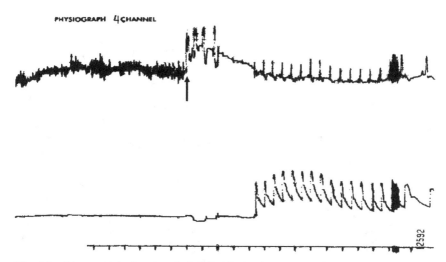

Fig. 2.1. Transventricular electrical defibrillation in an open-chest experimental dog. Top: ECG; Bottom: Arterial pressure. Time marks 1 sec apart. A direct shock restored activity. After a few ectopics and A-V block, pressure was also restored. Obtained by the author at the Physiology Dept, Baylor College Medicine, Houston, TX, USA. Also in Valentinuzzi *et al.*, 1986, with that publisher's kind permission.

directly on the ventricles, compressing them gently, and discharging a strong pulse. This is called *direct* or *transventricular defibrillation*. Figure 2.1 displays a couple of simultaneous records obtained from an open-chest medium-sized experimental dog. The upper channel shows the surface ECG, the middle one is blood pressure detected with an external transducer by cannulation of one carotid artery, and the bottom trace indicates time marks 1 s apart. Fibrillation had been triggered with a short train of pulses applied via hand electrodes directly to the epicardial surface and, less than a minute after, spoon electrodes were positioned laterally so that a good myocardial portion was embraced. The vertical arrow on the central part of the top channel marks the time of the electrical capacitor discharge, which was delivered from custom-made equipment. Arrest of fibrillation was immediate; three ectopics can be clearly seen followed by an AV total block resuming, thereafter, the normal sinus rhythm with full recovery of blood pressure, which during fibrillation had fell to zero level. The impedance seen by the electrodes was low and in the order of 25 ohms, the latter measured with a high-frequency constant-current Z-meter. Figure 2.2(a) shows how the spoons usually grab the ventricles.

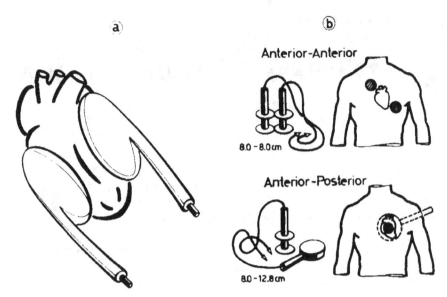

Fig. 2.2.   Defibrillating electrodes. Left (a) Transventricular spoon electrodes. Right (b) Transthoracic paddles: Anterior–anterior lead, both of 8 cm in diameter (above) and anterior (8 cm diameter)–posterior (12 cm diameter) lead (below).

### 2.3.2. *Transthoracic or Indirect*

It is the unexpected emergency, on a public place, at home or industrial, either due to myocardial pathology or to accidental electric shock. Electrodes are of the paddle type, placed over the anterior face of the thorax or as antero-posterior lead (Fig. 2.2(b)). Only a fraction of the delivered current crosses the myocardial mass and the success of the procedure depends on its intensity and distribution, for pathways not traversing the ventricles do not contribute to the depolarization process and, in fact, they may even damage other surrounding tissues. Location and electrode size are important parameters to take into account. The impedance faced by the generator is higher than in the direct case and lies in the order of 50 ohms, which may reach easily 70 or 80 ohms. The literature abounds and goes hand-in-hand with and as part of CPR.

### 2.4. Defibrillation Variables, Thresholds, and Concept of Dose

Conceptually, both types of defibrillation are influenced by the same variables, which can be grouped into *physiological* (or better, *physiopathological*) and *technological*. Since defibrillation is a *probabilistic* event, the condition of the heart (in itself the result of several variables) essentially determines how high or low that probability is. Physicians in their daily practice, based on clinical and biochemical information, precisely try to evaluate such probability when a patient is classified, say, as of low or high risk one to indicate or not his/her confinement in the Intensive Coronary Unit (ICU). No doubt, an ischemic or infarcted myocardium would have a lower probability of success, should it fall into fibrillation.

### 2.4.1. Physiological Variables

They are the same as those referred to in Sec. 1.6 and, therefore, as determining the probability of fibrillation, and will also play a similar role in setting the probability of stopping it. Critical defibrillatory mass, heart size, potassium, calcium, pH, oxygen concentration, and temperature are essential variables, besides, the patient may have had myocardial injury and received pharmacological agents that can change radically the situation. However, fibrillation time appears as important and significant added factor: the longer, the lower the probability of getting out, because damage to the tissues increases non-linearly with time.

(a) *Critical defibrillatory mass*

By definition, it is the minimal number of ventricular fibers that must be depolarized to stop fibrillation. A simple daily life example illustrates the concept: a school room full of $N$ talking and noisy children can be brought into silence by a teacher's shout if, and only if, the shout is heard by at least $M \leq N$ number of students who obey and hush; the relative silence produced by $M$ will drag the rest $(N-M)$ to silence, too. Of course, $M = N$ describes the trivial best case.

The basic goal in defibrillation is to interfere electrically with the reentry circuits (analog to children talking and making noise) to bring this activity to a halt. However, not all circuits need to be stopped. Zipes *et al.* (1975) concluded that about 28% of the ventricular mass would be enough. However, this figure sounds as too low and other authors have suggested a minimum in the order of 78%, which seems more plausible (Witkowski *et al.*, 1990; Malmivuo and Plonsey, 1995, see its Chap. 24).

Chen *et al.* (1991) concluded that often the shock intensity is not great enough (the teacher did not shout much) and, thus, fibrillation is reinitiated. First, typical shocks generate field strengths throughout the heart that are quite variable. Placing defibrillating electrodes on the right atrium and left ventricular apex of a dog, Ideker *et al.*, (1987) found the potential field gradient to vary over a 15:1 range on the epicardium. Second, the site of earliest measured activity following unsuccessful defibrillation coincided with the region with the lowest shock field strength. These conclusions support the idea that the goal of a defibrillating electrode system is the generation of a uniform field within the heart, which sounds sensible and quite acceptable. The minimum field for successful defibrillation was found by both groups to lie in the range of 3–9 V/cm (Witkowski *et al.*, 1990; Chen *et al.*, 1991).

While the aforementioned studies are valuable for a better understanding of fibrillation — defibrillation, they do not actually enlighten an electrophysiological *mechanism*. The only way a shock can influence the behavior of fibrillating cells is through the induced transmembrane potential, which could result in the activation of resting cells or of cells in relative refractory period. However, one has to keep in mind that fibrillating fibers do not behave in the same way as normal cells and in the way they interact with each other.

The concept of minimal defibrillatory mass is appealing and sounds as correct but, so far, no good percentage of the total ventricular mass has been determined and it does not seem to be an easy task to accomplish. The few figures found in the literature cover a wide range (28–78% of ventricular weight), the latter seemingly looking as more likely and even perhaps on the high side. Obviously, reaching all fibers should be the ideal situation, but inhomogeneities may lead to tissue damage because of too high field intensities. A more definitive answer is yet to be found regarding this matter.

(b) *Heart size*

In Chap. 1, the requirement of a minimal myocardial mass was mentioned to maintain fibrillation (critical fibrillation mass), meaning that small hearts could never, if ever, fall into the arrhythmia. Besides, reducing the size of a fibrillating heart may end up in the termination of the phenomenon. Garrey (1914) tested the hypothesis by cutting a fibrillating ventricle into smaller pieces to see, indeed, that they stopped. Besides, there is a correlation between heart size and the propensity to develop and maintain fibrillation. Atrial and ventricular fibrillation is more easily induced and sustained in large hearts than in small hearts (Johansson, 1984). This statement coincides with reports given by several other authors over the years (Zipes,

1975; Valentinuzzi *et al.*, 1986; Savino and Valentinuzzi, 1988; Ruiz and Valentinuzzi, 1994).

Conversely, when studying defibrillation, experience and experimentation demonstrated that bigger hearts are more difficult to halt requiring higher levels of current until, after a certain size, defibrillation becomes impossible. A horse heart falls mostly in the latter category. How would a fibrillating giraffe's or elephant's heart respond? Cardiac surgeons know well that big guys are always more problematic than smaller ones, should the need of defibrillation occur. Moreover, these bigger hearts appear as more sensitive to fibrillation. Since heart size is related to body size, the latter can also be considered as a determinant variable in the probability of defibrillation (see also the references given in the upper paragraph). There is a scarcity of data for children, especially grouping those by age, but hearsay among pediatric cardiologists during informal conversations seem to support the concept that fibrillation is rather uncommon in children and the few cases they witnessed or remembered presented no defibrillation difficulty. It appears, indeed, as an interesting statistics to collect. An interesting report we found is due to Pedrote *et al.* (2006), from Sevilla, Spain, with excellent reference material. They describe the case of a pediatric patient, 12 years old, with hypertrophic cardiomyopathy (HCM) who presented VF and to whom an implantable cardioverter defibrillator (ICD) was installed. Nine months later, the child experienced a recurrence of cardiac arrest during exercise, which was successfully treated with a defibrillator shock from the device. The stored electrograms demonstrated VF of abrupt onset following sinus tachycardia (Fig. 2.3). These authors confirm the notion of few reported cases of children with HCM resuscitated after cardiac arrest. The underlying arrhythmia is usually a polymorphic VT or VF. It is possible that in younger patients sudden death is more frequently related to myocardial ischemia rather than to a primary arrhythmogenic ventricular substrate. In the case described, the authors speculate that during strenuous exercise, sinus tachycardia combined with severe hypotension and decreased myocardial perfusion led to VF. This very young patient had two risk factors for sudden death at the time of cardiac arrest, the degree of wall thickness and the abnormal blood pressure response to exercise. An abnormal blood pressure response during exercise can be detected in 25% of HCM patients.

Attempts have been made to scale delivered shock energy (in joules) or delivered current (in Amps) either to heart size or for that matter to body size, so leading to the concept of *defibrillating dose*, analogous to established

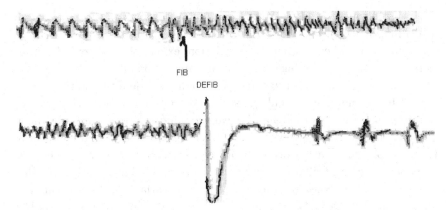

Fig. 2.3.    Fib-defib in a 12 year old child. Stored intracardiac electrogram from the ICD. Sinus tachycardia during exercise (upper left) followed by an onset of VF (upper right) terminated by a 27J shock from the device. Normal rhythm was thereafter normalized (lower right, three last beats). Modified after Pedrote, Morales *et al.*, 2006, with permission; downloaded from http://www.ncbi.nlm.nih.gov/pubmed/16687426).

medical practice when prescribing a given drug. The former would be stated in joules/kg *bw* or amps/kg *bw* while the latter is given in mg/kg *bw* (*bw* stands for "body weight"). Using a heart weight (HW)–body weight (BW) relationship (usually an empirical one that shows some dependence on the species and also on the size of the animal) would lead to whatever electrical unit is required scaled to grams of heart.

An old paper by Don R. Joseph, from the Department of Physiology and Pharmacology of the Rockefeller Institute for Medical Research, dated on May 6, 1908, published July 8 of the same year and downloaded from http://www.jem.org/cgi/reprint/10/4/521.pdf on January 6, 2008 (the original full reference is not given), reports interesting values for different species. Man, for example, lies between 5 and 6 g of *hw* per kg of *bw*, while pig, cattle, sheep, horse, hare, and dog spread between 4 and 9 g of *hw* per kg of *bw*. To illustrate, a normal person weighing 70 kg would be expected to have a heart of about 350–420 g. Armayor *et al.* (1979) found an average of 9 g/kg in 20 mongrel dogs averaging 13 kg of BW while another paper offers values within these ranges for horses and dogs (Gunn, 1989).

(c) *Potassium ion, calcium ion, pH, and oxygen blood levels*

Potassium is essential for the establishment of the diastolic membrane potential and for the degree of excitability. Calcium plays an electrophysiological role mainly related to the triggering threshold potential and to the plateau of the action potential; it is also a determinant factor in fiber contractility. The degree of acidity and the amount of oxygen in blood determine basic metabolic cell functions. All four variables influence profoundly the physiological condition of the myocardium and, thus, its probability of defibrillating when given an electric discharge. It should be emphasized that the electric shock, once applied, should bring an enough number of fibers to the refractory period. Let us review these variables in somewhat more detail.

*Potassium ion*

Assuming the electrophysiological behavior of ventricular fibers remain unchanged during fibrillation (and the assumption represents a big "if"), more $K^+$ outside would depolarize the membrane and further depolarization should be easier for an external discharge, that is, a lower voltage would be required. Specifically, the applied defibrillatory current (as any successfully expected stimulus) should need to be proportional to the difference between the resting membrane potential of the unexcited cells in a fibrillating myocardium and the threshold potential (critical triggering level) of those cells (Fig. 2.4; Valentinuzzi, 2004).

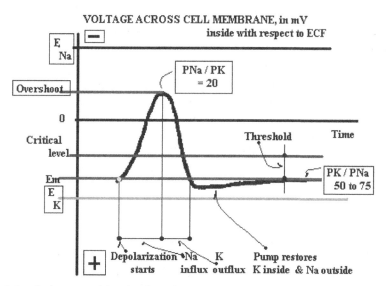

Fig. 2.4.   Action potential and its boundaries. The action potential is always bounded by the potassium potential, near the membrane potential, and the sodium potential above, which is a limiting unreachable value. The difference between the resting membrane potential $E_m$ and the critical or triggering level defines the threshold that a stimulus has to overcome in order to generate an action potential (after Valentinuzzi, 2004, with permission).

The extracellular to intracellular potassium concentration ratio, that is, $K_o^+/K_i^+$, is the determinant factor in the transmembrane resting potential. A first-order approximation of its value is given by Nernst equation, the so-called *potassium equilibrium potential*, or

$$E_K(\text{mV}) = -61.5 \log(K_o^+/K_i^+),$$

which is valid with the shown coefficient when the temperature $t = 37°\text{C}$. In physiological conditions, the actual resting potential is slightly less negative than the above given value because of some $Na^+$ influx (higher outside than inside the cell). Since $K_i^+ \gg K_o^+$, i.e. about 150 mEq/L against around 5 mEq/L, small changes in extracellular potassium can cause important variations in $E_K$ and, as a consequence, in the transmembrane potential without significant changes of intracellular potassium or, for that matter, of total potassium in the body.

Babbs *et al.* (1980) hypothesized that, since KCl injection brings the potassium potential $E_K$ toward the zero level because of depolarization while the triggering threshold gets lower, the defibrillation threshold (DT) should decrease. The latter was actually verified: with blood potassium concentrations of about 20 mEq/L, the DT tends to very low values. Besides, it was found that the amount of $K^+$ collected in the coronary sinus increased as fibrillation time increased explaining also the diastolic potential decrease in action potentials recorded with microelectrodes during fibrillation (Akiyama, 1981). This paper is to be commended because of the ingenious movement compensating technique employed.

Somewhat in line with the previous findings, Winecoff *et al.* (1997) postulated that if potassium conductance is a primary mechanism affecting DT values, then increasing potassium ion conductance, which enhances $K^+$ outflow and hyperpolarization, will increase defibrillation values. Conversely, inhibition of potassium ion conductance decreases DT, as mentioned above. The primary objective of this study was to determine if the ATP-dependent potassium (KATP) channel opener *pinacidil* would increase DT values. The second objective was to prove that the observed changes were due to potassium conductance by using the KATP inhibitor, *glyburide*, to reverse the electrophysiologic actions of *pinacidil*. The third objective was to determine if the electrophysiology actions of *pinacidil* correlate with changes in DT value. The study was carried out in 14 domestic farm swine, instrumented with monophasic action potential catheters and epicardial defibrillation patches. DT, action potential duration, effective refractory period, and VF cycle length were determined.

These authors concluded that *pinacidil* does not alter DT, but it reduces effective refractory period, action potential duration, and VF cycle length and does not increase electrical heterogeneity. Therefore, changes in potassium channel conductance as well as shortening repolarization are unlikely primary mechanisms for elevating DT.

> *Pinacidil* is a potassium channel opener that decreases blood pressure by reducing peripheral arterial resistance. It has significant cardioprotective effects, which are mediated primarily by the mitochondrial $K_{ATP}$ channel (Diodato *et al.*, 2004). The study was carried out in rabbits.
>
> *Glyburide* is in a class of drugs called sulfonylureas. It is used to treat Type 2 (non-insulin-dependent) diabetes, particularly in people whose diabetes cannot be controlled by diet alone. Glyburide manages to lower blood sugar levels by stimulating the pancreas to secrete insulin and helping the body use insulin efficiently. The pancreas must produce insulin for this medication to work. Glyburide is not used to treat Type 1 (insulin-dependent) diabetes (see http://www.lycos.com/info/glyburide.html).

Always dealing with cardiac effects of $K^+$ on the fibrillation–defibrillation process, Bradley and Salil (2003), referring to anodal excitation of cardiac tissue, distinguished between the classical *break* excitation and *make* excitation. The goal they set was to determine how an elevated extracellular potassium ion concentration affects the mechanism of anodal excitation. Computer simulations of unipolar stimulation were performed. They reported that diastolic threshold for anodal stimulation first decreased and then increased with increasing extracellular $[K]_o$, reaching a minimum value at $[K]_o = 12\,mM$, and concluding that high $[K]_o$ predisposes cardiac tissue to *break* excitation, which is thought to play an important role in reentry induction and defibrillation. Since fibrillation raises extracellular $[K]_o$ levels, *break* excitation may play a more important role in defibrillation than is suggested by simulations and experiments using normal $[K]_o$ values.

*Calcium ion*

Ca ion has several not well understood yet electrophysiological effects on the fibrillation–defibrillation process; in particular, it influences the critical or triggering potential. An increase in extracellular $Ca^{++}$, for example, decreases that potential bringing it closer to zero level and decreasing, in turn, the cell excitability. Conversely, raising its concentration leads to higher excitability because the triggering voltage is lowered, that is, it becomes more negative. Let us underline that threshold goes up when the triggering potential decreases (it gets closer to the zero level), that is, more depolarization is needed to bring the resting membrane potential to the critical triggering potential and so initiating the action potential (Hoffman and Cranefield, 1960). Thus, defibrillation changes are expected to occur with calcium concentration changes. However, predictions are difficult because the interactions are more complex than the simple explanation given above. Papers are often contradictory.

Merillat *et al.* (1990), for example, from Johns Hopkins University, developed a non-ischemic, isolated, perfused rabbit Langendorff preparation in which sustained VF could be induced by ac and which allowed changes in perfusate composition. Calcium channel blockade by *verapamil* or *nitrendipine* uniformly inhibited the initiation of VF, despite evidence of $Ca^{++}$ overload. Lowering extracellular calcium to $80\,\mu$M uniformly prevented the initiation of VF and resulted in defibrillation during VF whether induced by *ac* or by Na–K pump inhibition. *Verapamil* or *nitrendipine* also resulted in defibrillation regardless of the initiation method. Electrical defibrillation was successful only in *ac*-induced VF. The data suggest that increases in slow channel calcium flux were necessary for the initiation and maintenance of VF.

> *Verapamil* is a calcium ion influx inhibitor. Its mechanism of antiarrhythmic effects is believed to be related to its specific cellular action of selectively inhibiting transmembrane influx of calcium in cardiac muscle, coronary and systemic arteries, and in cells of the intracardiac conduction system. It blocks the transmembrane influx of calcium through the slow channel without affecting the influx of sodium through the fast channel. Thus, there is reduction of free calcium ions available within cells. Its action is brought about largely on the sinoatrial (SA) and atrioventricular (AV) nodes. It depresses AV nodal conduction and prolongs functional refractory periods; besides, it does not alter the normal atrial action potential or intraventricular conduction time, but depresses amplitude, velocity of depolarization and conduction in depressed atrial fibers. Through this action, it interrupts re-entrant pathways and slows ventricular rate (see http://www.mentalhealth.com/drug/p30-i03.html).
>
> *Nitrendipine* is also a calcium channel blocker and similar to other peripheral vasodilators. It inhibits the influx of extracellular calcium across the myocardial and vascular smooth muscle cell membranes possibly by deforming the channel, inhibiting ion-control gating mechanisms, and/or interfering with the release of calcium from the sarcoplasmic reticulum (SR). The decrease in intracellular calcium inhibits the contractile processes of the myocardial smooth muscle cells, causing dilation of the coronary and systemic arteries, increased oxygen delivery to the myocardial tissue, decreased total peripheral resistance,

decreased systemic blood pressure, and decreased afterload (see http://
www.mongabay.com/health/medications/Nitrendipine.html).

Possible drug interactions with electrical defibrillation were examined
by Krauthamer and Smith (2004) using adrenergic agents (epinephrine,
norepinephrine, isoproterenol) and a calcium channel blocker (*verapamil*;
see note above), when applied acutely and following a defibrillator shock.
Dissociated heart cells from 10-day chicken embryos were cultured to
form spherical aggregates and plated in Petri dishes. In the experiments,
the spheres were paced at $0.75\,\text{V/cm}$ above contraction threshold, and a
biphasic defibrillator shock was applied for 1 ms at $46\,\text{V/cm}$. The adrenergic
agents shortened the duration of arrest following a defibrillator shock, while
the calcium channel blocker lengthened the arrest time.

Complicating still further the calcium picture within the fibrillation–
defibrillation framework is the well-documented action of this ion on
cardiac fibers' contractility. In fact, calcium is an essential factor in that
respect. Suffice it to say that fibrillating cells rather quickly lose their
ability to contract, so worsening the recovery probability. Thus, calcium
possible arrhythmic actions via contractility effects become harder and more
complex to explain.

Abnormal sarcoplasmic reticulum (SR) calcium cycling is increasingly
recognized as an important mechanism for increased ventricular automaticity
that leads to lethal ventricular arrhythmias (Yuan *et al.*, 2007). According
to the latter authors, previous studies have linked lethal arrhythmogenic
disorders to mutations in the *ryanodine* receptor and *calsequestrin* genes,
which interact with *junctin* and *triadin* to form a macromolecular Ca-
signaling complex. The essential physiological effects of *junctin* and its
potential regulatory roles in SR Ca-cycling and Ca-dependent cardiac
functions, such as myocyte contractility and automaticity, are unknown. The
*junctin* gene was targeted in embryonic stem cells and a junctin-deficient
mouse was generated. Ablation of *junctin* was associated with enhanced
cardiac function *in vivo*, and junctin-deficient cardiomyocytes exhibited
increased contractile and Ca-cycling parameters. Short-term isoproterenol
stimulation elicited arrhythmias, including premature ventricular contractions, atrioventricular heart block, and VT. Long-term isoproterenol infusion
also induced premature ventricular contractions and atrioventricular heart
block in junctin-null mice. Further examination of the electrical activity
revealed a significant increase in the occurrence of delayed after depolariza-
tions; consistently, 25% of the junctin-null mice died by 3 months of age
with structurally normal hearts. These authors concluded that *junctin* is

an essential regulator of SR Ca release and contractility in normal hearts. Ablation of junctin is associated with aberrant Ca homeostasis, which leads to fatal arrhythmias. Thus, normal intracellular Ca-cycling relies on the maintenance of *junctin* levels and an intricate balance among the components in the SR quaternary Ca-signaling complex.

*Ryanodine* (molecular formula $C_{25}H_{35}NO_9$; molar mass 493.547 g/mol) is a poisonous alkaloid found in the South American plant *Ryania speciosa*. The compound has extremely high affinity to the ryanodine receptor, linked to calcium channels of skeletal and heart muscle cells. It binds with such high affinity to the receptor that it was used as a label for the first purification of that class of ionic channels and gave its name to it. At nanomolar concentrations, ryanodine locks the receptor in a half-open state, whereas it fully closes them at micromolar concentration. The effect of the nanomolar-level binding is that ryanodine causes release of $Ca^{++}$ from calcium stores in the SR leading to massive muscular contraction (Hille, 2001; retrieved from http://en.wikipedia.org/wiki/Ryanodine).

*Calsequestrin* is the main calcium-binding protein inside the SR of striated muscle. In mammals, the cardiac calsequestrin gene (*casq2*) mainly expresses in cardiac muscle and to a minor extent in slow-twitch skeletal muscle and it is not expressed in non-muscle tissues (Reyes-Juárez *et al.*, 2007).

*Junctin* is a 26-kDa integral membrane protein, which forms a quaternary protein complex with the *ryanodine* receptor, *calsequestrin* and *triadin* at the junctional SR membrane in cardiac and skeletal muscles. *Junctin* has been proposed to consist of a short N-terminal cytoplasmic domain, a single transmembrane domain, and a highly charged domain extending into the SR lumen. It has been hypothesized that *junctin* and *triadin* are calsequestrin-anchoring proteins that facilitate $Ca^{++}$ release. In fact, early studies on *junctin* indicated that it is important for the formation and/or stabilization of the junctional SR complex in intact cardiac muscle (Evangelina Kranias Lab, University of Cincinnati, see http://www.med.uc.edu/kranias/junctin.htm).

*Triadin*. The junction between the transverse tubules (T-tubules) and the SR of skeletal muscle is called the triad. At the triad, dihydropyridine (DHPR) receptors of the T-tubule serve as voltage sensors in excitation–contraction coupling, while *ryanodine* receptors (RyRs), the calcium release channels, exist in the membrane of the terminal cisternae of the SR. It is thought that during slow phase depolarization of the T-tubule, a third protein, *triadin* transmits electrochemical signals to the SR through direct interaction with both dihydropyridine receptors and RyRs. Though its exact role in this signaling process is unclear, *triadin* has been shown to play a role with both DHPR and RyR at the junctional face of the terminal cisternae (Györke *et al.*, 2004).

*Acidity (pH or ionic $H^+$ concentration), oxygen, and ischemia*

The three variables are intimately related and it is not easy to separate out the effects of each. Besides, effects are strongly interwoven with fibrillation itself which, in the end, always precedes the defibrillatory act. Thus, it is better to treat these variables as a group referring also, when needed, to fibrillation as the initial phenomenon so complementing the content of Chap. 1. Once again, reports appear as mixed and conflicting in some cases. Hydrogen cations $H^+$ play a role via the plasmatic pH. It has been demonstrated that under low pH conditions, ventricular contractility is severely depressed because it interacts with $Ca^{++}$ availability. Restoring the acid–base equilibrium, contractility returns to its normal values within minutes. The acidity degree affects excitability because it interferes with potassium exchange. Acidosis is usually accompanied by hyperkalemia plus a decrease in intracellular $K^+$ concentration. Moreover, it must be underlined that oxygen is carried by blood and, as a consequence, hypoxia and ischemia usually go hand-in-hand.

About 25 years ago, Kerber *et al.* (1983) carried out a study regarding this group reaching to somewhat unexpected results. The purpose was to assess the effect of myocardial ischemia, left ventricular hypertrophy, systemic hypoxia, and acid–base abnormalities on the energy requirements for defibrillation. They did not find significantly elevated values after left anterior descending coronary occlusion, nor was there a relationship between the size of the occluded coronary distribution area (coronary risk area) and the change in values in individual animals. Systemic hypoxia and acid–base abnormalities were also induced; only systemic hypoxia led to significant changes. Thus, they concluded that in dogs, myocardial ischemia, left ventricular hypertrophy, and acid–base abnormalities do not elevate defibrillation energy requirements, whereas hypoxia reduces the energy needed to defibrillate.

Echt *et al.* (1989), from Vanderbilt University, ran a well planned and detailed study of blood pH and its influence on lidocaine, in turn effecting defibrillation requirements. Excerpting from their paper is appropriate: "Lidocaine increases the energy required for ventricular defibrillation in dogs, thus, the pH dependence of this agent on internal defibrillation energy requirements was investigated in 28 dogs with atrial spring and left ventricular patch electrodes. Results of defibrillation testing were used to derive 50% and 90% successful energy requirements (ED50 and ED90) using logistic regression and were compared with analysis of variance. Acidosis produced by hydrochloric acid infusion decreased the arterial pH from

$7.40 \pm 0.05$ to $7.18 \pm 0.03$, but no significant change in ED90 was observed ($14\pm4$ to $16\pm6$ J). Lidocaine infusion to therapeutic levels ($4.2\pm0.07\,\mu g/ml$) at normal pH ($7.42 \pm 0.02$) increased ED90 from $13 \pm 3$ to $17 \pm 3$ J, and subsequent acidosis (pH $7.19 \pm 0.02$) exacerbated this effect of lidocaine on ED90 ($22\pm5$ J). Alkalosis produced by respirator hyperventilation increased the arterial pH from $7.41 \pm 0.03$ to $7.60 \pm 0.03$, with a fall in ED90 from $13 \pm 4$ to $8 \pm 3$ J."

Smith *et al.* (1995) tested the hypothesis that the loss of cell-to-cell electrical interaction during ischemia modulates the amplitude of ischemia-induced TQ-segment depression (i.e. the injury potential) and the occurrence of VF during the so-called Ib phase of ventricular arrhythmias. Sometimes, late tachycardia or fibrillation triggered, say, after 15–60 min of ischemia, is termed as Ib-type (Coronel *et al.*, 2002). In their own words: "Regional ischemia was induced by 60 minutes of mid-left anterior descending coronary artery ligation in open-chest swine. Cell-to-cell electrical uncoupling was defined as the onset of the terminal rise in whole-tissue resistivity ($R_t$). Local activation times and TQ-segment changes (injury potential) were determined from unipolar electrograms. Extracellular $[K^+]_e$ and pH were measured with plunge-wire ion-selective electrodes. VF occurred in 6 of 10 pigs during regional no-flow ischemia between 19 and 30 minutes after the arrest of perfusion. The occurrence of VF was positively correlated to the onset of cell-to-cell electrical uncoupling. Cell-to-cell electrical uncoupling superimposed on changes of $[K^+]_e$ and pH contributed to the failure of impulse propagation between 19 and 30 minutes after the arrest of perfusion. During ischemia, maximum TQ-segment depression was $-10$ mV at 19 minutes, after which TQ-segment depression slowly recovered. The onset of the TQ-segment recovery was correlated to the second rise in $R_t$. In conclusion, in the regionally ischemic *in situ* porcine heart, loss of cell-to-cell electrical interaction is related to the occurrence of VF and changes in the amplitude of the injury current. Cellular electrical uncoupling contributes to failure of impulse propagation in the setting of altered tissue excitability as a result of elevated $[K^+]_e$ and low pH. These data indicate that Ib arrhythmias and ECG changes during ischemia are influenced by the loss of cell-to-cell electrical interaction."

Perhaps, other ions have an influence too on the overall fibrillation-defibrillation picture (such as magnesium), however, they do not seem to be significant factors in this respect. Besides, terminology (such as *restitution hypothesis, type Ib-fibrillation,* or *tachycardia*) should be taken with a grain of salt; they are not widely used or clearly understood and tend to add confusion into an already complex subject. A similar comment ought to be said with respect to the excess use of acronyms; if not applied prudently, a single paragraph may become a cryptic piece!

*Duration of fibrillation*

It makes sense to state that the success of a defibrillation shock strongly depends on how long the myocardium was in fibrillation simply because the likelihood of cell damage is greater. Practical experience has well demonstrated this as it has also been shown in *ad hoc* studies, as for example, by Lerman and Engelstein (1995) who, opposite to other views, laterally claim that metabolic acidosis or alkalosis do not affect the outcome. The authors hypothesized that release of myocardial adenosine during VF could potentially mediate the time-dependent effects of VF duration on defibrillation. DT was therefore determined in dogs during concurrent infusion of adenosine and dipyridamole (a nucleoside transport blocker). Transthoracic DT increased by approximately 50%, whereas transmyocardial DT increased by approximately 100% in a separate group of dogs. These effects of adenosine on DT were abolished when the dogs were autonomically denervated, suggesting that the deleterious effects of adenosine on DT are due to its antiadrenergic mechanism of action. These data indicate that adenosine release during VF can markedly increase DT. Since adenosine myocardial release during VF is time dependent, it is likely that adenosine plays a significant role in mediating the increase in threshold that is dependent on the duration of VF.

*Temperature*

The effects of temperature on fibrillation–defibrillation should consider two different ways of introducing temperature changes: inhomogeneous sudden variations and slow decrease of temperature (hypothermia). The former would generate gradients and, thus, inhomogeneities (say, in conduction velocities or in refractory periods), that would tend to favor fibrillation. A corollary of the previous statements says that the velocity with which temperature changes appears as an added and probably significant factor. There are many studies on hypothermia but very few, if any, on the appearance of temperature gradients. Often, conclusions appear as conflicting and confusing.

Arredondo *et al.* (1980) found a significant decrease of DTs in hypothermic dogs when compared to normothermic animals (from 89.5 to 69.5 mA/g *hw*). Thereafter, the same group, Arredondo *et al.* (1982, 1984), determined a decrease, too, in hypothermic dogs after coronary occlusion (to 53.6 mA/g $hw$, where $hw$ stands for "heart weight"). Apparently, the effects of low temperature and ischemia are additive.

However, the results reported by Ujhelyi *et al.* (2001) were different while the methodology and conditions were not fully comparable. These authors experimented in domestic farm swine, all instrumented with a transvenous defibrillation system connected to a defibrillator that delivered a biphasic-truncated waveform. Values for defibrillation energy requirements were measured at baseline (normothermia, 38–40 °C) and during treatment with total body hypothermia (30 °C) or no temperature change (sham). Hypothermia was induced by circulating ice-water through anterior and posterior surgical thermal blankets. In the hypothermia group, defibrillation energy requirement values at baseline did not significantly change during hypothermia. Similarly, the defibrillation energy requirement values in the control group did not change from baseline to sham. Hypothermia profoundly affected cardiac electrophysiology, decreasing VF threshold by 72%, conduction velocity (CV) by 25%, and tissue excitability, while it prolonged ventricular repolarization and refractoriness by 7.5–15%, respectively. They concluded that total body cooling was highly arrhythmogenic, although this unstable electrophysiological state did not alter ventricular defibrillation energy requirements.

In opposition to the above-mentioned conclusion, the hypothesis of Chorro *et al.* (2002) was that a rapid and profound reduction of myocardial temperature impedes the maintenance of VF, leading to termination of the arrhythmia. High-resolution epicardial mapping and transmural recordings of ventricular activation were used to analyze VF modification during rapid myocardial cooling in Langendorff-perfused rabbit hearts. Myocardial cooling was produced by the injection of cold Tyrode into the left ventricle after induction of VF. Termination of the arrhythmia occurred preferentially in the left ventricle and was associated with a reduction in CV (60% in left ventricle and 54% in right ventricle). Their conclusion was that rapid reduction of temperature to <20°C terminates VF after producing an important depression in myocardial conduction. Once more, methodological differences must be pointed out. Besides, those papers using energy as the electrical evaluating parameter are not fully comparable with those using current. Thus, regarding the effects of temperature on the fibrillation–defibrillation process, no definite serious statement can be advanced yet and the only prudent advice would indicate another open area for more research.

*Previous myocardial damage*

Cardiac patients scheduled for open-chest surgery or confined in coronary units are usually classified as of *high risk* meaning, precisely, that their probability of dying is higher than other subjects because there is documented heart disease (say, ischemia, infarct, hypertrophy, dilatation, conduction blocks, valvulopathies, failure, unstable arrhythmias or the like). Often, the final event is VF and they become emergency defibrillation candidates. Regional ischemia, for example, encompasses a situation different than global ischemia; during the latter, the myocardium becomes hypoxic and acidotic, producing the release of potassium. Besides, there appear changes in the fiber action potentials so creating a functional electrophysiologic inhomogeneity which favors fibrillation. The amount of injury contributes to fiber resistivity modifications, fiber groups, ventricular areas and the ventricles at large, thus adding to the inhomogeneity. The electrical resistance of an ischemic myocardium is, in general, higher than the measured value in a normal one (Savino *et al.*, 1983; Arredondo *et al.*, 1984). The sensitivity to fibrillation and to defibrillation has been extensively studied in the injured heart, often reporting opposite results, although the overall contention indicates greater defibrillation difficulties. Since many times drugs are being used to ease the defibrillating situation, it becomes more difficult to compare values. For example, Ware *et al.*, (1993), based on previous studies on the effects of lidocaine and procainamide regarding the energy required for successful defibrillation, studied the effects of lidocaine and procainamide on the relationship between delivered voltage and defibrillation success in mongrel dogs $21 \pm 3$ days following ligation of the left anterior descending and first diagonal coronary arteries. Internal defibrillation testing using a patch–patch electrode configuration was performed before and during the administration of saline controls, lidocaine, and procainamide. The mean infarct size as determined by staining with tetrazolium was $13.4 \pm 8.3\%$ of right and left ventricles, and did not differ significantly between groups. The 50% effective defibrillation (ED50) voltage increased with infusions of saline ($16 \pm 15\%$), lidocaine ($40 \pm 22\%$), and procainamide ($13 \pm 15\%$) and the ED50 energy increased $41 \pm 44\%$, $104 \pm 62\%$, and $35 \pm 36\%$, respectively. Observe the very large coefficients of variation for the latter ($44/41$; $62/104$, and $36/35$). However, the increase in ED50 voltages and energies were significantly greater in animals receiving lidocaine compared to those receiving either saline control or procainamide. There were trends toward change of hemodynamic parameters in all animals following baseline defibrillation testing; stroke volume declined $21 \pm 16\%$; and mean pulmonary artery and aortic pressure increased by $22 \pm 25\%$ and $11 \pm 15\%$, respectively. In conclusion, unlike previous studies in dogs with normal hearts, in this model hemodynamic deterioration occurred with repeated fibrillation and defibrillation, and defibrillation voltage requirements increased in the control series. Taking into consideration the increase in defibrillation voltage requirements over the duration of the experiments, lidocaine increases and procainamide does not change ED50; thus, their effects are similar in normal and infarcted canine hearts.

Cheng *et al.* (2002) commented that shock-induced vulnerability and defibrillation have been mostly studied in normal hearts, rarely in clinical settings. Increased vulnerability has been reported during ischemia, which is likely to contribute to defibrillation failure. Their purpose was to examine the mechanism of increased vulnerability after myocardial infarction (MI). Ligation of the marginal branch of the left circumflex artery in rabbits was done 1–6 weeks before acute experiments. Epicardial electrical activity of Langendorff-perfused hearts was optically mapped before, during and after 8 ms monophasic shocks applied during T-wave from a right ventricular lead. Histology revealed that ligation consistently resulted in a discrete left ventricular apical infarction with a border zone characterized by action potential shortening. Cathodal shocks produced the virtual electrode polarization pattern with an area of positive polarization near the shock lead and an adjacent area of negative polarization (de-excitation area). Maximum transmembrane voltage gradient was located in the border zone. The resulting postshock break-excitation wavefronts consistently originated at this gradient and propagated toward the base, forming a sustained reentrant arrhythmia. It was concluded that regional MI provides the substrate for increased vulnerability via virtual electrode-induced phase singularity, which originates in the border zone. This may contribute to defibrillation failure.

### 2.4.2. *Technological Variables*

The electrical variables or parameters constitute determinant factors in the success of a defibrillating discharge. The manufacturer, the physician, the biomedical engineer and the intervening paramedics must have a clear understanding of them, their importance and of the estimated values to apply.

Such variables are *voltage* V, *current* I, and *resistance* R, respectively, measured in volts, amperes (or amps, for short) and ohms (sometimes indicated by the Greek letter $\Omega$). They are related by *Ohm's law* (Fig. 2.5), which states that,

$$R = V/I, \qquad (2.1)$$

that is, the ratio between the applied voltage across a load R and the current through it is a constant which precisely defines the resistance, or, in other words, the hindrance opposed to the circulation of the electric charges; that resistance R is the so-called load to the generator. *Ohm's law* was empirically discovered and later on it was demonstrated theoretically. It is valid for dc and for ac circuits and, in the latter case, only when sinusoidal signals are involved, otherwise a different approach is required.

The developed power P, and let us repeat to emphasize the concept, applying the voltage V across R to sustain the current I through it, is given by

$$P = VI, \qquad (2.2)$$

and it is expressed in watts ($= V \times A$). In turn, the energy dissipated in the load R when the power P is applied during a given time $t$ is,

$$E = P \times t, \qquad (2.3)$$

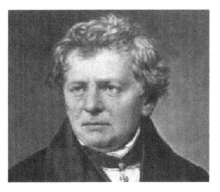

Fig. 2.5. *Ohm's law* was developed by Georg Simon Ohm (1787–1854) in 1827. Although he discovered one of the most fundamental laws of current electricity, he was virtually ignored for most of his life by scientists in his own country. Freely available in http://www.biografiasyvidas.com/biografia/o/fotos/ohm.jpg.

which is measured in joules J ($=$ W $\times$ s). Energy is equivalent to the work carried out by the intervening electrical forces, namely the above-mentioned voltage and current, and in the end, is dissipated as heat.

The thoracic cage or the ventricles, as they are embraced by the defibrillating electrodes, present respectively an electrical resistance R, the load to the generator, where the defibrillating energy E is dissipated. The literature often mentions values such as 200 or 300 J, for indirect defibrillation, or perhaps 20 or 30 J, for the direct situation. These figures refer precisely to the energy defined above.

So far, we have made a simple though quite valid description of the electrical parameters involved in a circuit formed by a generator which maintains a current through a resistive load. However, nothing was said about the nature of the voltage. Besides, choice of the most adequate parameter to define a defibrillatory discharge is not an easy task; there is still a controversial and not fully solved situation among users, unfortunately with a tendency toward energy. Commercial equipment indicate the stored energy probably because its determination is easier, however, recalling the definition of defibrillation, it is seen that "a critical current density $I_D$ (amps/cm$^2$) during a time $t$ (ms) is needed within the myocardial mass to depolarize a minimal critical number of cells". Thus, **current I, or perhaps better, current density $I_D$, is the most adequate parameter to describe defibrillation dose** (Valentinuzzi, 1995).

Let us somewhat deepen in this particular subject. The literature on defibrillation, either in clinical practice or in basic applied research, as said above, uses mainly energy (expressed by and large in joules) as the parameter to dose the discharge or to describe threshold. Manufacturers have followed the same trend and, traditionally, commercial cardiac defibrillators of any type are calibrated in terms of energy. The reasons to have chosen energy are inconclusive and, at best, weak and without good support. Even the concept of energy threshold should or could be questioned as such. Once the pulse duration and electrode lead system (with a given load impedance) are fixed, current is by far a much better parameter. This concept is also supported by Zimmerman *et al.* (1994). Any energy value, for example, 20 J, can be obtained with an infinite number of combinations of voltage, current, and duration of the applied pulse. Just for illustration, Table 2.1 displays an arbitrary collection of figures. By just eyeballing it, any experienced operator can anticipate what set of values are to be ruled out. Searching for the energy threshold simply means to change the voltage because the pulse duration is generally fixed (in the order of

Table 2.1. Combinations of voltage U, in volts [V], current I, in amps [A] and pulse duration D, in seconds [s], to obtain a constant energy E of 20 joules [J] with a rectangular pulse delivered over a load impedance Z = R, in ohms [Ω]. Reproduced from Valentinuzzi (1995), by permission.

| U[V] | I[A] | D[s] | E[J] | Z = R[Ω] | P[W] | COMMENTS |
|---|---|---|---|---|---|---|
| 20 | 1 | 1 | 20 | 20 | 20 | * |
| 100 | 2 | 0.1 | 20 | 50 | 200 | * |
| 200 | 4 | 0.025 | 20 | 50 | 800 | * |
| 400 | 5 | 0.010 | 20 | 80 | 2,000 | * |
| 500 | 10 | 0.004 | 20 | 50 | 5,000 | |
| 600 | 10 | 0.0033 | 20 | 60 | 6,000 | |
| 800 | 12 | 0.0021 | 20 | 66.67 | 9,600 | |
| 600 | 15 | 0.0022 | 20 | 40 | 9,000 | |
| 500 | 15 | 0.0027 | 20 | 33.33 | 7,500 | |
| 400 | 15 | 0.0033 | 20 | 26.67 | 6,000 | |
| 300 | 16 | 0.0042 | 20 | 18.75 | 4,800 | |
| 300 | 15 | 0.0044 | 20 | 20 | 4,500 | |
| 300 | 12 | 0.0055 | 20 | 25 | 3,600 | |
| 250 | 10 | 0.008 | 20 | 25 | 2,500 | * |
| 250 | 8 | 0.01 | 20 | 31.25 | 2,000 | * |

Those rows marked with an * are combinations which, in all likelihood, have no possibility of success.

3–5 ms) and the current will be determined by the impedance through the heart or the thorax, as the case may be (in the range of 20–60 ohms). By its very nature, energy does not arise as a good descriptor and the high values found in those unfavorable patients reported in the literature might well fall within some of the unacceptable combinations, as illustrated in Table 2.1. Current traversing the myocardium is by far more physiological. It is the ionic exchange through the excitable membrane responsible for its depolarization–repolarization sequence. It is the externally applied current that brings a number of fibers (the critical mass, as mentioned before) to an electrical halt in order to permit the regular rhythm to take over again.

Transventricular impedance was studied by Savino *et al.* (1983) and, in another article dealing with multiple pulse defibrillation (Puglisi *et al.*, 1989), it was concluded that peak current would be the best electrical parameter to assess DTs and efficacy of defibrillating methods. A multiple discharge applies the required energy keeping a beneficial low-peak current (high peaks may induce arrhythmias). Nonetheless, when shocks of different duration are to be compared, power would appear as a good parameter too to assess the defibrillatory act. Thus, the search to reduce the electrical parameters in defibrillators perhaps should be oriented toward a decrease in delivered power rather than in energy. Experiments carried out with a true constant current defibrillator clearly demonstrated its unequivocal results (Monzón and Guillén, 1985; Olivera *et al.*, 1991). In 1989, Charbonnier, Rockwell and Benvegar, from Hewlett-Packard Company, issued a current-based defibrillator patent (US 4,840,177) but apparently, this kind of instrument did not go into the market, probably because still poses technological and practical difficulties.

A challenging article by Irnich (1990) also partially supported the concepts herein discussed. This author said that "the weakness of the energy dose may be one of the reasons why results are so divergent. Energy is not a good predictor of defibrillation outcome; additionally, it may produce inconsistent results if the impedance seen by the electrodes is high or low. Whether peak current thresholds are superior to energy thresholds, as dose quantitative description, seems to be clear, but according to *Weiss' law* (Weiss, 1901), mean current and pulse duration must also be taken into consideration, as well as electrode surface area, to get an impression of which field strength is produced and its duration within the heart." Insistence in energy as the main criterion for defibrillation is perhaps producing data that are not true descriptors of reality and may lead into erroneous concepts and waste of time.

The electrical defibrillation parameters, current, energy, and charge (voltage could be added, too), are related by the experimental strength–duration curves shown in Fig. 2.6 (Koning *et al.*, 1975), in turn recognizing their origin in *Lapicque's contribution* (Lapicque, 1909). These authors found that defibrillation with a rectangular pulse led to a relationship

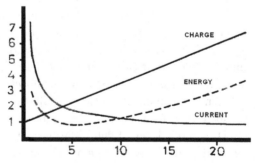

Fig. 2.6. Relative defibrillating threshold curves for current, energy and charge as functions of the defibrillatory pulse duration in ms. The minima do not coincide. A duration between 4 and 5 ms, which covers the region of minimum E, where current is low and the demanded charge is no yet too high, could be an acceptable compromise. Redrawn after Koning *et al.* (1975), with written permission from Springer.

between threshold current and pulse duration resembling a hyperbola. Charge Q is given by the integral of the current–duration relationship while energy E comes from the temporal integral of the squared current multiplied by the resistive load between electrodes. It is easily seen that there is no square wave showing coincident minima of the three parameters. At least from a theoretical viewpoint, high voltages and currents can damage the lipidic cell membranes; by the same token, high energies produce injury because of heating while excessive electric charges may lead to electrolysis in the body fluids and in the electrode–electrolyte interfaces. So far, none of the three parameters has been identified as the most dangerous culprit.

Besides, the defibrillating dose will depend also on the waveform, whether the shock is direct or indirect, on the size and type of electrodes and on their location; the latter factors determine the load impedance. These parameters are discussed in Chap. 3.

*Weiss Law.* In 1901, Georges Weiss published a paper trying to find out whether there are measures to make mutually comparable the different devices that physiologists used for nerve and muscle stimulation. Weiss was born on August 26, 1859 in Bischweiler (Alsace, France). He trained as an engineer in Paris and afterward began his medical studies reaching the doctorate in 1889. In the same year, he was appointed at the Department of Medical Physics, Medical School, in Paris. His main field of interest was electrophysiology. At the end of the nineteenth century the measuring capabilities for electrical stimulation pulses were limited and stimulation theories were based more on speculation than on measurements. Weiss found a fascinating method to produce short-lasting pulses of defined amplitude and duration. He constructed bridges by conducting threads within a circuit that were then destroyed by an air rifle bullet driven by liquid carbonic acid to produce short-lasting pulses. To investigate double pulses, the measuring system was expanded in the same manner, now with four bridging threads. The experiments were carried out with remarkable accuracy. The results included: (1) the threshold quantity for the voltage–time product is a linear function of the pulse duration; (2) there is always a minimum of the delivered energy dependent on pulse duration; and (3) pulse shape plays no role in electrostimulation. The physiologists were not impressed by Weiss' report, probably because technology was rather limited to repeat his measurements. It can be concluded that if there are statements in the literature contradicting one of the above three Weiss' theorems, one can infer that the investigation is questionable (Irnich, 2002). Weiss's law is mathematically described by:

$$Vt = \frac{1}{K}(h + kt), \qquad (2.4)$$

where $V$ is the applied voltage, $K$ and $k$ are constants, $t$ stands for pulse duration, and $h$ represents a local excitatory state (threshold) required to actually trigger excitation (Weiss, 1901; Blair, 1935; Irnich, 1990, 2002).

*Lapicque's strength–duration curve* leads to the important concepts of utilization time, rheobase, and chronaxy. This experimental relationship was introduced in 1909 by the French physiologist Louis Lapicque (1866–1952). In INTERNET, excellent and very didactic accounts can be found. Old beautiful theoretical and still valid in many respects descriptions were given by Nicholas Rashevsky in this classic books (Rashevsky, 1960; Defares and Sneddon, 1961). The interested reader is encouraged to at least take a look at some of them, as for example, Blair's Theory of Excitation. Notice that these theories were developed long before Hodgkin's, the latter made in the 1950s. Sometimes, Weiss and Lapicque's findings are collectively called Weiss–Lapicque law.

### 2.4.3. *Defibrillation Thresholds*

Up to here, we have used loosely and without introducing them, the terms *defibrillation thresholds* and *defibrillation dose*; both are related, as the latter is based on the former. It is time to define these concepts more precisely. First, let us say that defibrillation, defibrillating or defibrillatory thresholds, or doses are all linguistically acceptable terms. Thus, this subsection and the following deal with them.

Since the defibrillation procedure is probabilistic by nature and not free of risks, orienting values and safety margins are needed in order to guarantee success with a high confidence level while minimizing damages. Searching for such criterion, *electrical defibrillation threshold (EDT) is defined as the minimum value that leads to a successful outcome*. A series of measurements carried out in an experimental animal, following a step up–step down protocol searching for such limiting level, produces a cloud of points where successes and failures are mixed, as the trials proceed. There will always be a maximum value $DV_{max}$ which *did not* defibrillate and a minimum $DV_{min}$ which *did* defibrillate, thus, a band can be determined as the difference:

$$\Delta B = DV_{max} - DV_{min}, \qquad (2.5)$$

within which, at least ideally, the number $N_S$ of successful discharges should equal the number $N_F$ of failures (Fig. 2.7). The total number of discharges within the band is $N = N_S + N_F$, leaving above all the successes (black

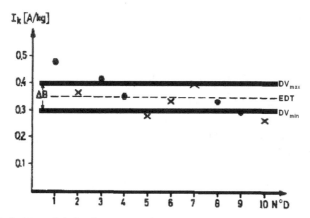

Fig. 2.7. Definition of defibrillation threshold. Maximum value $DV_{\max}$ which *did not* defibrillate and minimum $DV_{\min}$ which did defibrillate; electrical defibrillation threshold EDT is the average within the band or its middle value. Number of defibrillation shocks on the horizontal axis. Redrawn after Armayor, Savino, Valentinuzzi *et al.* (1979), with permission.

circles) and below all the failures (crosses). The mean value for $N$ within the band produces a figure near 50% that can be proposed as a better definition for the EDT, in whatever units one wishes depending on the chosen descriptor (voltage, current, energy, or charge), i.e.:

$$EDT = \frac{1}{N} \sum_{1}^{N} DV_i, \qquad (2.6)$$

where $DV_i$ stands for all values within the band and goes from 1 to obviously $N$. In practice, it was found that a numerically very close value, easier to calculate, is the middle band-value,

$$EDT = DV_{\min} + \frac{\Delta B}{2} \qquad (2.7)$$

also a good estimator of EDT. Hence, either definition is acceptable. The probability of successful defibrillation, obtained with any of the above expressions, is very near 50%, bringing us to another and more powerful definition of threshold, i.e. *that electrical value with a 50% probability of success.* Let us remind that the electrical fibrillation threshold has a similar definition, or, *the electrical value with 50% probability of triggering the arrhythmia* (Armayor *et al.*, 1979). A mechanical analogy can be represented by a man walking just on the border or edge of a ridge: a

small shift to one side, and he would fall down to the precipice; a small
step to the other side, and he would be safer.

### 2.4.4. *Concept of Defibrillation Dose*

The pharmacological definition of dose for a given agent represents the
amount needed to produce a certain effect. Usually, it is scaled to BW
considering also factors such as sex, age, and other pathologies. A similar
idea can be applied for defibrillation. With data from Armayor *et al.* (1979),
Fig. 2.8(a) displays the distribution of transventricular EDTs, expressed in
A/kg, in a population of 20 experimental dogs under conditions of relative
normothermia with an average of 0.82 A/kg (SD = 0.3) over a total of 761
discharges out of which only 346 were successful, thus giving a 346/761
= 0.455 probability of success. The curve shows the typical approximately
Gaussian bell-shape, with very few successes at low and high doses. The
cumulative curve, i.e. the integral of the former, is sigmoid (Fig. 2.8(b)) and
represents the probability of success for each shock value after dividing the
number of discharges by the total number of discharges. In it, the following
values are easily determined,

(1) *Effective dose* is that value with at least 90% probability of success;

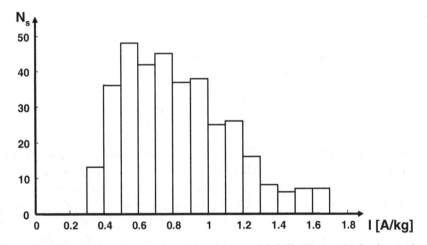

Fig. 2.8a.  Distribution of a number, $N_S$, of successful defibrillation shocks (vertical
axis) in 20 open-chest experimental dogs vs the current, I, scaled to body weight
[A/kg], that passed through the myocardium (horizontal axis). Redrawn after Armayor
*et al.* (1979).

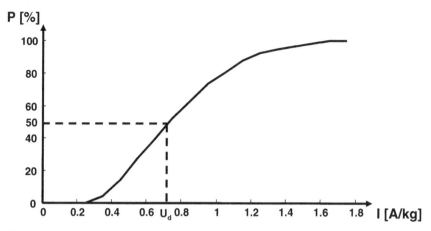

Fig. 2.8b. Dose–response curve, typically sigmoidal, showing the 50% probability for EDT. Lower values have lower probability of success wile a 90% level would require a higher current I.

(2) *Mean dose* is that value with 50% probability of success, that is, one-half of the population is expected to respond positively and is an estimate of the average EDT;

(3) Lower values to the left fall rapidly in their probability of success; and

(4) Higher values enter in the plateau region, where the probability does not increase any further and, in fact, it may even decrease because damage to the tissues is very likely to occur so becoming a toxic level.

If toxicity is defined as a discharge leading to detectable morphological injury to the myocardium (such as necrosis or epicardial lesions), a mean toxic dose can be determined, that is, $DTD_{50}$, which is a value able to produce damage at least in 50% of the cases. If the damage leads to post-defibrillatory death, a mean lethal dose, $DLD_{50}$, is also possible to define, or, one-half of cases would die, should this dose be applied. Babbs *et al.* (1980) clearly set up these concepts introducing the definitions of therapeutic and letal indices, which mathematically are expressed by,

$$I_{TT} = \frac{Mean\,ToxicDose}{EffectiveDose}, \qquad (2.8)$$

or, also,

$$I_{TL} = \frac{MeanLetalDose}{EffectiveDose}. \qquad (2.9)$$

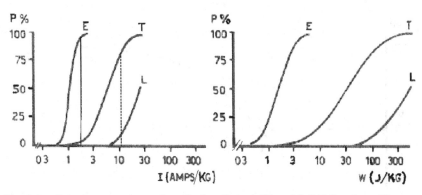

Fig. 2.9. Dose-response curves for effective E, toxic T and lethal L values. They are expressed as probability levels P, in percent, and referred to current (left), in amps/kg, or energy W, in joules/kg. The curves show the typical sigmoideal shape and shift to the right as the dose increases. Observe that values with high efficacy (vertical dotted line) may produce damage (toxicity) while, as the probability of damage goes up, so does the probability of death (vertical dashed line). Redrawn after Babbs *et al.* (1980), with permission from *Rightslink*.

These authors, using damped sinusoidal transthoracic shocks in experimental animals, plotted the dose–response curves scaled to BW for successful defibrillations without damage (effective E), with demonstrated damage (toxic T) and lethal (L). Figure 2.9 depicts the two sets, both for current and energy. The reported values were, respectively, $EDD_{50} = 1.1\,A/kg$ (effective), $TDD_{50} = 5.8\,A/kg$ (toxic), and $LDD_{50} = 24\,A/kg$ (lethal).

In 1979, Armayor *et al.* proposed the defibrillation dose concept based on the current delivered by the instrument after measuring the impedance of the fibrillating myocardium. An overall peak average of 0.82 A/kg of BW was found through a mean load of 25.9 ohms and a delivered energy of 23.7 mJ/g of heart. The method and doses reported in this paper were repeatedly and successfully applied in different experimental situations, such as body hypothermia, coronary occlusion, with quarter and half sinusoidal pulses, and after coronary occlusion and body hypothermia (Arredondo *et al.*, 1980, 1982, 1984; Monzón and Valentinuzzi, 1982). The latter article offered an empirical relationship between defibrillation current and BW:

$$I = 2.76 + 0.24\,BW \tag{2.10}$$

with a standard error of the estimate of 1.77, and I and BW given in amperes and kilograms, respectively.

In turn, Rattes *et al.* (1987) reported that a DT is achieved rapidly and would be better suited to study the effect of interventions on the ability to defibrillate patients. These authors assessed the relationship of DT to the defibrillation "dose–response curve" in 12 open chest, halothane anesthetized pigs. VF was induced electrically, and defibrillation was attempted by passing sequential pulse shocks through an indwelling catheter and plaque electrodes. DT was determined by decreasing the stored voltage of the initial shock until it failed to defibrillate the heart. Five different stored voltage levels distributed around defibrillation threshold were then randomly administered, six times for each level. A "dose–response curve" was obtained for each animal. DT superimposed on the "dose–response curve" at $76 \pm 7.2\%$ (mean $\pm$ SEM) defibrillation success. Energy delivered at 1.5 times average DT was predicted to achieve 100% defibrillation success for a single shock in all animals. They concluded that DT provides a simple and quantitative estimate of the ability to defibrillate with a predictable relationship to the "dose–response curve".

As a final paragraph of this section, it must underline the conceptual and numerical distinction and difference between defibrillatory threshold and electric dose for defibrillation. The former is defined as the minimum value (either expressed as current or energy) needed to defibrillate or, in other words, the electric value with a 50% probability of success. The latter, instead, corresponds to the value (again, either in current or energy terms) necessary to defibrillate with at least 90% probability of success and minimum or no damage to the myocardium. Threshold is a reference value while dose is a working quantity related to the previous one by a safety factor. These values should always be given per unit of BW or HW.

## 2.5. Cardiopulmonary Resuscitation (CPR)

As already referred to before (see Sec. 2.1), essentially, the concept introduced by the pioneers of CPR, mostly by William Kouwenhoven, can be summarized in the following two basic steps after fibrillation was established:

(1) Institute manual cardiac massage, directly on the myocardium if the patient is under open-chest surgery, or indirectly on the thorax in case of street or industrial emergency (precordial thumping). The objective is to produce enough ejection of blood from the ventricles to maintain

an acceptable minimum of blood flow to the brain and the coronary circulation at least.

(2) Institute artificial mouth-to-mouth respiration to keep an acceptable minimum oxygenation to the tissues. In the surgery room, a mechanical respirator is applied.

The two steps should alternate. When an out-of-hospital cardiac arrest is not witnessed by trained personnel, they may give about five cycles of CPR before checking the ECG rhythm and attempting defibrillation. One cycle of CPR consists of 30 compressions and two breaths. When compressions are delivered at a rate of about 80–100 per minute, five cycles of CPR should take roughly 2 min.

The patient must be in the supine position and the airways have to be fully clear of any obstruction (as mucus). Often, the procedure is performed by nurses who have attained adequate certification and, sometimes, even a lay person may do it in a public place. Several studies have documented the effects of time to defibrillation (see Sec. 2.4.1, Duration of fibrillation) and the effects of bystander CPR on survival from sudden cardiac death (SCD). For every minute that passes between collapse and defibrillation, survival rate decreases 7–10% if no CPR is provided. When bystander CPR is provided, the decrease in survival rates is more gradual and averages 3–4% per minute from collapse to defibrillation. CPR can double or triple survival from witnessed SCA at most intervals to defibrillation. The rescuer providing chest compressions should minimize interruptions in chest compressions for rhythm analysis and shock delivery and should be prepared to resume CPR, beginning with chest compressions, as soon as a shock is delivered. Basic CPR alone, however, is unlikely to eliminate VF and restore a perfusing rhythm, as spontaneous defibrillation in man very rarely, if ever, takes place. In children, though, it may occasionally happen.

After many years of research and experience in several countries, the Public Access Defibrillation (PAD) Trial was undertaken to determine whether deployment of automated external defibrillators (AEDs) in public locations would increase survival following out-of-hospital cardiac arrest (Fig. 2.10). The trial was sponsored by the National Heart, Lung, and Blood Institute with additional financial and material support from several federal and private institutions.

Between July 2000 and January 2002, 993 public facilities were enrolled to participate in the study in 21 centers in the United States and three centers in Canada. Volunteers at participating centers received training

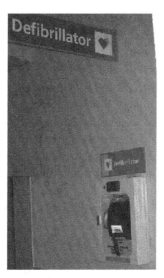

Fig. 2.10. Public defibrillator placed at Newark Liberty International Airport, New Jersey, USA, close to Gate 57. Picture taken by the author in October 2006. Similar equipment is currently seen, too, at Buenos Aires Domestic Airport, called *Aeroparque*, in Argentina.

in CPR. In addition, volunteers in one-half of the facilities (randomly chosen) received access to, and training in, the use of AEDs. Approximately 20,000 volunteers were initially trained (average 20/facility). Of these, 48% were retrained after an average of 5.5 months, and 20% received a second retraining at an average of 9.8 months from the first retraining. A total of ∼1500 AEDs were deployed (average 3/facility). Follow-up in the study ended September 30, 2003.

Preliminary results were based on a total of 292 attempted resuscitations, yielding an approximate rate per facility per year of 0.15. This means that a typical facility that participated in the PAD Trial could expect to see one treatable cardiac arrest every 6.7 years. There were 44 survivors from among these cardiac arrest patients. Serious adverse effects were rarely reported. No volunteers received inadvertent shocks, and no patients were shocked unnecessarily. AED maintenance problems were infrequent. A few participating volunteers reported severe stress responding to emergency situations.

The interference originated in the CPR movements modifies the ventricular fibrillation signal; its reduction in order to allow ECG analysis *during ongoing chest compression* could be beneficial relative to analysis only during "hands-off" intervals as such interruptions impair the perfusion of the fibrillating heart. We know of a group in Innsbruck, Austria, led by Amann and Klotz, that works in this direction.

Summarizing this section on CPR: For any victim of cardiac arrest, good CPR — push hard, push fast, allow complete chest recoil, and minimize interruptions in chest compressions — are essential musts. Some victims of VF-SCA may benefit from a short period of CPR before attempted defibrillation. Whenever defibrillation is attempted, rescuers must coordinate good CPR with defibrillation to minimize interruptions in chest compressions and to ensure immediate resumption of chest compressions after shock delivery.

This information, even with much more detail, is freely available in the WEB (see http://circ.ahajournals.org/cgi/content/full/112/22_suppl/ III-17, *Circulation* 2005; 112:III-17–III-24, American Heart Association) or check the 2005 *International Consensus Conference on Cardiopulmonary Resuscitation and Emergency Cardiovascular Care Science with Treatment Recommendations* (see also http://www.americanheart.org).

## 2.6. Cardioversion or Atrial Defibrillation

In Chap. 1 (Sec. 1.4.2), atrial fibrillation was introduced as an arrhythmia that can take place while the ventricles continue their beating, although irregular and tachycardic in their action because of the electrical bombardment from the upper chambers. By and large, atrial fibrillation (AF) and its variant, flutter, are treated pharmacologically. Sometimes, when response is not as expected or when atrial hypertrophy becomes too large, electrotherapy may be recommended and the shock **must be** synchronized with the QRS complex to avoid triggering of VF. The procedure is called *synchronized cardioversion* (version: turning of an organ, thus, it turns from one condition into another). The energy used for a synchronized shock is lower than that used for unsynchronized ventricular defibrillation. Unfortunately and relatively often, programmed cardioversion has not lasting results and the patient may return to the arrhythmia because the etiological causes are still there (Mittal *et al.*, 2000; Adgey and Walsh, 2004; Koster *et al.*, 2004; Alatawi *et al.*, 2005).

Various antiarrhythmic agents can be used to return the heart to normal sinus control. Amiodarone, cardizem, and metoprol are frequently given before cardioversion to decrease the heart rate, stabilize the patient, and increase the chance that cardioversion is successful. If the patient is stable, adenosine may be administered first, as the medicine performs a sort of "chemical cardioversion" and may stabilize the heart and let it resume normal function on its own without using electricity.

The subject, however, remains somewhat unsettled yet as to the long term efficacy of electrical cardioversion and also as to its relative success with respect to the pharmacological approach. Valencia Martín *et al.* (2002), from Alicante, Spain, assessed the efficacy of scheduled cardioversion by comparing the electrical vs the pharmacological cardioversion. For that matter, 230 patients with AF of more than 48 hours duration and requiring sinus rhythm restoration were included. One hundred forty-four patients underwent external electrical cardioversion and 86 patients received quinidine. These authors analyzed the rate of success, duration of hospital stay, complications, and clinical and echocardiographic variables that might predict success as well. Sinus rhythm was restored in 181 of 230 patients (79%). The rate of success was 77% (111/144 patients) in the electrical group and 81% (70 of 86 patients) in the pharmacological group. In 13 pharmacological patients for whom the first attempt failed, a second attempt with electrical cardioversion was applied; 8 out of the 13 responded favorably (61%). Only AF lasting less than 8 weeks was associated with a higher success rate. They concluded that scheduled cardioversion in AF is an effective technique with a high success rate and a very low rate of complication. Electrical cardioversion and pharmacological cardioversion with quinidine are similarly effective, although the latter involves a longer hospital stay. Similarly, de Paola *et al.* (2003), in Brazil, assessed the effectiveness and costs of chemical vs electrical therapy. In turn, Koster *et al.* (2004) compared monophasic and biphasic waveform shocks for external cardioversion of AF.

## 2.7. Are there other methods? Ablation

AF and VT can also be treated by radiofrequency (RF) catheter ablation techniques, which have had a dramatic impact. In the USA alone, about 2 million people are affected by some form of AF and each year about 200,000 patients are treated for VT. Cardiac surgery has been used for curing AF in patients undergoing open-chest surgery for other cardiac conditions. Although this procedure can achieve sinus rhythm, it is associated with significant morbidity because of its high invasive level. RF catheter ablation has the potential of becoming the therapy of choice for AF. Preliminary studies report that the RF ablation approach has already had some success, even though the procedure continues to pose a major challenge. Basic conditions require,

(a) Optimal electrode/catheter geometry;
(b) Optimal placement of inner temperature sensors for the purpose of efficient temperature-controlled RF ablation; and
(c) Optimal power application and ablation procedure duration.

All these should lead to an adequate electrical–thermal response of the catheter–tissue system during RF ablation. Localization of arrhythmias, however, still appears as a major difficulty. This stems from limitations of fluoroscopy and conventional catheter-based mapping techniques that limit the accurate anatomic localization of complex arrhythmogenic substrates. The physical principles of a newly catheter-based endocardial mapping techniques and their clinical applicability for treatment of complex arrhythmias were discussed by Darbar *et al.* (2001), from the Mayo Clinic in Rochester, MN, who also considered intracardiac echocardiography as an additional tool to facilitate mapping.

Sometimes, ablation fails in its antiarrhythmic effect. Himel *et al.* (2007) introduced an intraoperative index to assess the quality of the procedure. They hypothesized that a rise in the translesion stimulus–excitation delay (TED) can indicate a continuous, transmural, linear lesion, and that the TED is related to the path length in the viable tissue around the lesion. Rabbit hearts were isolated, perfused with a warm physiological solution and stained with transmembrane potential-sensitive fluorescent dye. RF ablation was performed on ventricular epicardium with a vacuum-assisted coagulation device to produce either a complete or incomplete lesion. Complete lesions were both transmural and continuous. Incomplete lesions were non-continuous or non-transmural. The TED was determined with bipolar stimulation at one side of the lesion and either a bipolar electrogram at the other side or optical mapping on both sides. Hearts were then stained with tetrazolium chloride and examined histologically to estimate minimum path lengths of viable tissue from the stimulation site to the recording site. Complete lesions increased significantly the TED by factors of 2.6–3.1, whereas incomplete lesions did not significantly increase the TED. Larger minimum path lengths were found for cases that had an increased TED. The TED was quantitatively predictable based on a CV of $0.38$–$0.49\,\mathrm{m\,s^{-1}}$, which is typical of rabbit hearts. The TED significantly increases when a linear lesion is complete, suggesting that an intraoperative measurement of the TED may help to improve ablation lesions and outcomes. Predictability of the TED based on the viable tissue path suggests that quantitative TEDs for clinical lesions may be anticipated provided that the CV is considered.

## 2.8. Conclusions and Review Questions

The first important concept to keep in mind underlines that once VF is triggered, it must be stopped within a very short time (if possible, not longer than 3 min) because, otherwise, the risk of death ensues due to lack of perfusion to the essential organs. This emergency medical act is called *defibrillation* and frequently is associated with artificial respiration, too, the whole procedure encompassed under the term CPR. Chemical defibrillation appears revived and as a potential possibility still opened, although for the time being the electrical counterpart is the only widely accepted procedure showing much better probability of success, either in cardiac surgery or in cases of domestic, street, or industrial emergencies. Successful defibrillation depends strongly on a cross-lateral transventricular current density large enough to depolarize a myocardial mass equal to or bigger than the *critical defibrillatory mass* (which is different and not related to the *critical fibrillatory mass*). Besides, defibrillation variables are grouped in physiopathological and technological, and all them play a role in the probability of the arrhythmia reversion sometimes heavily biasing the outcome, as for example acidosis or, most important, the time spent by the patient in fibrillation. After introducing and discussing such variables, it is concluded that current is the best descriptor although power should not be fully dismissed, even when practice has imposed the use of energy without offering convincing evidence in its favor. Thereafter, EDT is defined as the minimum value that leads to a successful outcome or, for short, as that electrical value with a 50% probability of success. Effective dose, instead, is that value with at least 90% probability of success and minimum or no tissue damage at all. If toxicity is defined as a discharge leading to detectable morphological injury to the myocardium, a mean toxic dose is a value able to produce damage at least in 50% of the cases. Threshold is a reference value while dose is a working quantity related to the previous one by a safety factor. These values should always be given per unit of BW or HW. Finally, cardiopulmonary resuscitation (CPR) and its essential steps, synchronized defibrillation and ablation are described and discussed to close the chapter.

*Review questions* (T = True; F = False)

1. Defibrillation in its practical terms consists of a
   controlled electrical discharge when the ventricles are
   in a state of uncoordinated pulseless activity.                    T     F
2. The longer the myocardium is in VF or VT, the more
   damage, and the lesser the chance of survival.                     T     F
3. An electric current can lead the cardiac chambers into
   fibrillation and another similar, but much higher one,
   may be able to stop it.                                            T     F
4. A sudden injection of a potassium-rich solution into
   the coronary circulation, thereafter followed by a
   wash-out solution, may massively depolarize cardiac
   cells giving them the chance to resume their natural
   rhythm.                                                            T     F
5. Critical defibrillatory mass is, by definition, the
   minimal number of ventricular fibers that must be
   depolarized to stop fibrillation.                                  T     F
6. Bigger hearts are more difficult to defibrillate
   requiring higher levels of current until, after a certain
   size, defibrillation becomes impossible.                           T     F
7. Fibrillation is rather uncommon in children.                       T     F
8. *Pinacidil* is a potassium channel opener that decreases
   blood pressure by reducing peripheral arterial
   resistance.                                                        T     F
9. *Verapamil* selectively inhibits transmembrane influx of
   calcium in cardiac muscle, coronary and systemic
   arteries, and in cells of the intracardiac conduction
   system.                                                            T     F
10. *Nitrendipine* is potassium channel blocker.                      T     F
11. Blood pH and oxygen levels have no influence on the
    probability of defibrillation.                                    T     F
12. Cardiac patients scheduled for open-chest surgery or
    confined in coronary units are usually classified as of
    *low-risk* patients.                                              T     F
13. Voltage, current, and resistance in a dc or ac circuit
    are related by (select one),
    Weiss' Law ............... Poiseuille's Law ...............
    Ohm's Law .............. Bell–Magendie Law

14. Energy is the best parameter to specify defibrillation thresholds or dose.                                  T      F
15. *Effective defibrillation dose* is that value with 50% probability of success.                             T      F
16. Manual cardiac massage before application of the defibrillating shock is not mandatory.               T      F
17. Atrial defibrillation, as ventricular defibrillation, does not have to be synchronized with cardiac electrical or mechanical activity.                                    T      F

18. Ablation consists of a short low-frequency discharge.       T      F

19. The first true experimental electrical defibrillation was carried out by, GEORGE OHM    PREVOST AND BATELLI    GUIDO BECK
20. The restitution hypothesis refers to,

    (A) the relationship between the voltage and its duration applied to the heart.
    (B) the relationship between voltage and current.
    (C) the relationship between the action potential duration and the preceding diastolic interval.

# Chapter 3

# DEFIBRILLATORS

*Always beware of lose connections and faulty leads...*

After a very brief historical review, this chapter deals with the defibrillator as an electrical–electronic machine without entering into technical details because technology advances so rapidly that, when published, soon it is superseded by newer one. Thus, only general principles are discussed. A defibrillator is an instrument designed to deliver an electric discharge able to terminate the arrhythmia. It can be characterized *technologically* and *functionally*, i.e. first, by defining energy and output current ranges, power source, and other specifications of its hardware and software (block diagram and general equations are given), and, second, by the circumstances of its intended use, such as place and operational settings, which lead to the external units, nowadays mostly automated, and internal models, exclusively for implantation and obviously also automated. Thereafter, the pulsed waveforms are presented: simple capacitor discharge, damped sinusoidal discharge, fractional sinusoidal shocks, truncated and rectangular pulses, and biphasic and triphasic discharges. Because of its better efficacy, in addition to biphasic waveforms, virtually all new units have added some type of impedance compensation that changes the shock based on the measured value of the patient impedance. This chapter ends with a very short discussion of cardiac pacemakers, which are devices akin of defibrillators and sometimes even combined with them.

## 3.1. Introduction

The preceding Chap. 2 dealt with defibrillation as a procedure, including the variables influencing its possible outcome; this chapter, instead, takes care of the device, as an electrical–electronic machine that actually generates and delivers the discharge. However, we are not going to enter into technical details and their intricacies because technology advances by leaps and bounds and what is written today, when published, very likely becomes obsolete and is superseded by newer and better technology. Thus, only general principles and basic concepts will be discussed while the design engineer's duty is to keep updated with the several know-hows. Besides, and unavoidable, there will be some degree of repetition and superposition between these chapters and such a thing, rather than being distasteful, should be taken as acceptable from the didactic point of view.

Electrical stimulation, as part of the wider area called electrotherapy, goes deep into history many centuries back, when the generator used was an *electric fish*, which is able to deliver a nice and shaking couple of hundred volts, followed in the eighteenth century by the Leyden bottle (a capacitor) previously charged up, either by means of Benjamin Franklin's kite (the first rudimentary *lightning rod*, introduced in 1752) which, in turn, depended on the weather conditions and on the operator's skill (who put his own life at risk in the procedure) or by an electrostatic manual machine, until Alessandro Volta, inspired probably by Luigi Galvani's first experiments with frogs, produced the pile, which is to be considered the first fully controllable electric generator. In electrophysiology, however, Faraday's electromagnetic induction and his practical consequence, the *inductorium* (in modern terminology, the transformer), connected to the *dc* voltaic pile and to an on–off switch in series with the primary coil, has to be considered the stimulator that for decades dominated the field. Full details regarding all of the above-mentioned subjects along with many fascinating stories, including artifacts of different kind, can be found at the Bakken Museum and Library, in Minneapolis, MN, and also in its website. A good account was published by Geddes (1984), as a monograph, after a period spent in Minneapolis. Another, more specifically referred to early development of defibrillation devices, was given by Troup (1990), of the University of Wisconsin, at Milwaukee. Keeping within defibrillation, the interested reader may also consult Lown (1967a, 1967b, 2002; Verrier and Lown, 1982) and Eisenberg (2006).

> *Electric fish* (order *Torpediniformes*) are fish with specialized organs capable of producing an electric discharge (between 10 and 250 volts), depending on the species, which the animal uses to stun or kill prey. The most known members are those of the genus *Torpedo* (from Latin, "torpere", to be stiffened). These shocks were somehow noticed by the ancient Greeks and Romans.

## 3.2. Characterization

In nowadays terms, a defibrillator is an instrument for medical use, designed to deliver an electric discharge able to terminate the arrhythmia. For its characterization, two aspects need to be considered: one is *technological* and the other is *functional*. The former defines the energy and output current ranges, power source, and other specifications related to its hardware and software design. The latter, instead, refers to the different circumstances of its intended use, such as place and operational settings.

### 3.2.1. *Technological Aspects*

A typical basic defibrillator may be represented by a set of blocks (Fig. 3.1), that is, a power source (PS), a voltage or current generator (G), and a discharge circuit which includes the patient are considered as the main parts of the load. Besides, there is a manual control, MC, an optional synchronizing circuit, S, and a monitor, M, also optional. The generator G presents at its output terminals a voltage $V_G$, which, when the switch SW1 is closed, sustains the current $i(t)$ that circulates through the internal resistance $R_I$ of the equipment and also through the load $Z_L$. Hence, $V_G$ splits into a smaller portion $V_R$ lost across the internal resistance $R_I$ (in a good design it is much lower than the load) and a much larger portion $V_L$ across $Z_L$, which stands for the total impedance seen by the electrodes when applied to the patient, i.e. the electrode–electrolyte interface impedance $Z_{INT}$ and the biological impedance $Z_B \approx R_B$ (essentially resistive) either of the thorax or the myocardium. Clearly, the current $i(t)$, a function of time, is described by:

$$i(t) = \frac{V_G}{R_I + Z_L},\qquad(3.1)$$

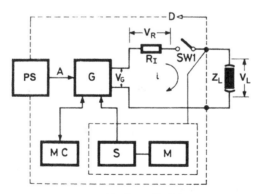

Fig. 3.1. Block diagram of a basic defibrillator D. PS = power source; G = generator; $R_I$ = generator internal resistance; $Z_L$ = load impedance; MC = manual control; S = synchronization (optional); and M = monitor (optional); and SW1 = switch. The load impedance includes the patient, essentially resistive, and the electrode–electrolyte interfaces, i.e. $Z_L = R_B + Z_{INT}$, the latter $Z_{INT}$ stands for the interfaces.

which is obtained after the first Kirchhoff's law (the sum of the voltage drops around any closed loop in a network equals zero). The energy delivered by the generator is given by the current–voltage product integrated over the duration $T_\mathrm{D}$ of the discharge, that is,

$$E_\mathrm{G} = \int_0^{T_\mathrm{D}} V_\mathrm{G}(t)i(t)dt, \qquad (3.2)$$

while the energy dissipated over the load $Z_\mathrm{L}$ is described by,

$$E_\mathrm{L} = \int_0^{T_\mathrm{D}} V_\mathrm{L}(t)i(t)dt, \qquad (3.3)$$

always recalling that the load of interest is the resistive part of $Z_\mathrm{L}$, the so-called *biological resistance* $R_\mathrm{B}$, represented either by the thorax or the heart. Besides, it must be underlined, too, that both, voltage $V_\mathrm{G}(t)$ and current $i(t)$, are functions of time.

The power source can be either the public power line (say, 110 V or 220 V, at 60 or 50 Hz, respectively), when the equipment is within the hospital or industrial environment, or an adequate battery for the portable pieces, which might also be found in health institutions and many other places and tends to be the current trend for safety and practical reasons. The generator is always an electronic circuit, from very simple design to rather complex and sophisticated ones, which usually include software to reach a decision, depending on the manufacturer and model.

The ideal requirements that, at least in principle, the defibrillating machine should meet are the following:

(1) current intensity, in amperes, and duration of shock, in milliseconds, ought to be specified by the operator from the control panel (in fully automated equipment this information is preconditioned); and
(2) both variables ought to be independent of the load faced by the generator.

Even though recent equipment satisfy relatively well such conditions, full compliance to them still pose practical difficulties.

### 3.2.2. *Functional Aspects*

From this viewpoint, the first classification speaks of the *external* and *internal* types, that is, *external* are those equipment intended for indirect or transthoracic use and also those to be applied directly on the myocardium, which obviously refer nowadays only to the operating room during open thorax surgery. It is underlined that both belong to the external type, even though the double use of the word "external" may look as misleading in the second case, and for either case, an operator always applies the electrodes. The term *internal defibrillator*, instead, is unequivocally and exclusively reserved for the implantable type, to be described further down in the text.

## External defibrillators

Traditionally, and since the beginning of the antiarrthymic saga, this kind of equipment is manual, however, and relatively in recent times, automated external defibrillators (AEDs) detect first the arrhythmia delivering thereafter the shock. There are even types simple enough for the use of the layman. In other more sophisticated manual and semi-automatic defibrillators, a professional can act as a pacemaker, should the cardiac frequency be too slow, and perform other functions (such as reading the ECG). AEDs are generally either held by trained personnel or are Public Access Units (PAU). The location of a public access AED takes into account the number of people who usually gathers in that place because it directly relates to the probability of the event. Emergency vehicles are likely to carry AEDs, in addition to manual defibrillators, as police or fire vehicles do. A recent trend is that of AEDs for home use, particularly in households where a family member has a known heart condition. Some physicians have objected these home users claiming that they do not have appropriate training while others advocate the more widespread use of community responders, who can be appropriately trained. Time and more experience will very likely have the final word in this respect.

Typically, an AED kit will contain a face or mouth shield for providing a barrier between patient and aider during rescue breathing, a pair of rubber gloves, a pair of shears for cutting through a patient's clothing if needed, a small towel for wiping away any moisture on the chest, and a razor for shaving those with hairy chests. Some units need to be switched on in order to perform a self-check; other models have a self check system built in with an indicator.

When turned on, the AED will instruct the user to connect the electrodes or pads to the patient. The pads allow the AED to examine the electrical output from the heart and determine if the patient is in a shockable rhythm (ventricular fibrillation (VF) or ventricular tachycardia (VT)). If the device determines that a shock is warranted, it will use the battery to charge its internal capacitor. After that, the device instructs the user to ensure no one is touching the victim and then to press a button to deliver the shock; human intervention is usually required to deliver the shock in order to avoid possible accidental injury to other people. Depending on the manufacturer and model, after the shock, most devices will analyze the victim and either instruct that CPR be given, or administer another shock. Many units have a memory to store the ECG of the patient along with details of the time the unit was activated and the number and strength of the shocks delivered.

Summarizing, unlike regular defibrillators, an AED requires very little training to use. It automatically diagnoses the heart rhythm and determines if a shock is needed. Automatic models will administer the shock without the user's command. Semi-automatic models will tell the user that a shock is needed, but the user must tell the machine to do so. In most circumstances, the user cannot override a "no shock" advise. Most states in the US now include the "good faith" use of an AED by any person under the Good Samaritan laws, meaning that a volunteer responder cannot be held liable for the harm or death of a victim (for more details, see http://en.wikipedia.org/wiki/Automated_external_defibrillator).

### 3.2.3. *Implantable Defibrillators*

An implantable cardioverter defibrillator (ICD) is a small device that is placed in the chest or abdomen. An ICD has electrodes connected to the chambers of the heart and continually monitors its rhythm. When the device detects an irregular signal, the ICD delivers a shock similar to those applied by the external counterparts. An ICD is akin to a pacemaker, although there are some differences. Pacemakers only give off low-energy electrical pulses and are used to treat less dangerous arrhythmias. New ICDs can pacemake and defibrillate (http://www.nhlbi.nih.gov/health/dci/Diseases/icd/icd_whatis.html).

Michael Mirowski (1924–1990) was the inventor, developer, and main promoter of the device briefly outlined above (Fig. 3.2). If long was the saga of the several external defibrillator developers, shorter but harder was indeed his with the implantable cousin. He was born in Poland and, after suffering antisemitic persecution by the Nazi regime during World War II and many years of wandering through Europe, he managed to finish medical school in France moving, thereafter, to the USA. Impressed by the sudden death of a fellow physician in Israel, where he also spent some time, he decided to work on the idea of the automatic implantable defibrillator. The

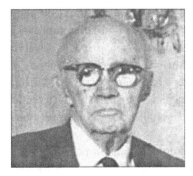
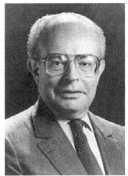

Below, Michael Mirowski, 1924–1990.
Inventor of the internal implantable
defibrillator, in 1969.

Fig. 3.2. Defibrillator inventors. Above left, William Bennett Kouwenhoven (1886–1975). Between 1928 and 1950s, he developed three external defibrillators: the open-chest defibrillator, the Hopkins AC Defibrillator, and the Mine Safety Portable. Both, he and Mirowski, carried out their pioneering work at Johns Hopkins, Baltimore.

first equipment was built in Baltimore, in 1969, in the basement of the Sinai Hospital, with the collaboration of his intimate friend, Morton M. Mower. Other people also teamed up with them, Stephen Heilman, Alois Langer, Mir Imran, the latter a young engineer. After four years of animal experimentation and considerable opposition from the medical community, in February 1980, the first implantation was carried out on a female patient at Johns Hopkins Hospital, also in Baltimore, paradigmatically the same place where Kouwenhoven did his pioneering studies on external defibrillation (Fig. 3.2). The device weighed 295 g and occupied a volume of 145 cc for which reason, it had to be placed in the abdomen; battery life hardly reached one year. Currently, weight is below 50 g and volume less than 50 cc, not thicker than about 13 mm, with a life span in the order of eight years (I have known people with equipment which easily surpassed 10 years). The ICD was approved for use by the FDA in 1985. Modern ICDs do not require a thoracotomy and often possess pacing and cardioversion capabilities, too. The ICD has since evolved into a multi-programmable antiarrhythmic device capable of treating bradyarrhythmias, VT, and VF. Thanks to technology advances, the current devices are significantly smaller and offer tiered therapy with programmable anti-tachycardia pacing schemes, as well as low and high-energy shocks in multiple ranges of tachycardia rates. In addition to cardioversion and defibrillation, some devices are capable of single or dual-chamber rate-responsive bradycardia pacing or biventricular pacing. Sophisticated discrimination algorithms are available to minimize shocks for non-life-threatening supraventricular tachycardias. Improvements in endocardial and epicardial lead systems have resulted in ICDs that can deliver a variety of shock patterns in different intracardiac and extracardiac locations. Defibrillation thresholds have been reduced with the use of biphasic shocks, particularly with endocardial lead placement. Diagnostic functions, including stored electrograms, allow verification of shock appropriateness.

Mirowski and his group encountered strong opposition when their results were submitted to the medical community and also to specialized journals, and he was even accused of unethical practice. For example, and surprisingly, Bernard Lown, an outstanding contributor to the development of external defibrillators (so much that there is one type named after him, which delivers a damped sinusoidal waveform with a half-cycle time of approximately 5 ms), published in 1972, in a prestigious journal, *Circulation*, that *"the very rare patient who has frequent bouts of ventricular fibrillation is best treated in a coronary care unit and is better served by an effective antiarrhythmic program or surgical correction of inadequate coronary blood flow or ventricular malfunction. In fact, the implanted defibrillator system represents an imperfect solution in search of a plausible and practical application"*. In fact, a letter exchange was triggered whose details can be found in the same journal (1973, 47:1135–1136, downloaded from *circ.ahajournals.org* on March 20, 2008). By no means does such statement detract from its author's intrinsic values, after all similar examples are found in other fields (such as computers and, much earlier, in microbiology when Louis Pasteur proposed the bacterial existence), which usually are stained by a grain of silly arrogance. Historical perspective teaches us never in science or technological development to prevent a young motivated guy to test an idea or theory for we, no matter how impressive our accomplishments might be, are fallible as any human being can be, and our jumpy, hasty, and lightly outspoken opinion may do a lot of harm, without mentioning the risk of making a fool of ourselves. Nonetheless, and in spite of those human problems, several papers were able to cross the barriers remaining in the early specialized literature as unerasable hallmarks (Mirowski, 1971; Mirowski *et al.*, 1978, 1980a, 1980b, 1981; Veltri *et al.*, 1988). The latter paper, with Veltri as first author, was perhaps the last published by Michael before his untimely and premature death in 1990. His close collaborator, Mower, published several articles reviewing and updating the subject (Mower, 1993, 1995; Mower and Hause, 1993).

A quick search in PubMed shows easily the many papers published by the group over the years and since the ICD's birth.

There is a huge literature on the subject, touching all conceivable aspects. Larson *et al.* (2003) produced a well-documented report, up to that year, of the current status of ICDs while clinical trials and over 27 years of increasing worldwide experience have demonstrated the superiority of the ICD over antiarrhythmic drug therapy in the prevention of death from malignant arrhythmias. Congestive heart failure (CHF) patients, as one example, implanted with an ICD showed a death risk lower than placebo or amiodarone patients (Bardy *et al.*, 2005). Other apparently lateral but not less significant aspects have been also analyzed; Carlsson *et al.* (2002) studied the psychosocial adjustments for both, patients and relatives, involved in an ICD implantation, and even though this departs from the purely technological bias of the chapter, it deserves a few lines taken verbatim from the referred to paper. Thus, "the aim of this pilot study was to design a plan of education and to follow a selected group of patients with interviews, observations and a questionnaire. The goals included seeing how well they accepted their situation after the operation when they had ongoing support of the nurse, in comparison to a control group who received conventional patient education by the physician. The patients were randomly allocated into two groups. Twenty patients were recruited, 10 in the study group and 10 in the control group, between February, 1997 and April, 1998. There were 16 men (average age, 63) and four women (average age, 57). The Nottingham Health Profile was used to measure health-related quality of life. Sleep disturbances were the greatest problem in both the study group and the control group before ICD implantation. In the study group, there was a significant improvement after ICD implantation in four patients. The study also revealed a difference between men and women, with women having more sleep disturbances before ICD implantation than men. In both groups, there was a lack of energy and emotional reactions, both before and after ICD implantation. Few considered family life a problem before or after the study. In the control group, the patients missed the lack of contact with health care personnel more than in the study group. There was also a greater need for group meetings after the hospital stay. By means of the questionnaire, interviews, and observations, it became evident that there was a great need for information, and a plan of patient education in addition to follow-up by the nurse was felt to be very important". It should be also underlined that the shock delivered by an ICD, if the patient does not have time to lose consciousness due to the fastness of the equipment response, produces a well-documented strong pain, which has been described as a "kick in the back" that may lead the patient to request removal of the machine, and such information may be passed on to other potential implant receivers who, in turn, might reject implantation when advised. They may need psychological support. However, and in spite of a few drawbacks, now the success and health recovery impact of the electrical internal procedure has well passed the tests.

Initially ICDs were implanted via thoracotomy with defibrillator patches applied to the epicardium or pericardium. The device was attached via subcutaneous and transvenous leads to the device contained in a subcutaneous abdominal wall pocket. The device itself acts as an electrode. Most ICDs nowadays are implanted transvenously with the devices placed in the left pectoral region similar to pacemakers. Intravascular spring or coil electrodes are used to defibrillate. The devices have become smaller and less invasive as the technology advances (for further details, see http://en.wikipedia.org/wiki/Implantable_cardioverter-defibrillator).

The subject calls for public attention, so much that rather often comments of different kind appear in the press, as for example one by a prominent cardiologist (Dr. Robert G. Hauser, Minneapolis Heart Institute), who warned about potential problems involved in a new way of connecting defibrillators to the leads. The article states that, "Food and Drug Administration (FDA) officials said they expected the first products containing the new connectors to reach the market early in 2009. Dr. Hauser presents his argument in *The New England Journal of Medicine*, coauthored with another cardiologist, Dr. Adrian K. Almquist. The new wiring would allow the use of smaller heart devices, intended to be more comfortable for patients. Questions about the adequacy of component testing emerged in late 2007, after *Medtronic* recalled a relatively new electronic lead for defibrillators called the *Sprint Fidelis*. The FDA had let the *Fidelis* leads onto the market in 2004 on the basis of stress tests and animal studies, rather than the human trials that are usually required. But the new leads, which were thinner than the type previously used, began to fracture and fail at an unexpectedly high rate. By the time they were recalled, they had been implanted in some 235,000 patients. Scores of patients underwent procedures to have the *Fidelis* leads replaced. Currently, the two high-voltage defibrillator wires enter the housing of a device through separate channels that are insulated from each other. In the new design, they effectively enter together and are insulated in a different way, which Dr. Hauser said could increase the risk of short-circuiting" (extracted from *The New York Times*, Dec. 11, 2008, page B2, electronic edition).

### 3.2.4. *Generator Types*

This section deals with the generator block of a defibrillator, from which a pulse of predetermined amplitude, waveform and duration will be delivered either manually or automatically. It is the core of the machine where much effort, development, and tests have been invested on. The criterion to classify it is the pulse shape, thus, we find the *capacitive discharge* and the *damped sinusoidal discharge*, the *sinusoidal and the fractional sinusoidal discharges*, the *trapezoidal* and the *rectangular* shapes, and the *biphasic pulses*. Even, multiphasic pulses have been tested and proposed. Observe that these waveforms are somewhat related, as it will become clear in the sections below.

*Simple capacitive and damped discharges*

Perhaps the simplest and also historical arrangement (remember the Leyden bottle) is based on charging a capacitor by an adequate dc supply (a battery or an electronic rectifying unit, in turn fed from the public ac line) and, thereafter, discharging the charged capacitor through the patient (Fig. 3.3). The switch SW1, when in position C, enables the charging circuit $V_G$–$R_G$–C, and, when in position D, allows the discharge via $R_I$ and $Z_L$. The middle position E places the circuit in stand-by. Let us first assume that

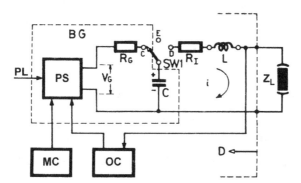

Fig. 3.3. Capacitive and damped discharge generators. The whole defibrillator $D$ is encompassed by the right-hand unfinished dashed line. On the far right, there is the load impedance (electrodes and patient). The closed dashed lined section surrounds the generator itself, including the power source (can be a battery) or an electronic source fed from the public power line PL. MC: manual control; OC: optional controls. $R_G$ and $R_I$ stand, respectively, for the generator's internal resistance and for an added limiting resistance. The inductance $L$ can be either short-circuited or removed by appropriate construction.

the inductance L is short-circuited so that we are left with the capacitor discharge case that collects Q coulombs in C at a voltage V, that is,

$$Q\,(\text{coulombs}) = C\,(\text{Farads})V\,(\text{volts}), \tag{3.4}$$

where $V \approx V_G$ represents the voltage across C, if $R_G$ can be neglected when compared with the load. Since the capacitor keeps its charge for a rather long time, depending on its losses, it becomes the effective generator when the SW1 is switched to position D, so that the current through $Z_L$ is expressed by,

$$i(t) = \frac{V_G}{R_I + Z_L} e^{-[t/(R_I + Z_L)C]}, \tag{3.5}$$

where $(R_I + Z_L)C$, or better, $(R_I + R_B)C$, stands for the time constant $T_D$ of the capacitive discharge, clearly depending on the patient for the other resistance belongs to the equipment. In other words, the duration of the shock is mainly determined by the biological load. Let us insist that $Z_L \approx R_L \approx R_B$ (see Chap. 5 on electrodes and pastes, where this impedance is dissected out in detail).

Figure 3.4 is a didactic graphic non-scaled description of the time-dependent events, which are well-mastered by any electrical engineering student in his/her early years. Let us quickly review them: The left side

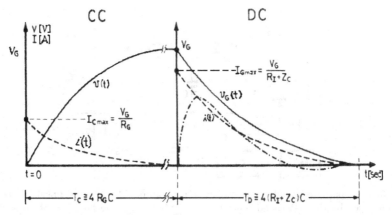

Fig. 3.4. Electric time-dependent non-scaled events during the charge–discharge of a capacitor. CC (left): charge, displaying the increasing voltage $v(t)$ across C and the decreasing current $i(t)$ through it. DC (right): discharge, showing the decreasing voltage $v_G(t)$ and the decreasing current, the latter with dashed lines. A damped voltage discharge of the Lown type is also shown on the right with dashed-dotted line. See text for further details.

of the figure displays the growing voltage across the capacitor C up to essentially the maximum value $V_G$ (disregarding the minor drop on $R_G$) and the decaying charging current $i(t)$, which starts at the maximum initial value $V_G/R_G$ (hence, its protective function). Four time constants $R_G C$ cover practically all the phenomena. Obviously, SW1 must be on C. The right side DC takes care of the discharge, that is, the switch is moved to position D (Fig. 3.3). Starting at the initial value $V_G$, the voltage across C drops exponentially to zero at the far right end of the graph, while the current (dashed middle line) also decays to zero starting at $V_G/(R_I + R_L)$. On purpose, we are using $Z_L$, $R_L$, and $R_B$ interchangeably (not to confuse the reader, but to make him familiar with the daily loose use of the terminology) understanding that, as already mentioned before, from a conceptual viewpoint, they are different even though in absolute numerical terms they may be rather close, for the former includes the electrode–electrolyte interface impedance and any other resistive load component, including the biological resistance $R_B$. Finally, the only load we are interested in is the latter, because *that is the site where fibrillation takes place.* A corollary out of all this is that the duration of the exponential sharp pulse is not fully controllable by the operator because of $R_B$ variability; he/she may only guess. Bernard Lown, in 1967, published a beautiful account about electrical reversion of cardiac arrhythmias, from which we have reproduced a photograph displaying clearly the voltage and current time course during a capacitor discharge (Fig. 3.5).

The manufacturer of a capacitor discharge (or *dc* equipment, as often as it is also-called) indicates in a panel instrument the *stored energy* (not equal to *delivered energy*) applying the also known equation,

$$E_G = (1/2)CV_G \tag{3.6}$$

so that, by changing the charging voltage $V_G$, usually the 20–450 W-S (or joule) range is covered. It is easily seen that the relationship between delivered energy over the load and stored energy depends on the impedance ratio (see Fig. 3.3),

$$E_L/E_G = Z_L/(Z_L + R_I), \tag{3.7}$$

from where we come back to current intensity, in amperes, as a better indicator. In the past, tests were carried out on commercial equipment uncovering that many of them delivered considerable less energy than the

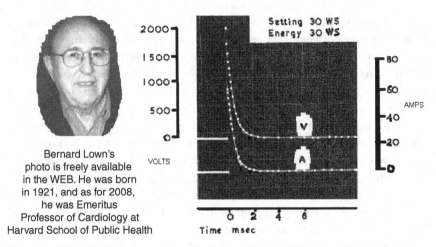

Fig. 3.5. Waveform of a capacitor discharge without inductance. Single discharge set at 30 watt-seconds across the intact chest evokes ventricular arrhythmia. Median energy required for transthoracic defib is about 70 ws. After Lown B (1967) Electrical reversion of cardiac arrhythmias. *British Heart J* 29:469–489. Downloaded from www.heart.bmj.com on 20 March 2008; with permission from *Br Heart J* through *Rightslink*. Slightly retouched to improve its resolution.

stored value given by their respective meters. Such situation has improved, but one task of clinical engineering technicians is to check it.

Often, after an unsuccessful shock, a second one of similar strength results in recovery of the rhythm. Very likely, this phenomenon is associated with the decrease in either transthoracic or myocardial impedance with a sequence of successive shocks (Geddes, Tacker *et al.*, 1975; Savino, Tirado and Valentinuzzi, 1986), a phenomenon that leads to a larger current so that it improves the efficacy of the shock. Mathematically, this is verified by reordering the equations in terms of the stored energy after considering Eq. (3.6),

$$i(t) = \frac{1}{R_I + Z_L}\sqrt{\frac{2E_G}{C}}[e^{-t(R_I+Z_L)C}], \qquad (3.8)$$

where the factor before the bracketed exponential is the maximum current $I_{Gmax}$ for each value of $Z_L$. Figure 3.6 displays parametrically such maximum current, in amperes, as a function of the energy $E_G$, in W-S, as the load impedance $Z_L$ decreases in successive shocks from $Z_{C1}$ to $Z_{C4}$. Observe how the sustained current goes up. The right-hand side of Fig. 3.6 shows the exponential decrease of the currents starting at the previously indicated maxima and also with $Z_L$ as parameter; the overall discharge

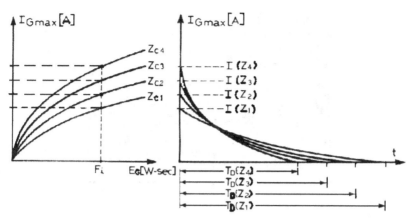

Fig. 3.6. Parametric curves of the maximum capacitive discharge currents as functions of the stored energy $E_G$ and time $t$. The load impedance $Z_L$ decreases from value 1 to value 4 as the number of shocks increases. The curves on the right show a clear crossing point. See text for details. After Valentinuzzi *et al.*, 1986, with permission.

duration $T_D$ in each curve, as expected, decreases from the first shock 1 to the last fourth shock 4. Interestingly enough, all curves have a single crossing point.

Most of the commercial equipment add an inductance in series (Fig. 3.3) to produce the damped sinusoidal discharge (Fig. 3.4, right side, dashed–dotted curve) and so having the *Lown defibrillator* (Alexander *et al.*, 1961; Lown *et al.*, 1962), or sometimes named, too, the *Lown–Gurvich defibrillator* because Gurvich and Yuniev (1946, 1947), in the Soviet Union, also contributed to its development. It is now widely used, especially as external piece. In his 1967 account, Lown very clearly tells the story and gives a photograph of a typical damped discharge (Fig. 3.7). It is eventually also called *dc* defibrillator generating some confusion in the terminology because neither the damped waveform nor the capacitor discharges are direct current in the strict meaning of the words so that we do not encourage such names. More precise use of the language is mandatory in biomedical engineering. The inclusion of an inductance in the discharge circuit of the capacitor decreases the peak voltage and peak current and lengthens the duration of discharge. The reduction in energy dissipation per unit time lessens the damage to subjacent tissues. Even so, such attenuated capacitor discharges may disrupt cardiac rhythm, impair conduction, and induce other deleterious biological effects.

Equation (3.8) and Fig. 3.4 summarize the expected limitations: for a given stored energy, current pulse and duration depend on the impedance

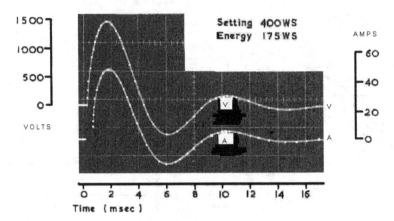

Fig. 3.7. Lown's damped discharge, both in voltage and current. After Lown (1967) Electrical reversion of cardiac arrhythmias. *Heart* 29: 469–489. Downloaded from www.heart.bmj.com on 20 March 2008. The delivered energy was lower than the set energy. With permission from BHJ through *Rightslink*.

seen by the electrodes; the internal resistance introduces a loss and the biological load is never known exactly. Besides, both types of discharge may produce myocardial damage, especially if the circulating current is too high or if the delivered energy is too high or if the latter takes place along with a low current (see Chap. 2, Sec. 2.4.2, Technological variables). For that reason, efforts are being invested, searching for ways of reducing the electrical parameters' amplitudes.

The interested reader, as a complementing exercise, is invited to review the equations that describe the damped discharge in an LCR series circuit, making zero the driving signal on the right-hand side of Eq. (3.9) or replacing the latter by the Dirac delta function. The differential equation to start with is,

$$L d^2 q / dt_2 + R dq / dt + qC = V_0 \cos \omega t, \qquad (3.9)$$

where $q$ stands for the electric charge in coulombs. The rest can be found in any electrical engineering textbook.

*Bernard Lown*, in 1959, being aware of 1956 Zoll's paper, and perhaps also of Claude Beck's in 1947, began animal studies trying to define a less traumatic and more effective form of electric shock. This work resulted in the *Lown defibrillator* described above. Following the research findings, Lown contacted an engineer, Barouh Berkovits, of the American Optical Company, who produced a clinical prototype. The original machine weighed some 27 kg delivering shocks at energy levels up to 100 J for exposed heart applications and 200–400 J for transthoracic use. Lown, who graduated from the University of Maine in 1942 and as physician from Johns Hopkins in Baltimore, no doubt a paradigmatic place in the defibrillation history, is also a peace activist. Born in Lithuania in 1921, he emigrated in 1935 at the age of 13 with his parents to the USA undergoing, as many others, racial persecution. Bernard Lown is currently Professor of Cardiology Emeritus at the Harvard School of Public Health, in Boston, MA. No doubt, he was one of the great driving forces in the development of defibrillators.

*Naum Lazarevich Gurvich* (1905–1981) was born near the capital of Byelorussia, Minsk. He received his MD from Saratov Medical School, in 1928, and then worked as a family physician for four years near Moscow. In 1932, he was enrolled into graduate school at the Institute of Physiology, also in Moscow. His PhD advisor and director, L.S. Schtern, was a former trainee and associate of Prevost in Geneva (good ancestry, indeed), who was one of the discoverers of defibrillation in 1899, along with Batelli. His doctoral dissertation, presented in 1939, titled "On excitation of intramural system by sinusoidal current of low frequency". The same year he coauthored a paper with G.S. Yuniev, in which they proposed the use of capacitor discharge for defibrillation instead of an alternating current and, in 1940, Gurvich also proposed, well in advance of much later tendencies, the use of

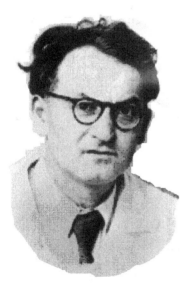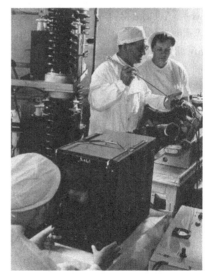

Fig. 3.8.   Naum Lazarevich Gurvich (1905–1981) and also in a picture during one of his experiments in Moscow. From http://efimov.wustl.edu/defibrillation/history/ Naum_Lazarevich_Gurvich.htm, with permission from Dr. Igor Efimov and with the author's book recognition.

biphasic waveforms for defibrillation (Fig. 3.8). Gurvich moved to the Laboratory of Experimental Physiology of Resuscitation, at the Academy of Medical Sciences of USSR, Moscow, in 1948. The main focus of his entire research career was on the mechanisms of fibrillation and defibrillation. He also introduced the concept of spatial heterogeneity and the concept of "mother-reentry", as foundations of the development and sustenance of fibrillation. In the early 1950s, Gurvich designed one of the first commercially available transthoracic defibrillators in the world. Biphasic waveforms are now becoming commonly accepted in defibrillation therapy, replacing monophasic waveforms used up to now in some of the transthoracic defibrillators. Abstracted note originally written by Igor Efimov, PhD, on Dec 14, 2001 (see http:// efimov.wustl.edu/defibrillation/history/Naum_Lazarevich_Gurvich.htm).

*Alternating sinusoidal current*

In 1947, *Claude Beck* (1894–1971) successfully defibrillated a 14-year-old boy whose heart went into fibrillation after an operation and reported it to the American Medical Association. This defibrillator was made by James Rand, a friend of Beck. The silver paddles (the size of a large tablespoon) were for open-chest use. The circuit connected the heart to the 110 V power line through an ammeter, a switch, and a resistance adjustable between 10 and 35 ohms (Fig. 3.9). Quite interestingly, Beck trained also at Johns Hopkins, as Lown did in turn, and where Kouwenhoven and Mirowski carried out tests and first implantations, respectively. Maybe

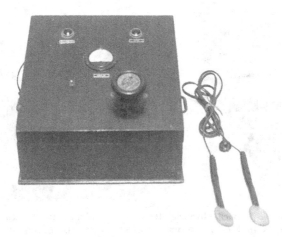

Fig. 3.9.   Beck and Rand's first ac defibrillator used in a human being. Rand made two equipment that year of 1947: one is in the Smithsonian and one in The Bakken's collections. Courtesy: The Bakken, Minneapolis, MN.

the place encompasses a favorable intellectual culture broth or there is a particular *karma* (immeasurable and invisible energy) surrounding it, as someone might like to say. (Corollary for students: Always be very careful and choosy when searching for a school). Thereafter, Paul Maurice Zoll (1911–1999) published another daring paper describing resuscitation of open-heart surgery patients by means of a 110 V alternating current electric shock (derived from a wall socket) and conducted to the sides of the exposed heart by metal plate "paddles" (Zoll, 1956). While being an advance in emergency resuscitation, the technique was later shown to be both damaging to the heart muscle and of unpredictable effectiveness in reverting VF. Many people used the sinusoid, including Kouwenhoven in his early trials, but soon it was abandoned due to its many risks, among them the induction of atrial fibrillation.

One apparent improvement is the limitation of the number of cycles to just one, one-half or even one-fourth of a cycle by means of an electronic switch, so actually transforming the discharge into a biphasic one or a single short pulse of either 10 or 5 ms, if the line frequency is 50 Hz (Moore *et al.*, 1977; Monzón and Valentinuzzi, 1982).

In the first paper, the standard Lown-type capacitor discharge waveform was compared with a single half-cycle 60 Hz sinusoid for effectiveness of defibrillation. Both shock types were used in attempts to defibrillate a series of dogs over a range of intensities from that below the minimum required for defibrillation to values well above those which were consistently successful. The half-cycle sinusoid required 18% more energy but 20% less peak current and 15% less peak voltage for 80% probability of success at these intensity levels. These results indicate that the half-cycle 60 Hz sinusoid is a reasonable alternative as a defibrillating waveform for low-energy applications, say, open-chest surgery, some pediatric cases, and small animal applications (Moore *et al.*, 1977). The waveform and the duration of the delivered pulse is fully independent of the load, however, even when its efficacy was similar to the damped shock (one-half sinusoidal cycle), the technology of the time was still too gross and cumbersome.

*Trapezoidal and rectangular pulses*

A truncated exponential or capacitor discharge produces a trapezoidal-shaped pulse (Fig. 3.10), so saving useless energy for defibrillation at the tail of the discharge which, besides, dissipates in the cardiac tissues potentially

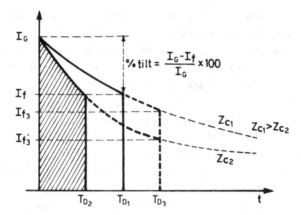

Fig. 3.10.  Truncated exponential pulses derived from discharges on different loads and by cutting them at different times. The shaded area represents the ampere-millisecond product actually delivering defibrillating energy to the tissues.

damaging heat. The tilt of the pulse is defined as,

$$TILT\% = \frac{I_G - I_f}{I_G}100, \qquad (3.10)$$

where $I_G$ is the maximum initial current value and $I_f$ represents the cutting or truncating value that takes place at time $T_{D1}$, defining also the duration of the pulse. Another parameter to characterize this kind of pulse is the slope of the tilt, that is, $(I_G - I_f)/T_{D1}$. The latter would be expressed in amperes/ms. A zero tilt or a zero slope would describe a rectangular pulse and, as the tilt or the slope increases, the pulse tends to a sharp spike. Obviously, the latter is not advisable for defibrillation. Rectangular pulses are, by and large, generated by adequate electronic circuits and they are sometimes used in the biphasic mode (see section below). Implantable devices generate both types, either trapezoidal or rectangular pulses.

Bardy, Zaghi *et al.* (1994) carried out a prospective randomized comparison of defibrillation efficacy of truncated pulses and damped sine wave pulses in humans. Their purpose was to determine whether damped pulses have a role in implantable defibrillators. For that matter, in 21 survivors of cardiac arrest, defibrillation efficacy of a standard truncated capacitor (RC) monophasic pulse was compared with a damped sine wave inductor–capacitor (LRC) pulse using a right ventricular–left ventricular epicardial patch–patch electrode system. The RC pulse was a standard 65% tilt monophasic waveform generated from a 120 $\mu$F capacitor. The LRC pulse was designed to simulate the waveform currently used in transthoracic defibrillators and was generated by passing the charge stored on a $40\,\mu F$ capacitor through a 37 mH inductor. Capacitor voltage, peak delivered voltage, peak delivered current, discharge pathway resistance, delivered energy, and stored energy were compared for the two waveforms at the defibrillation threshold. There was no difference in defibrillation efficacy for the two waveforms. Peak delivered voltage was similar at the defibrillation threshold: $313 \pm 101$ V for the RC pulse and $342 \pm 119$ V for the LRC pulse. Similarly, no differences were found in defibrillation threshold peak delivered current: $8.6 \pm 2.5$ (RC) vs $9.3 \pm 2.7$ (LRC) amperes; discharge pathway resistance: $37 \pm 11$ (RC) vs $38 \pm 13$ (LRC) ohms; delivered energy: $7.0 \pm 4.5$ (RC) vs $7.0 \pm 4.0$ (LRC) J; and stored energy: $8.7 \pm 5.7$ (RC) vs $9.8 \pm 5.4$ (LRC) J. Although both waveforms performed the same, it was necessary to use substantially higher stored voltages with the damped sine wave delivery system than with the truncated waveform delivery system: $356 \pm 110$ V for the RC pulse and $675 \pm 192$ V for the LRC pulse. They concluded that RC monophasic pulses provide equally effective epicardial defibrillation as LRC pulses with respect to delivered voltage and current and stored and delivered energy. However, in order for LRC pulses to provide comparable delivered voltage, current, and energy to that of RC pulses, nearly twice the voltage must be stored on the capacitor to accomplish the same task. These findings suggest that despite the nearly 50-year experience with damped sine wave pulses with transthoracic defibrillators, there is no need to begin using damped sine wave pulses for implantable defibrillators. Moreover, these data raise a question regarding the need for inductors in transthoracic defibrillators. The same group, Bardy *et al.* (1995), among others, have added studies of truncated biphasic pulses for transthoracic defibrillation.

*Biphasic pulses*

For years and by many investigators, two pulses of opposite polarity and short sequence were claimed as more efficient for defibrillation than any monophasic pulse (Jones, Jones and Balasky, 1987; Bardy, Marchlinski and Sharma, 1996; Keener and Lewis, 1999). Such two pulses are usually of the trapezoidal or truncated form, as described in the preceding section (see Fig. 3.11).

Out of those many papers, Tang *et al.* (2001), from Palm Springs, CA, compared biphasic and monophasic waveforms after prolonged VF in domestic experimental pigs. For a better grasp, it is worthwhile to shortly quote from them: "Defibrillation was attempted transthoracically

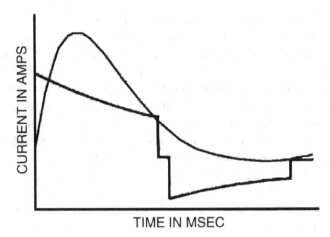

**TIME IN MSEC**

Fig. 3.11. Didactic figure comparing a monophasic damped discharge with biphasic trapezoidal pulses. Current is in the order of 40–50 amps (vertical axis) while each monophasic pulse lasts about 4–5 ms.

with up to three 150 J biphasic shocks or a conventional sequence of 200 J, 300 J, and 360 J monophasic discharges. When reversal of VF was unsuccessful, precordial compression was performed for 1 min, with or without administration of epinephrine. It was concluded that lower-energy biphasic shocks were as effective as conventional higher-energy monophasic shocks for restoration of spontaneous circulation after 10 min of untreated VF. Significantly better post-resuscitation myocardial function was observed after biphasic defibrillation".

The monophasic waveforms used in commercial defibrillators over the last 40 years were either monophasic damped sine (MDS) or monophasic truncated exponential (MTE) waveforms. It is generally assumed that patient impedance is 50 ohms. The biphasic truncated exponential (BTE) waveform was developed initially for implantable defibrillators and became the standard for these devices in the late 1980s. The advantage of this waveform is that it defibrillates at lower energies. The desire to produce a smaller and lighter AED led designers to pursue this waveform for external applications in the mid-1990s. The BTE waveform also has an advantage related to the shape of the defibrillation response or efficacy curve (Fig. 3.12). With the gradual slope of the MDS waveform, it is apparent that as current increases, the defibrillation efficacy also increases. This explains why escalating energy is needed: the probability of defibrillation increases with an increase in peak current. The steeper slope of the BTE waveform, however, results in a curve where the efficacy changes very little

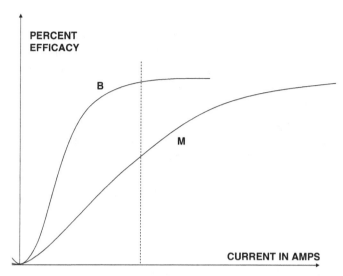

Fig. 3.12. The percent defibrillation efficacy of biphasic pulses B is higher than for monophasic M at the same current intensity (vertical dashed line).

with an increase in current, past a certain level. It means, then, that if the current level is chosen appropriately, escalating is not required to increase the efficacy. This fact, combined with the lower energy requirements of BTE, leads to the feasibility of choosing a fixed current for effective and safe defibrillation. Biphasic waveforms, so far, have no standards to comply with (as for example those of the American Association for Medical Instrumentation, AAMI), and thus, each defibrillator manufacturer has designed its own system and many patents have been issued that protect the individual designs. As a result, the user needs to follow the manufacturer's recommendation for energy protocol since what may be appropriate for one, may not be appropriate for another. Reference to the supplier's recommendations is mandatory.

Not long ago, triphasic pulses were advocated (Zhang *et al.*, 2003), in Iowa University; it is Richard E. Kerber's group (a long standing specialist in the subject). The study was carried out on swines based on the hypothesis that triphasic shocks caused less post-shock dysfunction than biphasic shocks in chick embryo studies. "After 30 s of electrically induced ventricular fibrillation (VF), each pig in part I ($n = 32$) received truncated exponential biphasic (7.2/7.2 ms) and triphasic (4.8/4.8/4.8 ms) transthoracic shocks. Each pig in part II ($n = 14$) received biphasic (5/5 ms) and triphasic shocks (5/5/5 ms). Three selected energy levels (50, 100, and 150 J) were tested for parts I and II. Pigs in part III ($n = 13$) received biphasic (5/5 ms) and triphasic (5/5/5 ms) shocks at a higher energy (200 and 300 J). Although the individual pulse durations of these shocks were equal, the energy of each pulse varied. Nine pigs in part I also received shocks where each individual pulse contained equal energy but was of a different duration (biphasic 3.3/11.1 ms; triphasic 2.0/3.2/9.2 ms). Triphasic shocks of equal duration pulses achieved higher success than biphasic shocks at delivered low energies: $< 40$ J: $38 \pm 5\%$ triphasic vs $19 \pm 4\%$ biphasic ($p < 0.01$); 40 to $< 50$ J: $66 \pm 7\%$ vs $42 \pm 7\%$ ($p < 0.01$); and 50 to $< 65$ J: $78 \pm 4\%$ vs $54 \pm 5\%$ ($p < 0.05$). Shocks of equal energy but different duration pulses achieved relatively poor success for both triphasic and biphasic waveforms. Shock-induced ventricular tachycardia (VT) and asystole occurred less often after triphasic shocks. It was concluded that triphasic transthoracic shocks composed of equal duration pulses were superior to biphasic shocks for VF termination at low energies and caused less VT and asystole." Years ago, even multiple shocks and different angles for electrodes directly applied to the myocardium were tested in experimental dogs (Puglisi *et al.*, 1989) with results that, at most, were only encouraging. In a similar but much better based line of thought, Brooks *et al.* (2009) proposed that a defibrillation shock would achieve higher success if the shock vector was oriented along the largest of the VF amplitudes measured simultaneously in three orthogonal ECG leads, and that this axis could be determined near-instantaneously in real time. Quite a good idea, indeed, for they demonstrated in pigs that choosing the defibrillation vector based on that concept the probability of success improved.

*Impedance compensation*

As early as 1977, this author and his group (Armayor *et al.*, 1978, 1979) dosed and searched current defibrillation thresholds for direct myocardial shocks based on the impedance modulus measured with an impedance meter at high frequency, *before delivering the discharge*. The voltage and the myocardial impedance determine the current flow. Factors that influence impedance include voltage, electrode size, paddle–tissue coupling material, number and time interval of previous shocks (as already mentioned before), and distance between electrodes and paddle pressure. When impedance is too high, a low-voltage shock will not generate enough current to achieve defibrillation. The procedure demonstrated to be quite efficient, because it allowed the application of the necessary voltage to sustain the prescribed current intensity, so that other experimental series under different conditions were undertaken (Arredondo *et al.*, 1980; Arredondo *et al.*, 1982;

Monzón and Valentinuzzi, 1982; Arredondo *et al.*, 1984). Later on, Kerber *et al.* (1984), of Iowa University, in an excellent series carried out in patients, applied successfully a similar concept but this time in the transthoracic situation. They concluded that transthoracic impedance (TTI) can be accurately predicted in advance of defibrillation and cardioversion and that the method permits preshock identification of patients with high impedance in whom attempts to defibrillate with low-energy shocks are inappropriate.

We have detected at least two patents (but there seems to be more) on the now called *impedance compensation procedure for defibrillation*. One of them, Lopin and Ayati (1998), says verbatim in its abstract: "An electrotherapy circuit administers to a patient a current waveform. The electrotherapy circuit includes a charge storage device, at least two discharge electrodes connected by electrical circuitry to opposite poles of the charge storage device, a sensor that senses a patient-dependent electrical parameter (such as a patient impedance sensor), and a control circuit. The control circuit is connected to the sensor and the charge storage device and controls discharge of the charge storage device through the electrodes, based on the patient-dependent electrical parameter (such as the patient impedance) as sensed by the sensor. The discharge is controlled in a manner so as to reduce the dependence of peak discharge current on the electrical parameter (such as patient impedance) for a given amount of charge stored by the charge storage device".

The other (Elabbady *et al.*, 1999) says: "A defibrillator method and apparatus wherein a patient's measured TTI is used to control the amount of energy contained in a defibrillation pulse applied to the patient. Prior to delivering a defibrillation pulse, the patient's TTI is measured by an impedance measuring circuit. The patient's TTI may also be measured during delivery of a prior defibrillation pulse. A microprocessor uses the measured patient TTI to control the shape of the defibrillation pulse by controlling: (i) the *phase duration* of the defibrillation pulse; and (ii) the voltage level to which the defibrillator's capacitor bank is charged. The defibrillation pulse shape is controlled so that the energy conveyed by the defibrillation pulse to the patient is near or exceeds a desired value. The desired value may be set by an operator via an energy selector. A switch controls the connection of defibrillator electrodes to the impedance measuring circuit and the capacitor bank". Note: The term *phase duration* is not explained.

In addition to transitioning to biphasic waveforms, virtually all new waveforms have added some type of impedance compensation that changes the waveform based on the measured value of the patient impedance.

Although this has been implemented differently by various defibrillator manufacturers, it has allowed each new waveform to tailor how the energy is delivered to each patient to maximize the effectiveness of the waveform. Instead of treating each patient the same, impedance compensation allows low impedance patients to receive a different wave-shape than high impedance patients. This contributes to safer and more effective waveforms, regardless of the load impedance (see http://www.touchcardiology.com/biphasic-waveform-technology-a308-1.html). The number of articles abounds and reviewing them is beyond our scope (Poole *et al.*, 1997; White, 1997; Gliner *et al.*, 1998).

### 3.3. Pacemakers

Pacemakers are only laterally and briefly discussed here because they do not fit the central subject of the book. They belong to the general area of electric cardiac stimulation and often, if not always, modern units now include pacemaking and defibrillation capabilities, the so-called implantable cardioverter defibrillator (ICD).

Already by the end of the nineteenth century, it was known that the heart could respond to external stimuli, either mechanical or electrical, and several researchers tested and even reported their results. The historical development, including highly attractive technical details, have been told and written in many places (Schechter, 1983; Geddes, 1984; Westrum, 1993; see also, http://en.wikipedia.org/wiki/Artificial_pacemaker#History_of_the_artificial_pacemaker). Quite obviously, the transistor first and later on the integrated circuit played an essential role in further and dramatic improvements, so that the 1950s decade and the early 1960s saw the appearance of truly acceptable pieces from the viewpoint of size and life expectancy. Earl Bakken, Walton Lillehei, Seymour Furman and Wilson Greatbach, in the USA, Rune Elmquist and Åke Senning, in Sweden, where a patient named Arne Larsson received 26 different pacemakers during his lifetime, passing away in 2001, at 81. Jorge Reynolds Pombo, an electronics engineer, in Colombia (http://es.wikipedia.org/wiki/Jorge_Reynolds_Pombo), and Orestes Fiandra and Roberto Rubio, two physicians, in Uruguay (http://www.ccc.com.uy/company/director.htm), made significant contributions, too, both groups starting around 1958–1959 and still active, the latter founding a company, CCC (meaning in Spanish *Centro de Construcción de Cardioestimuladores del Uruguay*), which continues in development and production. This is not the proper place to try to determine the first to build and implant the device, for that is a matter better left to historians (Geddes and Bakken, 2007). Most important is to say that painful and long animal experiments and clinical trials, full of difficulties, made around those years by several pioneers paved in more than one place the way for the more reliable units that started to show up in the 1970s. As Mirowski stated, *the bumps in the road are not bumps, they ARE the road.*

The lithium–iodide battery, introduced by Greatbach in 1970, was a significant step forward to extend duration. Electrodes used to be a problem too and, in fact, there is another history, not well documented and almost hidden that parallels the improvements of the core circuitry. Another obstacle to reliability was the diffusion of water vapor from the body fluids through the epoxy encapsulation that tended to damage the electronics of the pacemaker. Hermetically metallic sealed encasing was the solution, started in Australia and continued in the USA, which eventually became the standard.

Pacemaking can be divided into three types: *transcutaneous*, *transvenous*, and *permanent*. The former is external; it constitutes a temporary means of pacing the heart during an emergency. It is accomplished by delivering pulses of electric current through the patient's chest, which, as may be expected, is usually uncomfortable for the patient, so that some kind of tranquilizer should be considered. Prolonged transcutaneous pacing may cause burns on the skin and it is meant only to stabilize the patient until a more permanent procedure is obtained. The second one, instead, is endocardial and used primarily to correct profound bradycardia, when the patient does not respond to transcutaneous pacing or to drug therapy. It requires threading of an electrode through a vein into the right atrium, right ventricle, or both. The latter belongs to the transvenous group, but the unit and its electrodes are implanted by means of a nowadays relatively minor surgical procedure in the patient's thorax.

Cardiac pacemakers are designed and produced nowadays in a rather wide variety of models according to specific rhythm disturbances. Cardiac arrest and bradychardia lie on one end while tachyarrhythmias and fibrillation are on the other. Controlled and well-dosed electrotherapy has been shown to be the solution in a large percentage of cases, thus, it is considered as reliable. This is why many models combine both therapies: defibrillation and pacemaking.

We need to mention dyssynchronization of the two ventricles as a potentially serious condition in cases of heart failure, that is, the left and right ventricles do not contract simultaneously. Comparing with a malfunctioning car gas engine, when the mixture within the cylinders do not explode at the prescribed time (timing is out of phase), the heart behaves also as "out of phase". As a mechanics can diagnose the faulty timing just by listening to the running engine, a cardiologist also hear split heart sounds and can detect other signs, as for example, a too long QRS complex. Normally it is 60 to 90 ms and when out of synchronism it may reach 150 or more. This parameter, precisely, can be used as one criterion to install what it is called Cardiac Resynchronization Therapy (CRT), that is, a pacemaker that anticipates the contraction of one of the ventricles in order to put the two of them back into synchrony. Usually, the procedure requires biventricular pacing. The device has three leads, one in the atrium, one in the right ventricle, and a third in the coronary sinus to stimulate the left ventricle. They can be combined, too, with automatic defibrillation possibilities.

The conclusion, so far, is that in patients with heart failure and cardiac dyssynchrony, cardiac resynchronization improves symptoms and the quality of life and reduces complications and the risk of death. These benefits are in addition to those afforded by standard pharmacologic therapy. The implantation of a cardiac resynchronization device should routinely be considered in such patients (Bristow, Saxon *et al.*, 2004; Cleland, Daubert *et al.*, 2005).

### 3.4. Defibrillator Analyzers

One piece of accessory equipment that should be mentioned as a must in any Clinical Engineering Department is the Defibrillator Analyzer. It is intended to test the different technological characteristics, such as voltage, current and energy outputs, calibration, internal impedance, possible leaks, faulty connections, and software that might be included (see, for example, http://www.defibrillatoranalyzer.com/products_Delta2000.htm; or, with no listed author, Defibrillator analyzers, in *Health Devices*, Dec 1999, 28(12):477–501, at http://www.ncbi.nlm.nih.gov/pubmed/ 10604089?dopt=Abstract, for further information).

### 3.5. Conclusions and Review Questions

A basic defibrillator may be represented by a power source, a voltage or current generator, and a discharge circuit which includes the patient, considered as the main part of the load. Besides, there is a manual control, an optional synchronizing circuit, and a monitor, also optional.

The generator presents at its output terminals a voltage, which, when a switch is closed, sustains the current that circulates through the internal resistance of the equipment and also through the load. Ideal requirements are: (1) current intensity, in amperes, and duration of shock, in milliseconds, ought to be specified by the operator from the control panel (in fully automated equipment this information is preconditioned); and (2) both variables ought to be independent of the load faced by the generator. Even though recent equipment satisfy relatively well such conditions, full compliance to them still pose practical difficulties. From the functional viewpoint, there are *external* and *internal* defibrillators. The former are those equipment intended for transthoracic use and also those to be applied on the myocardium, while the term *internal defibrillator*, instead, is exclusively reserved for the implantable type. Unlike manual defibrillators, an automated external unit diagnoses the heart rhythm and determines if a shock is needed. Automatic models administer the shock without the user's command. Semi-automatic models tell the user that a shock is needed, but the user must tell the machine to do so. In most circumstances, the user cannot override a "no shock" advise. Most states in the USA protect against liability any person that volunteers to rescue a victim in case of his/her death. An ICD is a device that is placed in the chest or abdomen with electrodes connected to the chambers of the heart; it continually monitors its rhythm. When it detects an irregular signal, the ICD delivers a shock similar to those applied by the external counterparts. New ICDs can pacemake and defibrillate. The pulse shapes that have been tested are the *capacitive discharge* and the *damped sinusoidal discharge*, the *sinusoidal and the fractional sinusoidal discharges*, the *trapezoidal* and the *rectangular* shapes, the *biphasic pulses* and even *triphasic pulses*. The tendency nowadays favors biphasic discharges with impedance compensating programs because their better defibrillation efficacy has been demonstrated.

*Review questions* (T = True; F = False)

1. The first biomedical electrical stimulator was the
   Leyden bottle.                                      T      F
2. The total load impedance of a defibrillator includes
   the electrode–electrolyte interface.                T      F

3. The energy delivered by the generator is given by the current–voltage product integrated over the duration $T_D$ of the discharge.                                    T        F

4. It is not possible to defibrillate with 110 V at 60 Hz.          T        F

5. An internal defibrillator is typical of the surgery room.                                                               T        F

6. Emergency vehicles are likely to carry AEDs, in addition to manual defibrillators, as police or fire vehicles do.                                                      T        F

7. Implantable defibrillators may not produce any kind of uncomfortable sensation in a patient at the moment of the discharge.                                          T        F

8. The waveform mostly used in defibrillation is the fractional sinusoidal discharge.                              T        F

9. The number of discharges does not affect the biological impedance, neither of the myocardium nor of the thorax.                                                    T        F

10. A typical myocardial impedance can be in the order of 20–30 ohms.                                                 T        F

11. Biphasic pulses for defibrillation are gaining more and more favor.                                                 T        F

12. Current flow is a better parameter for dosing defibrillation, especially if combined with load impedance compensation.                                        T        F

13. Current intensity and duration of shock ought to be specified by the operator from the control panel while in fully automated equipment this information is preconditioned.                                          T        F

14. Contributors to defibrillation knowledge were...
    Pavlov   Kouwenhoven   Mirowski   Volta
    Galvani

15. Chemical defibrillation is much more efficacious than electrical defibrillation.                                      T        F

16. Tilt of a truncated waveform is defined as...
    (A) the slope of the rising phase of the pulse.
    (B) the slope of the upper phase.
    (C) the slope of the falling phase.

17. A biphasic defibrillating pulse is composed of ...
    (A) two pulses of opposite polarity.
    (B) two pulses of the same polarity.
    (C) neither of the above.
    (D) either (A) or (B).
18. A shock based on impedance compensation adjusts the discharge according to the measured load impedance during fibrillation.      T     F
19. Resynchronization therapy is a type of cardiac stimulation based on the concept of
    (A) the atria do not pump enough blood into the ventricles.
    (B) one ventricle contracts significantly before the other.
    (C) the excitation wave spreads from apex to base instead of from base to apex.
    (D) the P–R interval is too long.
    (E) none of the above.
20. In case of VF, CPR must be applied as soon as possible, the sooner, the better    T    F      INDIFFERENT

# Chapter 4

# VENTRICULAR FIBRILLATION DETECTION

*As soon as possible try to know for sure whether the crazy worms have taken over the well-behaved movement ...*

**Eric Laciar Leber and Max E. Valentinuzzi**

In automatic defibrillation, early detection of the arrhythmia constitutes an essential and extremely sensitive task. Its failure means no shock delivery and, hence, no possible reversal leading to the patient's death. Besides, as Golden Rule, a shock should not be delivered to a collapsed patient not in cardiac arrest and a successfully defibrillated patient should not be defibrillated again. After defining basic evaluating parameters (*sensitivity, specificity, receiver operating curve, positive predictivity,* and *accuracy*), several algorithms are reviewed comparing them at the end of the chapter in an attempt to help the designing engineer in his/her selection. Acronyms are used along the text for the sake of space knowing the risk of confusion, although frequently their full identification is repeated and realizing that occasionally the same algorithm shares two abbreviations. To make navigation in this chapter easier, find here listed the seven algorithms treated plus other nine mentioned in the discussion, including also two algorithms for QRS complex detection, and calling attention to some overlapping between the two sets, that is: Probability Density Function (PDF), Threshold Crossing Intervals (TCI), Cardiac Frequency (CF), Signal Morphology (SM) or Correlation Waveform Analysis (CWA), Time–Frequency Analysis (TFA), Wavelet Transform (WT), and Phase Space Analysis (PSA), in the first group, followed by Threshold Crossing Intervals (TCI), described in Sect. 4.2.2, AutoCorrelation Fischer (ACF$_{95}$) algorithm, based on Correlation Waveform Analysis (CWA), explained in Sect. 4.2.4, VF Filter algorithm, after Kuo and Dillman (1978); Spectral (SPEC) algorithm based on Fourier Transform analysis, described in Sect. 4.2.5, Complexity (CPLX) algorithm, the Standard Exponential (STE) algorithm, the Modified Exponential Algorithm (MEA), an STE akin, the Signal Comparison Algorithm (SCA), the Wavelet (WVL) Algorithm, also explained in Sect. 4.2.6. Likewise, two QRS complex detection algorithms are considered: Tompkins (TOMP, see Sect. 4.2.3) and LI algorithm (see Sect. 4.2.6).

## 4.1. Introduction

Either in automatic external or in implantable cardiac defibrillators, early detection of the arrhythmia constitutes an essential and extremely sensitive task. Its failure means no shock delivery and, hence, no possible reversal leading to the patient's death. There exists a wide variety of methods and ideas for handling this task. Such algorithms should have a high detection quality, be easily implementable, and work in real time. Their testing poses a not easy task.

In early defibrillators, when detecting algorithms were still in their infancy, the solution was the *brute force criterion*, that is, even facing a doubtful ventricular fibrillation (VF) episode, the discharge was applied just in case. However, the criterion was far from being sensible and could produce unnecessary shocks with at least three types of drawbacks (Jenkins and Caswell, 1996): (a) inflicting needless pain; (b) possible triggering of a previously non-existing ventricular tachycardia or fibrillation; and (c) battery charge reduction for future real events. A Golden Defibrillation Rule clearly states that **an automatic defibrillator should not deliver a shock to a collapsed patient not in cardiac arrest; moreover, a successfully defibrillated patient should not be defibrillated again.**

Current digital electronic devices (microprocessors, A/D converters, memories) along with advances in signal processing techniques and pattern recognition strategies have led to the development of a wealth of automatic algorithms able to quickly and efficiently detect the establishment of VF or tachycardia. Basic requirements include the following:

(a) they must be fully automatic, which in simple words mean without human intervention;
(b) they must operate in real time, that is, permanent monitoring of cardiac electrical activity should pick out as fast as possible the eventual appearance of the arryhthmia;
(c) they must have high sensitivity, i.e. they must be able to correctly detect all of these kinds of cardiac events;
(d) the number of false discharges must be minimized, or better, must be zero; and
(e) energy consumption and response time must be minimized, too.

The following parameters are often defined to assess the performance of automated algorithms for VF detection:

*Sensitivity* $S_e$, as the ability (or probability) to correctly detect ventricular fibrillation, or

$$S_e = \frac{TP}{TP + FN} \qquad (4.1)$$

Table 4.1. Truth table to assess the performance of automated algorithms for ventricular fibrillation (VF) detection.

| Clinical Diagnosis | | |
| --- | --- | --- |
| Algorithm Detection | VF | All Others |
| VF | True Positive (TP) | False Positive (FP) |
| All Others | False Negative (FN) | True Negative (TN) |

where TP stands for the number of True Positive decisions or the number of correctly detected cases of VF, and FN is the number of False Negatives (that is, no detection, or cases given as negative when they actually were fibrillations). Obviously, the sum in the denominator represents the total number of VFs. Both values are defined schematically in Table 4.1, where columns give the true clinical diagnosis and rows present the algorithm decision.

*Specificity* $S_p$, instead, is the probability to correctly identify the absence of VF or, in mathematical terms,

$$S_p = \frac{TN}{TN + FP} \tag{4.2}$$

where TN stands for the number of True Negative events or of "no VF" correctly not reported as fibrillation and FP is the number of False-Positive decisions (that is, unnecessary shocks were perhaps delivered to the patient). In other words, the denominator collects all the cases of "no VF" (see Table 4.1).

For example, a sensitivity of 91% and a specificity of 98% describe equipment which 91% of the time detects a rhythm that should be defibrillated and 98% of the time does not deliver a shock when defibrillation is actually not indicated. Hence, it is a technologically and medically acceptable unit. A given algorithm may show high sensitivity but low specificity, or just the opposite. In fact, there is a tradeoff between the two parameters. To arrive at a common and single quality parameter, the Receiver or Relative Operating Characteristic (ROC) is frequently used, i.e. **sensitivity $S_e$ is plotted as function of $(1 - S_p)$**. By calculating the area under the ROC curve, it is possible to compare different algorithms by one single value (Fig. 4.1). In medical diagnosis, ROC curves have become standard tool for this purpose and its use is becoming increasingly common in other fields, too. The ROC can also be represented by plotting the fraction of TP

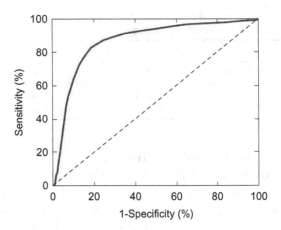

Fig. 4.1.   The relative operating characteristic (ROC) curve obtained by changing the threshold test. See text for mathematical definitions. The diagonal marks the equal value geometrical locus.

as function of the fraction of FP since, after Eq. (4.2), $(1 - S_p)$ = $1 - TN/(TN + FP) = (TN + FP - TN)/(TN + FP) = FP/(TN + FP)$.

Other algorithm evaluating parameters are *Positive Predictivity* $P_{re}$ and *Accuracy* $A_{cc}$; the former defined as the number of detected cases of VF divided by all cases given as VF, or, in quantitative terms,

$$P_{re} = \frac{TP}{TP + FP} \qquad (4.3)$$

which describes the probability that classified VF is truly VF. The latter, in turn,

$$A_{cc} = \frac{TP + TN}{TP + FP + TN + FN} \qquad (4.4)$$

is the probability to obtain a correct decision, for it relates all true decisions to all decisions.

Observe that specificity and sensitivity always depend on the chosen critical threshold. The ROC curve removes such dependence and allows comparison of different algorithms when choosing a given specificity (Amann *et al.*, 2005).

Summarizing, sensitivity measures how good the test is at picking out VF. It is simply the True Positive Fraction (TPF). Specificity describes the ability of the test to pick out cases where there is no VF. This is synonymous with the True Negative Fraction (TNF). The ROC curve is an exploration of what happens to TPF and FPF as we vary the position of an arbitrary test threshold. The closer the ROC curve is to the diagonal, the less useful the test is at discriminating between the two populations. The steeper the curve moves up and then across leveling off, the better the test. A more precise way of characterizing the "closeness to the diagonal" is to look at the Area Under the ROC Curve (AUC), which behaves as non-parametric. The closer the area is to 0.5 (it covers only $\frac{1}{2}$ of the square surface area), the worse the test, and the closer it is to 1.0 (it tends to cover the whole square), the better the test (see also http://www.anaesthetist.com/mnm/stats/roc/ Findex.htm, The Magnificent ROC or Receiver Operating Characteristic curve, where dynamic demonstrations are available).

## 4.2. Algorithms for the Detection of Ventricular Fibrillation (VF)

There is a good variety of automatic algorithms able to flag the presence of this lethal arrhythmia. Pannizo *et al.* (1988), Lang and Bach (1990), and Jenkins and Caswell (1996) well reviewed the subject while more recent techniques have been updated by Schuckers (2006) and Gillberg (2007). Most of them, however, deal with the detection of malignant arrhythmias to be handled by implantable cardiac defibrillators, even though the majority, if not all, are easily adaptable to external defibrillators.

Such algorithms explore either the electrogram (EGM) or the electrocardiogram (ECG) and are based in one or more of the following aspects or information always contained in the signal:

— Probability Density Function (PDF)
— Threshold Crossing Intervals (TCI)
— Cardiac Frequency (CF)
— Signal Morphology (SM)
— Time–Frequency Analysis (TFA)
— Wavelet Transform (WT)
— Phase Space Analysis (PSA)

Hence, computational means should be developed to look into the numerical features characterizing such aspects.

### 4.2.1. *Probability Density Function (PDF)*

A histogram is a graphical description of how frequent (say, how probable) the values of a random variable or variate $x$ take place. Height or weight of a given population, for example, will produce a distribution from which usually the average and the spread are calculated. From such distribution stems the concept of PDF (Mandel, 1964).

Perhaps, it was the first criterion used in the early generation of defibrillators. The main idea lies on the fact that the heart electrical activity most of the time rests on the isoelectric line and only briefly (during the P, QRS, and T waves) deviates from it (Mirowski *et al.*, 1980a, 1980b; Jenkins and Caswell, 1996). Figure 4.2(a) illustrates a sinus rhythm (SR) with amplitudes near the baseline during significant periods, especially for the PR and ST segments and between the end of T and the following beginning of P. Instead, in VF (Fig. 4.2(b)), the ECG signal has an oscillatory nature so that, most of the time, it lies either above or below the baseline. The corresponding PDFs (Figs. 4.2(c) and 4.2(d)) clearly show the differences, where amplitudes are represented on the $x$-axis and their probabilities are

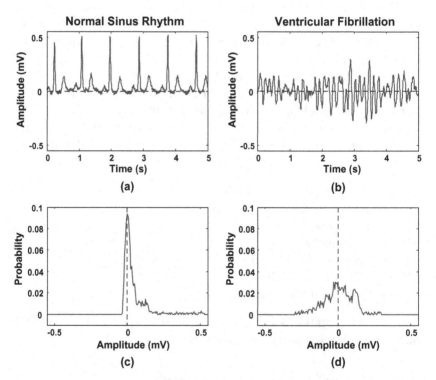

Fig. 4.2. VF detection by PDF. (a) ECG during normal sinus rhythm. (b) ECG during VF. (c) and (d) PDFs of the signals above, respectively. Downloaded from http://www. physionet.org/physiobank/database/vfdb/, taking different segments of record #426, *MIT-BIH Malignant Ventricular Arrhythmia Database*, freely available.

marked on the $y$-axis. Obviously, the normal rhythm has a high peak around zero amplitude while it falls to almost nothing during VF. Thus, the decision criterion (with a given threshold) is the sharp decrease of the PDF at zero amplitude.

Even though the method is extremely simple and works acceptably, it has limitations; for example, it cannot distinguish sinus tachycardia, supraventricular tachycardia, ventricular tachycardia (VT), and VF (Toivonen *et al.*, 1992), thus, it has been replaced by other more powerful ones.

### 4.2.2. *Threshold Crossing Intervals (TCI)*

With the objective of solving some of the PDF method limitations, Thakor *et al.* (1990) developed a simple temporal algorithm to distinguish SR, VT, and VF, based on the ECG binarization and a few sequential hypotheses.

In a first stage and after filtration, the ECG is compared against a predetermined threshold to generate a binary sequence that takes level 1 if the ECG amplitude lies above the threshold and becomes 0 when the signal is below it (Fig. 4.3). The duration of each pulse in the generated

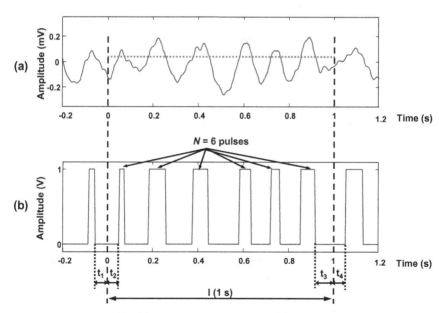

Fig. 4.3.   TCI algorithm. (a) ECG segment during VF. (b) Pulse sequence after applying the threshold crossing criterion.

sequence varies according to the time the signal stays above or below the cutting value. The threshold is chosen as 20% of the ECG maximum peak value within an interval $I = 1$ s and is recalculated in each of the following intervals, that means a threshold adaptation to the signal amplitude changes supplying also some noise immunity.

The number $N$ of pulses related to the ECG threshold crossings within the 1 s segment $I$ is counted while the average interval $TCI$ between crossings is determined applying Thakor *et al.*'s formula (1990),

$$TCI = \frac{1000}{(N-1) + \frac{t_2}{t_1+t_2} + \frac{t_3}{t_3+t_4}}[ms], \qquad (4.5)$$

where $N$ stands for the number of pulses within $I$ and $t_1$ is the time from the beginning of $I$ back to the falling edge of the preceding pulse (which belongs to the preceding segment); $t_2$ is the time from the beginning of the segment to the rising edge of the first pulse in the segment; $t_3$ and $t_4$, located at the end of the segment, are some kind of mirror image of the first two distances for, respectively, they measure the time from the falling edge of the last pulse within the segment to the end of the segment and the time from the segments end to the rising edge of the first pulse in the subsequent segment (Fig. 4.3, bottom).

Once the $TCI$ is obtained, several hypotheses must be used to screen out SR, VT, and VF. For example, if $TCI \geq TCI_0 = 400$ ms, the ECG is classified as SR. Others of the kind are usually applied to separate out VT from VF. Seven to eight segments (that is, 7–8 s) are recommended to check so that a better robustness is reached, however, detecting speed can be improved by somewhat lowering those numbers, always at the expense of less sensitivity and specificity. As always, there is a trade off.

### 4.2.3. Cardiac Frequency (CF)

It is perhaps the most widely used criterion that showed up after the PDF method. The normal resting fundamental heart rate, governed by the sinus node, covers roughly the 60–100 beats/min range, that is, in the order of 1–2 Hz (Bayés de Luna, 1999). VT, instead, go well beyond the 120 beats/min mark (2 Hz), reaching easily values of about 240 beats/min (4 Hz) or even more for VF (Fig. 4.4). In other words, heart rate appears as excellent criterion to quickly flag the establishment of either tachycardia or fibrillation. The algorithm must first pick out each ventricular beat (the QRS complex) and, thereafter, compute its frequency. The QRS frequency

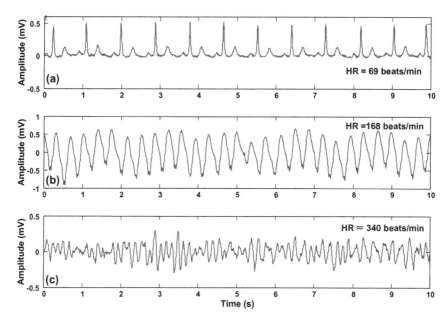

Fig. 4.4. Human ECGs during, (a) normal sinus rhythm (NSR), top; (b) ventricular tachycardia (VT), middle; and, (c) ventricular fibrillation (VF), bottom. Observe the cardiac frequency increase. Record #426, from the *MIT-BIH Malignant Ventricular Arrhythmia Database*, http://www.physionet.org/physiobank/database/vfdb/, freely available.

content is, by and large, greater than that of the other ECG components (P and T) because it is sharper than the latter two.

Köhler *et al.* (2002) produced a rather comprehensive review of QRS detecting algorithms. One of them, often applied, was proposed by Pan and Tompkins (1985) and described in detail by Afonso (1993). Its implementation is simple reaching high levels of sensitivity and predictivity (both >99.5%). Bandwidth, slope, and pulse duration are the three criteria used by the algorithm. Figure 4.5 displays a block diagram with their respective expected outputs. A bandpass filter keeps the spectral portion where most of the QRS energy concentrates, attenuating the P and T low-frequency components, removing baseline slow changes or drifts and reducing 50/60 Hz line interference and electromyographic high-frequency noise. A differentiator picks out the steep QRS edges, obviously much different that the other components' smoother edges. Thereafter, the mean quadratic value of each signal sample is computed by a non-linear unit to obtain only positive values and to emphasize the QRS high-frequency

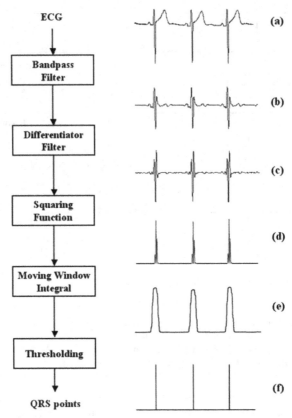

Fig. 4.5. Block diagram with the respective expected signals for QRS detection, as proposed by Pan and Tompkins (1985). (a) original ECG; (b) output from bandpass filter; (c) differentiator output; (d) squaring function output; (e) integrator moving window output; and (f) detected QRS pulses.

components. A moving window integrator adds up the areas under the quadratic signal to produce pulses and to remove short-duration artifacts. Such output goes to the decision unit where each pulse is compared with the pre-established threshold singling it out or not and locating it in its proper relative temporal place. The overall output is composed of the temporal marks or spikes each corresponding to the detected QRSs.

Another method uses the algorithm proposed by Li *et al.* (1995), which applies the Quadratic Spline Wavelet Transform. It will be explained in Sec. 4.2.6, where this transform is defined. Once the QRSs are detected, the RR intervals are measured calculating thereafter the instantaneous frequencies by the well-known,

$$F_c = 60/RR, \tag{4.6}$$

where $F_c$ stands for the instantaneous CF in beats/min and $RR$ represents the distance between two consecutive QRS complexes, in seconds. Finally, since sporadic ectopics might activate the detection algorithm, a safety condition is set requiring that the average $F_c$ after a given number of beats (say, 12 or 14) must be higher than a pre-established threshold before a rhythm is declared either VT or VF.

### 4.2.4. *Signal Morphology (SM) or Correlation Waveform Analysis (CWA)*

It is another technique for the recognition of ventricular arrhythmias many years ago described by Feldman *et al.* (1970), Hulting and Nygards (1976), and Thakor (1984), using surface ECG, or endocardial EGM, by Lin *et al.* (1986). The correlation coefficient $\rho$ (Eq. (4.7), below) between a normal sinus template previously stored and the analyzed sequence is calculated, i.e.:

$$\rho = \frac{\sum_{i=1}^{i=N} (t_i - \bar{t})(s_i - \bar{s})}{\sqrt{\sum_{i=1}^{i=N} (t_i - \bar{t})^2 \sum_{i=1}^{i=N} (s_i - \bar{s})^2}}, \tag{4.7}$$

where $N$ = number of data points in the template; $t_i$ = template point $i$; $s_i$ = analyzed signal point $i$; $\bar{t}$ = average of the template points; and $\bar{s}$ = average of the signal points. The correlation coefficient varies from $-1$ to $+1$, being $+1$ if the template and the signal show exactly the same morphology and are perfectly aligned. Instead, $\rho = -1$ when both show identical morphology but are opposite in phase, that is, at $180°$. Finally, $\rho = 0$ if the template and the signal are not related at all.

An example is displayed in Fig. 4.6: on top, a normal rhythm averaged template is seen, while on the bottom left a typical normal detected beat appears showing high correlation with the former. The bottom right-hand panel, instead, shows a ventricular beat during fibrillation and, thus, correlation is much lower. An adequate correlation threshold provides the detection criterion.

In summary, high correlations mean normal rhythm while low consecutive correlations flag the presence of arrhythmia. The technique calls first for each QRS complex either in the ECG or the EGM and,

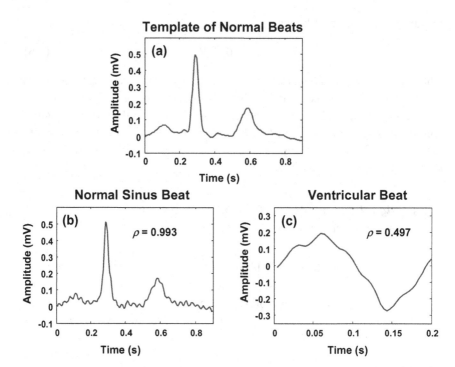

Fig. 4.6.  Ventricular arrhythmias detected by correlation waveform analysis (CWA). (a) Normal template by averaging. (b) Normal sinus rhythm showing high correlation. (c) Ventricular beat during VF with low correlation. Downloaded from record #426 of the already referred to *MIT-BIH Malignant Ventricular Arrhythmia Database.*

thereafter, for the alignment of all recorded beats to get the averaging. The QRS detector is similar usually to that described in the previous section while alignment makes use of the QRS peak value. However, the latter is rather noise sensitive and other alternative more elaborate alignment methods have been suggested (Jané *et al.*, 1991; Laguna *et al.*, 1997; Laciar *et al.*, 2003). A salient advantage of the CWA technique lies on the correlation insensitivity to baseline fluctuations and to beat amplitude changes. However, the computational cost involved in Eq. (4.7) is relatively high leading to other possible solutions (Throne *et al.*, 1991).

### 4.2.5. *Time–Frequency Analysis (TFA)*

The Fourier Transform (FT), as defined by Eq. (4.8), or any of its variants, the Discrete Fourier Transform (DFT) or the Fast Fourier Transform

(FFT), represents the essential tool for this kind of analysis, that is,

$$X(f) = \int_{-\infty}^{+\infty} x(t)e^{-j2\pi ft}dt. \tag{4.8}$$

In it, $x(t)$ stands for either the EGM or ECG signal in the time domain, $X(f)$ represents its Fourier Transform and $f$ is frequency in Hz. The squared function $|X(f)|^2$ describes the power spectral density (PSD), often called simply the *signal spectrum*, for short, along the frequency axis.

Figure 4.7 illustrates the differences obtained from a patient when the rhythm was normal and during spontaneous VF. The former has a wide spectrum with a central frequency of 1.2 Hz and several harmonics below 10 Hz (Fig. 4.7(c)), while the latter shows a sharp peak at a frequency

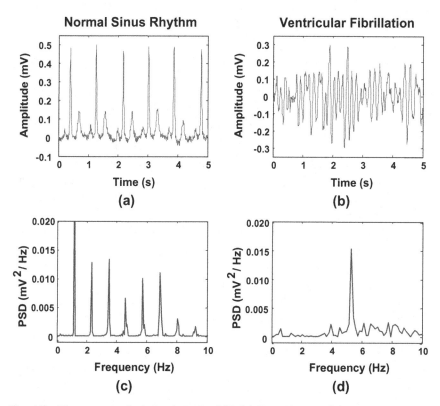

Fig. 4.7. Frequency analysis for detecting VF. (a) Normal ECG. (b) ECG during VF. (c) Normal ECG spectrum. (d) VF Frequency spectrum.

beyond 5 Hz (Fig. 4.7(d)), so reflecting a CF higher than 300 Hz (Clayton *et al.*, 1995).

Frequency analysis, however, is plagued with limitations, unfortunately. It can only be applied to stationary signals, a condition which is not met usually by the electrical cardiac activity. Besides, such frequency analysis requires a minimum signal length, if a reasonable resolution is to be obtained. That segment complicates the determination of the exact VF starting instant.

Several time–frequency distributions have been proposed to circumvent the difficulties mentioned before (Afonso and Tompkins, 1995; Clayton and Murray, 1998; Millet-Roig *et al.*, 1999). TFA allows examining the signal energy distribution (by and large non-stationary) simultaneously in time and in frequency. The simplest form is represented by the Short Time Fourier Transform (STFT), which basically applies a finite length moving window shifted along the signal and computing, for each instant, the FT of the piece within the window. The definition of the STFT is given by Eq. (4.9), or

$$X(t, f) = \int_{-\infty}^{+\infty} x(\tau)w^*(t - \tau)e^{-j2\pi f\tau}d\tau, \qquad (4.9)$$

where $x(t)$ is the ECG, $X(t, f)$ represents its STFT, $w(t)$ is the moving window, the symbol $*$ means *complex conjugate*, $t$ is time in seconds, and $f$ stands for frequency in Hz. The STFT can be interpreted as a *local signal spectrum* around instant $t$ (Fig. 4.8). The two bottom panels display time, in seconds, in abscissae and frequency, in Hz, on the vertical axis. For ventricular fibrillation, most of the energy concentrates around a dominant frequency at about 7 Hz (Fig. 4.8(d)), which, when compared with panel (c), shows more dispersion.

To quantify the STFT differences between normal heart rhythm and VF, several parameters have been suggested, such as modal frequency, mean frequency, and peak size (Clayton and Murray, 1998). Specifically, modal frequency increases during the beginning of VF, it may abruptly change during the arrhythmia and eventually may even decrease after a few minutes. Such parameters offer the possibility of following dynamic changes of ventricular fibrillation.

Nonetheless, the method is not free of some limitations when dealing with its temporal and frequency resolutions. For that matter, modifications such as the Wigner–Ville and Choi–Williams distributions appear as alternatives (Afonso and Tompkins, 1995; Clayton and Murray, 1998), which lead to similar results as before and, thus, do not mean a clear-cut improvement.

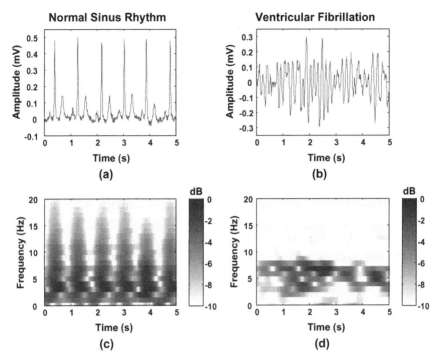

Fig. 4.8. Time–frequency analysis for VF detection. (a) Normal ECG. (b) VF (c) time–frequency distribution by STFT for normal rhythm. (d) Same as in (c) but for VF. The scale on the right represents frequency intensity in a black–white range, with 0 equated to black and intermediate grays down to the $-10$ dB level or white. Panel (d), for example, shows between 2 and 3 s a high intensity at about 6–7 Hz.

## 4.2.6. *Wavelet Transform (WT)*

This transform has been proposed as one way out of the problems encountered by the STFT previously described (Addison *et al.*, 2000; Ruiz de Gauna *et al.*, 2004). Basically, a *wavelet*, as the name indicates, is a small wave with its energy concentrated in time that permits analysis of transient and non-transient phenomena (Burrus *et al.*, 1998).

A temporal signal $x(t)$ containing finite energy has a Continuous Wavelet Transform (CWT), which was described by Akay (1996), as

$$X_{\mathrm{CWT}}(a,b) = \int_{-\infty}^{+\infty} x(t)\psi_{a,b}^*(t)dt = \langle x(t), \psi_{a,b}(t)\rangle, \qquad (4.10)$$

where the asterisk * means that the function below is a *complex conjugated* quantity, $a$ is a scale factor inversely proportional to frequency, and $b$ stands for a temporal shifting parameter. Hence, the CWT of a function $x(t)$ can be expressed as the internal product between the two vectors $x(t)$ and $\psi_{a,b}(t)$, the latter obtained by scaling and temporal shifting of a prototype or mother wavelet $\psi(t)$, which is defined as,

$$\psi_{a,b}(t) = \frac{1}{\sqrt{|a|}} \psi\left(\frac{t-b}{a}\right). \qquad (4.11)$$

In the latter Eq. (4.11), the following conditions must be met: $a \in \Re^+, b \in \Re$. With different values for $a$ and $b$, this transform supplies a representation of the signal in the time-scale domain leading to a description of the $x(t)$ characteristics in different temporal and frequency resolutions, as opposed to the STFT, where both resolutions are constant. Something should be underlined: this transform goes from the time domain to an arbitrary scale domain expressed in abstract numbers. Such concept is similar to the scales used in geographic maps, where so many centimeters correspond to so many kilometers. The factor scale $a$, as anticipated above, is inversely proportional to frequency in the Fourier Transform, so the WT region corresponding to high values of $a$ are related to low-frequency content in the signal and, conversely, the WT region corresponding to low values of $a$ scale reflect the high frequencies present in the signal.

Due to the relatively high frequencies involved in VF, the CWT appears as particularly useful in the detection of such arrhythmias. Addison *et al.* (2000) applied this transform in pigs identifying VF patterns at the high-frequency region of the WT. Figure 4.9 depicts an example from a human ECG. In VF, energy concentrates at the lower scale values ($20 < a < 40$), so reflecting the high-frequency components in the electrical cardiac signal. Besides, in normal rhythm, energy spreads more, reaching values of $a$ bigger than 80, indicating low-frequency content in the signal.

Once the CWT is computed, calculations of several parameters, such as total energy within a predetermined scale range, or median frequency, or maximum energy frequency, lead to VF detection. Other parameters have also been proposed to distinguish tachycardia from fibrillation (Ruiz de Gauna *et al.*, 2004).

However, the CWT is not free of difficulties: computing time may be longer than desirable because energy must be obtained in all scales and all instants. The Discrete Wavelet Transform (DWT) improves computing time by running the transform algorithm only for specific $a$ values, which are often chosen as integer powers of 2, that is, $a = 2^j$, with $j \in Z$. In this way,

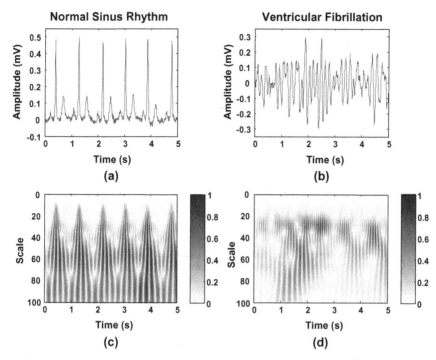

Fig. 4.9. VF detection by CWT. (a) Normal rhythm. (b) VF. (c) CWT for the normal rhythm, above. (d) CWT during VF. For convenience, vertical axes in (c) and (d) are inverted, so that the lower scale values appear in the upper part and the higher values at the lower part. Note that these numbers are NOT in dB as in Figure 4.8 before.

the DWT provides a dyadic decomposition that can be easily implemented by Mallat's (1989) algorithm, which is equivalent to an octave filter bank. The DWT of a signal $x(n)$ is defined as,

$$X_{DWT}(j,k) = \sum_{n=-\infty}^{+\infty} x(n)\psi_{j,k}^*(n) = \langle x(n), \psi_{j,k}(n) \rangle \qquad (4.12)$$

with

$$\psi_{j,k}(n) = 2^{-j/2}\psi(2^{-j}n - k), \qquad (4.13)$$

where $\psi_{j,k}(t)$ represents the scaled and shifted versions of the mother wavelet $\psi(t)$.

One of the most used mother or prototype DWT functions is the so-called *Quadratic Spline Wavelet*, proposed by Mallat and Zhong (1992). It

132              *Cardiac Fibrillation-Defibrillation*

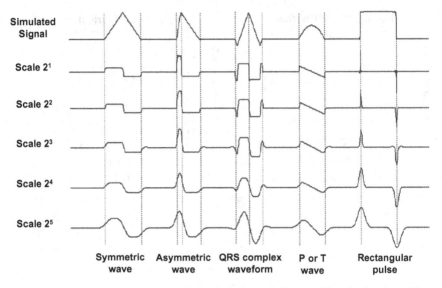

Fig. 4.10.   Sequence of different simulated waves and their multi-scale decomposition obtained by the Quadratic Spline Wavelet.

can be easily implemented by linear phase filters producing a time invariant decomposition for different scales, the latter representing smoothed versions of the signal first derivative. Figure 4.10 illustrates a simulated sequence with shapes that resemble some ECG components treated with this wavelet. Due to its characteristic derivative, this wavelet transforms the signal maxima and minima into zero crossings at the different scales, thus making it quite appropriate to detecting the ECG's P and T waves and QRS complex (Li *et al.*, 1995) and also for picking out the beginning and end of such electrocardiographic components (Martinez *et al.*, 2004). In the algorithm proposed by Li *et al.* (denoted as LI Algorithm), the scales $2^1$ to $2^4$ are selected to carry out the search for QRS complexes. Such waves are found by comparing energies from the ECG signal in the scale $2^3$ with the energies in the scale $2^4$. Redundant modulus maximum lines are eliminated by different rules and the $R$ detected peaks.

### 4.2.7. *Phase Space Analysis (PSA)*

Not long ago, the concept named in this section title was introduced as a powerful tool for the purpose studied in this chapter (Amann *et al.*, 2007). Given a time signal $x(t)$, as the ECG, its phase space is a bidimensional diagram plotting on the $x$-axis the $x(t)$ amplitudes and on the $y$-axis the values for $x(t + \tau)$, where $\tau$ is a time constant conveniently chosen. Such phase diagram permits the identification of either a dynamic or random behavior of the signal under study. Figure 4.11 shows the differences when those plots are obtained from a regular cardiac rhythm and from ventricular fibrillation. The lower left panel (c) shows a regular structure covering just a very small region while the right-hand lower panel (d), derived from the upper fibrillatory pattern, spreads chaotically all over the area (Amann *et al.*, 2007). All the surface area is divided with a grid formed by 40 × 40 squares (Figs. 4.11(c) and 4.11(d)), counting those squares visited as the signal runs the diagram. Immediately thereafter, the parameter $d$ is

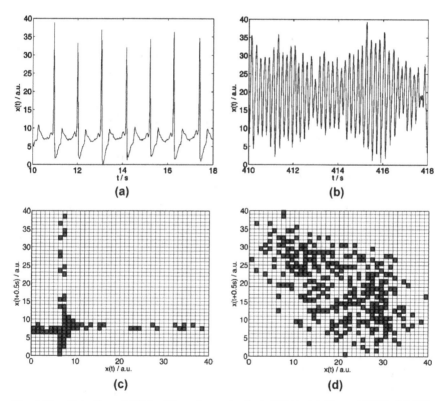

Fig. 4.11.   Detection of VF by Phase Space Analysis (PSA). (a) Normal ECG. (b) VF. (c) y (d) Phase Space representations for (a) and (b), respectively. Observe the sharp concentration aroun 6–8 horizontal value for (c) as opposed to the spread seen in (d). From Amann *et al.* (2007), with permission.

computed as,

$$d = \frac{\text{number of visited boxes}}{\text{number of all boxes}}. \tag{4.14}$$

If $d$ is greater than a threshold $d_0$, the algorithm classifies the rhythm as VF. After tests with 123 ECG records from different databases, it has been determined that optimal values for the time constant and for the threshold are, respectively, $\tau = 0.5$ s and $d_0 = 0.15$, considering a total number of boxes equal to 1,600 (or $40 \times 40$). Such values produced a sensitivity of 79%, specificity of 97.8%, predictivity of 77.3% and an accuracy of 96.2%. The computational cost of the method is low as compared to other algorithms.

### 4.3. Discussion

In the sections above, several detection algorithms were briefly described and illustrated using information available in the current abundant literature on the subject. This last section draws from Amann *et al.* (2005), who in a long, detailed and very well-done paper compared nine VF detection and two QRS complex algorithms in a standardized way. Some of them can be classified within the groups already presented here. For this study, ECG records were downloaded from recognized and validated databases, such as the Boston's Beth Israel Hospital and MIT (BIH-MIT), Creighton University (CU), and the American Heart Association (AHA). For each algorithm, approximately 330,000 decisions were calculated. The quality parameters of NO/VF-VF/DECISIONS were tested against the annotated diagnosis made by cardiologists. Ventricular tachycardia was not considered. The ROC curve was applied as evaluation criterion.

The VF detection algorithms studied in the above-mentioned paper are the following:

(1) Threshold Crossing Intervals (TCI), described in this book in Sec. 4.2.2;
(2) AutoCorrelation Fischer ($ACF_{95}$) algorithm, based on CWA, explained in Sec. 4.2.4;
(3) VF Filter algorithm, after Kuo and Dillman (1978), which applies a narrow band elimination filter in the mean frequency region of the ECG signal;
(4) Spectral (SPEC) algorithm based on Fourier Transform analysis, described here in Sec. 4.2.5;
(5) Complexity (CPLX) algorithm, proposed by Zhang *et al.* (1999), which transforms the ECG signal into a binary sequence and uses a complexity measure in order to find repeating patterns;

(6) The Standard Exponential (STE) algorithm counts the number of the signal crossing points with an exponential curve decreasing on both sides. The decision for the defibrillation is made by counting the number of crossings;

(7) The Modified Exponential Algorithm (MEA), an STE akin, lifts the decreasing exponential curve at the crossing points onto the following relative maximum. This modification gives rise to better detection results;

(8) The Signal Comparison Algorithm (SCA) compares the ECG with four predefined reference signals (three sinus rhythms containing one PQRST segment and one VF signal) and makes its decision by calculation of the residuals with respect to the reference signals;

(9) The Wavelet (WVL) Algorithm is based on the WT explained in Sec. 4.2.6; likewise, the paper studied two QRS complex detection algorithms: Tompkins (TOMP) algorithm, explained in Sec. 4.2.3, and LI algorithm, described in Sec. 4.2.6.

Figure 12, reproduced from that paper, collects the ROC curves of the analyzed algorithms listed above. Besides, Table 4.2 summarizes the results so that easily the different parameters can be compared. The last two columns give, respectively, the area under the ROC curve (AUC), as a number, and the computation time, expressed as percent of the record real duration.

TCI reaches the highest sensitivity (75.1%) while the VF Filter, SPEC, SCA, and WVL algorithms show best specificity (>98%). However, after

Table 4.2. Performance of ventricular fibrillation detection algorithms (sensitivity ($S_e$), specificity ($S_p$), positive predictivity ($P_{re}$), accuracy ($A_{cc}$), Area Under the ROC Curve (AUC), Calculation Time CT) (Data extracted from Amann *et al.*, 2005).

| Parameter | $S_e$ | $S_p$ | $P_{re}$ | $A_{cc}$ | AUC | CT |
|---|---|---|---|---|---|---|
| TCI | 75.1 | 84.4 | 31.1 | 83.6 | 82 | 2.1 |
| ACF$_{95}$ | 49.6 | 49.0 | 8.3 | 49.0 | 49 | 3.6 |
| VF | 18.8 | 100.0 | 97.7 | 93.0 | 87 | 1.9 |
| SPEC | 29.1 | 99.9 | 96.1 | 93.8 | 89 | 1.9 |
| CPLX | 59.2 | 92.0 | 40.8 | 89.2 | 87 | 2.5 |
| STE | 50.1 | 81.7 | 20.4 | 79.0 | 67 | 1.9 |
| MEA | 51.2 | 84.1 | 23.2 | 81.3 | 82 | 2.5 |
| SCA | 71.2 | 98.5 | 81.6 | 96.2 | 92 | 5.9 |
| WVL | 26.7 | 99.7 | 90.5 | 93.5 | 80 | 1.9 |
| LI | 9.0 | 93.9 | 12.1 | 86.6 | 58 | 15 |
| TOMP | 92.5 | 40.6 | 12.7 | 45.0 | 67 | 0.84 |

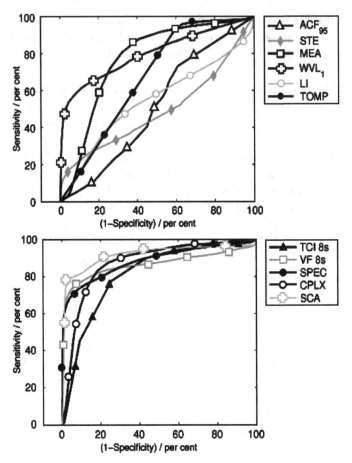

Fig. 4.12.   ROC curves for different VF detection algorithms. From Amann *et al.* (2005), with permission.

the parameter AUC, the Signal Comparison Algorithm (SCA) gave the highest value (92%), followed by SPEC (89%), VF Filter (87%), and CPLX (87%). All of the latter in line with Fig. 4.12, because these four algorithms obtained ROC curves well bent toward the upper left region, tending to the (0, 1) coordinate, which clearly would depict the ideal 100% $S_p$ y $S_e$. Out of the latter four algorithms for VF detection, the Spectral (SPEC) and the VF Filter algorithms produced the shortest computing time CT (1.9%), followed by CPLX (2.5%) and SCA (5.9%). Regarding QRS detection, TOMP gave a better AUC (67% vs 58%), with a far shorter computing time CT (0.84% vs 15%), as compared to LIs.

## 4.4. Conclusions and Review Questions

Without having exhausted the literature, a rather good sample of the most important VF algorithms has been described trying to show their main characteristics and advantages. A few require computational costs that may play a role in their time response when facing the emergency. The evaluating values offered here should serve as orientation for their possible choice. As engineers, we should keep always in mind that simplicity is not to be forgotten. Medical emergency personnel, as ultimate users, have the final word.

*Review questions* (T = true; F = False)

1. Early defibrillators decided whether the arrhythmia was present by the *brute force* criterion meaning that false shocks were relatively frequent.      T      F

2. After the Defibrillation Golden Rule, an automatic defibrillator must always deliver a discharge to an unconscious patient.      T      F

3. Computing time and energy consumption are parameters to take into account in choosing a given detection algorithm.      T      F

4. An algorithm sensitivity measures the probability of correctly detecting VF, while specificity refers to the probability of identifying events that are not VF.      T      F

5. An ideal algorithm shows the ROC curve tending to the diagonal.      T      F

6. The ECG PDF during VF clearly shows a sharp peak around zero amplitude.      T      F

7. The Threshold Crossing Interval (TCI) algorithm relies on the number of pulses going beyond a predetermined level.      T      F

8. Algorithms based on cardiac frequency take into account that rhythm usually is lower during VF than during sinus arrhythmia.      T      F

9. Correlation Waveform Analysis (CWA) compares the morphology of each beat against a template obtained by averaging a series of normal beats.      T      F

10. Time–Frequency Analysis examines the ECG energy distribution simultaneously in the time and in the frequency domains.      T      F

11. The Wavelet Transform has a scale factor $a$ which is directly proportional to the Fourier Transform.        T        F
12. Phase Space Analysis relates the ECG as a time signal against a version of the same signal but shifted in time.        T        F
13. Most of the current VF detection algorithms produce better sensitivity than specificity.        T        F
14. If you are in the surgery room, how would you best detect VF?
15. If you are in a coronary care unit (CCU), how would you detect VF or VT?

   (A) with an algorithm
   (B) checking the monitor
   (C) an alarm activated by an algorithm
   (D) looking at the patient.

# Chapter 5

# ELECTRODES AND PASTES

*The in-between of the sandwich gives its true very taste...*

The main objective here is to develop the overall concept of the impedance faced by the defibrillator clearly separating out its components: the electrode–electrolyte interface impedance and the biological load impedance as main actor. A second objective aims at the defibrillating electrodes (both internal and external) along with contact impedance decreasing agents (pastes), which are only employed in the latter situation. Finally, since the connecting system (wiring) represents a weak link in the overall chain, possible failures are discussed, including also failures of other origins. A better tuning of the subject leads us to a single main idea: the biological load impedance, which is mostly resistive and represented either by the myocardial mass or the thorax, must be as low as possible in order to guarantee that all current efficiently traverses it to depolarize a maximum number of cardiac fibers. This requires the electrode contacts offer minimum hindrance to current flow.

## 5.1. Introduction

A defibrillator is a high-energy stimulator, not like other types used in electrophysiology, which mostly deliver pulses in the millivolt–milliampere range. Similar to the latter, however, its physical link with cardiac tissue, either directly (when the thorax is opened) or indirectly (transthoracic), is also and not surprisingly obtained by a couple of cables each connected to an electrode. Thus, there is always some hindrance to the current flow termed the *electrode–electrolyte interface impedance* (EEI). In the case of systems recording small electrical signals (such as the ECG, EMG, or EEG), such interface often plays a significant disturbing role (Valentinuzzi, 2004, see Chap. 4). When current is injected into the tissues, instead, the interface loses importance, especially if the amplitude is large, and defibrillation always handles in the order of several amperes along with tens or even hundreds of volts. For this reason, we refer to it below only briefly.

The main objective here is to develop the overall concept of the impedance faced by the defibrillator clearly separating out its components:

the EEI mentioned above and the biological load impedance as main actor. A second objective aims at the description of defibrillating electrodes (both internal and external) along with impedance decreasing agents (pastes), which are only employed in the latter situation. Finally, since the connecting system represents a weak link in the overall chain, possible failures in it are discussed. A better tuning of the subject leads us to a single main idea: the biological load impedance (mostly resistive and represented either by the myocardial mass or the thorax) must be as low as possible in order to guarantee that all current efficiently traverses it to depolarize a maximum number of cardiac fibers.

## 5.2. Electrode/Tissue Impedance and the Biological Load Impedance

### 5.2.1. *The Electrode–Electrolyte Interface Impedance (EEI)*

Over a period of about one hundred years, say, roughly from 1899 to 1997, with many contributions in-between, abundant electrochemical research has produced models to at least partially elucidate the real interfacing system. Remember that models are neither right nor wrong; they are just approximations that may describe better or worse the system under study depending on the specific conditions of the latter. The contact region between an electrode and the surrounding medium is ill-defined; since it is located in the midst of two entirely different regions, namely the electrolytic environment and the electronic side, that is, a solution or a wet side and a metallic face, it was named *electrode–electrolyte interface*, the latter word meaning literally "between faces", which colloquially speaking, can be thought of as two faces looking at each other and exchanging kisses.

There is an exchange phenomenon that consists of ions either receiving or delivering electrons. An interface is formed spontaneously the very moment an electrode is immersed in an electrolytic solution, or when it touches the epicardium or endocardium via a catheter tip or just when placed over the naked skin surface (always there is NaCl dissolved in small amounts of sweat or because a conductive paste is added). The metal can be considered as a cloud of free electrons around positive fixed ions or attached to a crystalline network. Instead, free positive and negative ions and polar molecules that behave as orientable dipoles usually form the wet face. Once the electrode is installed, a redistribution of charges takes place on both sides of the limiting faces building up a metal-solution difference of potential. Two basic phenomena account for it,

(1) *appearance of superficial either free or induced charges, in excess or defect, with respect to the bulk of each face*; or
(2) *formation of a layer of oriented dipoles toward the electrode surface.*

The complex system of charges and oriented dipoles has been named the double electric layer or simply the double layer. Another name is *Helmholtz double layer*, for it was this German scientist who first studied it in 1879. Now, however, it is well documented that the charge distribution is much more complex and only exceptionally formed by just two layers. The interface region keeps an overall electrical balance in accordance to the principle of neutrality, but it is far from being static, for there is *transference of charges* while several other electrochemical reactions take place. Say that we look at the solution side: an ion must first arrive in the interface region. Such arrival can be due to any of three different transport processes,

— *migration* or *drift*, when the driving cause is an electric field;
— *diffusion*, when concentration gradients are present, irrespective of the particle having or not an electric charge; and
— *convection*, which happens when movement is due to temperature gradients or to mechanical stirring of the medium. Combinations of the three phenomena are also possible.

Once at the interface, ions either deliver electrons to the electrode or receive electrons from it. The exchange is collectively called the *oxidation–reduction process* (oxidation refers to loss of electrons and reduction to gain of electrons). In the case of sodium, potassium, or chloride, reduction or gain of an electron is a simple reaction. When proteins are involved, the situation appears as more complex.

An array of parallel RC circuits that for simplicity are usually lumped into one RC network is frequently used to model the electrode–electrolyte interface (Fig. 5.1). Its main components are the *electrolytic medium resistance* $R_m$, (which in our case is represented by the biological load), accounting for ionic conduction in the solution bulk, the *double layer capacitance* $C_{dl}$ formed by ionic accumulation and/or by polarized particles which give rise to the half-cell potential (the other half is located at the companion electrode completing the circuit), the *charge transference resistance* $R_{ct}$ to model the hindrance faced by the electrons when moving

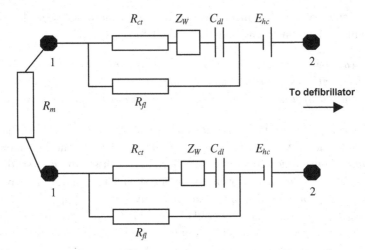

Fig. 5.1. Electrode–electrolyte interface equivalent circuit. $R_{ct}$ or *charge transfer resistance*; $C_{dl}$ or *double layer capacitance*. These components together are called *polarization elements*. $E_{hc}$ or *half-cell potential* and $R_{fl}$ or *resistive faradic leak*. $Z_w$ stands for the Warburg impedance. The return electrode is similar and the two points 1 see the load resistance $R_m$.

to and from the electrodes, and the *diffusion impedance $Z_w$*, also called the *Warburg impedance* after the investigator who proposed it back in 1899; the latter considers how difficult is for the charges to diffuse toward the interface or away from it. Often, the electric elements of similar kind are lumped into a single one (say, the Warburg resistance is combined with the transference resistance) but conceptually this is not quite correct because different phenomena are being mixed even though it is electrically simpler. The Warburg impedance has a complex nature, for a resistance in series with a capacitance form it. These components vary with the frequency of the signal applied to the interface. Besides, it must be underlined that the half-cell potential is characteristic of each metal–electrolyte combination and is not able to sustain any current. The total voltage between a pair of electrode terminals is the algebraic sum of the two half-cell potentials; usually, they are numerically different, and they may even display opposite signs depending on the metals the electrodes are made of. If the metal is the same for both electrodes and since the half-cell potentials appear in series, at least theoretically, they should tend to cancel out. Changes in acidity (a desired signal in pH meters), bacterial growth (also a desired change in impedance microbiology), movement of the electrodes (undesired in ECG or in EMG records) modify the half-cell potentials, which are detected and amplified by the recording system. To measure a single half-cell potential is impossible; thus, an arbitrary standard electrode has been chosen (the *hydrogen electrode*) and electrode potentials are measured and tested against it in electrochemistry laboratories. There are other types of reference electrodes. The bibliography describing constructive and technical details is abundant (Geddes and Baker, 1989).

When a small sinusoidal potential of a given frequency is applied to the interface, the circulating current is also of the same frequency with amplitude proportional to the applied potential. Thus, the current is predictable if the interface impedance is known; the system is said to have a linear behavior. However, if the potential increases, beyond a given level the circulating current is distorted showing harmonics at the interface. Thus, the behavior becomes non-linear. Besides, EEI decreases as the applied potential increases. The proportional relationship between potential and current is lost. Figure 5.2 describes such situation, where the impedance drop is dramatic beyond 0.7–0.8 mA. The origin of this behavior is still subject of research and it is believed that, at least partially, is due to the charge transference phenomenon (McAdams *et al.*, 1995). Leslie Geddes, Herman Schwan and their collaborators carefully studied the EEI as function of current density. Their many contributions, classics in the literature, are frequently used for bioinstrumentation design (Schwan, 1968; Ragheb and Geddes, 1991, 1997; Mayer *et al.*, 1992; Geddes and Roeder,

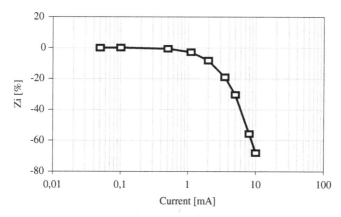

Fig. 5.2. Interface impedance modulus vs applied current. Stainless steel electrodes (area = 0.3 cm²) immersed in *Brain Heart Infusion* at 37°C. The impedance decrease is shown as percentage of the initial value at low current. Experimental data obtained at the Department of Bioengineering, UNT. After Valentinuzzi (2004), with permission.

2001). More recent reports have expanded the subject introducing newer approaches, especially underlining the non-linear behavior (Ruiz *et al.*, 2005).

The important conclusion out of this brief account is that whatever the effects of the EEI, they are fully overcome in the special case of defibrillation because, first, the applied amplitudes of voltages and currents are very high (compare them with the much lower values shown in Fig. 5.2), and second, the duration of pulses is very short (in the range of a few milliseconds and never more than 10 or so), so that there is not enough time to show any detectable phenomenon.

However, if the electrode impedance is higher than a given level due to poor conductive contact, the success of the procedure may be hampered to the extent of failure because it seriously limits the delivered current. Thus, Fig. 5.1 should include an added series resistor to account for the contact itself, say between points 2 and the half-cell battery on each side. Such contact resistance (the two sides are collected into a single unit), which depends on the electrode type, size, and surface area, must be minimized. Measurements previous to the defibrillation discharge usually carried out injecting a high frequency–low amplitude sinusoidal constant current (say, at 10–20 kHz and 20–30 $\mu$A), produce a modulus value where the interface components are negligible relative to the load impedance. The electrode contact resistance, however, may not be negligible, and such situation must be prevented.

### 5.2.2. *The Biological Load Impedance*

This is the main actor during the defibrillation procedure and, even though it may show a minor capacitive component, its significance is unimportant and we can refer to it as simply the biological load resistance $R_B$.

In the case of direct defibrillation, it is the resistance offered by the ventricles when embraced with the defibrillating paddles, often covered with gauze but many times used as naked metal. The electrolyte is the body fluids, rich in conductive ions. Armayor *et al.* (1978, 1979) found an average of 25.9 ohms (SD = 4.9), with a maximum of 44 ohms and a minimum of 17 ohms, in measurements made on 20 experimental normothermic dogs after 346 successful defibrillations. As mentioned above, the measurements were made with an impedance meter at 12 kHz injecting very low current (20 $\mu$A). This value can be considered as typical for the described condition and it does not vary much in other animal species, including man.

The same group of authors, employing the same measuring technique during fibrillation, reported average values for the myocardium under conditions of hypothermia (Arredondo *et al.*, 1980), ischemia by acute coronary occlusion (Arredondo *et al.*, 1982), and hypothermic coronary occlusion (Arredondo *et al.*, 1984), reaching the following figures: 28.5 ± 6.0 ohms, 27.5 ± 5.7 ohms, and 36.2 ± 5.5 ohms, respectively, where second values stand for standard deviations. The combined effect of hypothermia and ischemia might account for the increased resistance as compared with the others. Dispersions, including the normothermic case, maintained similar levels, which speaks in favor of the measuring technique and its stability.

Different is the situation when the electrodes are inside the heart, as with implantable defibrillators, or when they are externally applied over the thoracic cage. In all cases though, the electrode size and their actual surface contact area play an essential and determinant role and, for this reason, values may cover a relative wide range, reaching a maximum of may be 100 or 110 ohms for the latter. For transthoracic resistance in humans, 50 ohms can be quoted as typical. A quick tour through several relevant contributions published in the last 25 years or so is appropriate; in them, useful numerical values are reported. In spite of many advances, the subject always calls attention and interest, especially of manufacturers developing new electrodes, catheters, and electrolytic bridges.

One of the earliest papers is that of Ewy *et al.* (1972); apparently two families became interested in the canine thoracic resistance. Kerber *et al.* (1984) studied the importance of the load impedance in determining the success of low-energy shocks. Via defibrillator electrodes, they applied 31 kHz current to the chest during the defibrillator charge cycle, before the defibrillating shock was actually delivered. The current flow was limited by the transthoracic impedance (TTI); a microprocessor monitored the predischarge current flow and determined the predischarge impedance by calibration against known resistance values. Actual impedance to the defibrillating shock was also determined and compared with the predicted impedance. With this approach, they predicted impedance in 19 patients who received 66 shocks for ventricular and atrial arrhythmias. Predicted impedance ($y$) correlated very well with actual impedance ($x$), using,

$$y = 0.90x + 11.3,$$

with a high correlation coefficient ($r = 0.97$). To determine the importance of impedance in defibrillation and cardioversion, they prospectively gathered data from 96 patients who received shocks of various energies for ventricular or atrial arrhythmias. In patients with high TTI (greater than 97 ohms), low-energy shocks (less than or equal to 100 J) for ventricular defibrillation had only a 20% success rate as opposed to a 70% success rate for low-energy shocks in patients with low or average impedance. It was concluded that TTI can be accurately predicted in advance of defibrillation and cardioversion. This method permits the pre-shock identification of patients with high impedance in whom attempts to defibrillate with low-energy shocks are inappropriate.

Sternotomy may have a post-surgery effect on chest impedance. Kerber *et al.* (1992) ran a series of tests in order to explore such possibility. For that matter, TTI was determined by using a validated test-pulse technique that does not require actual shocks. Seventeen patients undergoing median sternotomy were studied prospectively. TTI was determined before operation, 3–5 days after operation and (in eight patients) greater than or equal to 1 month after operation. When measured using paddle electrodes placed in the standard apex-right parasternal defibrillating position, TTI declined after sternotomy in all patients, from $77 \pm 18$ to $59 \pm 17$ ohms; smaller declines were demonstrated by using other electrode positions. TTI remained below the preoperative level in the eight patients who underwent a second set of measurements at least 1 month after operation. Six normal subjects not undergoing sternotomy underwent serial TTI measurements at least 5 days apart; mean TTI did not change. It was concluded that TTI declines after sternotomy.

Kontos *et al.* (1997) also recognized that peak current flow across the heart determines the success of defibrillation and is inversely dependent on impedance between defibrillation electrodes. Since factors associated with elevated impedance in patients with implantable defibrillators using non-thoracotomy lead systems had not been well described, these authors undertook the analysis of clinical and echocardiographically derived variables in 41 patients in whom implantation of a non-thoracotomy lead system was attempted. Lead impedance was measured at end-expiration with 5 J monophasic shocks. Successful defibrillation with or without addition of a subcutaneous patch with $< 20$ J, monophasic waveform, was required for non-thoracotomy lead placement. Patients were divided into two groups based on impedance: low ($\leq 47$ ohms, $n = 30$) and high ($> 47$ ohms, $n = 11$). Twenty-four patients had successful defibrillator implantation using a transvenous lead alone, 13 required placement of a subcutaneous patch, and four required epicardial patch placement. The mean left ventricular end-diastolic and end-systolic volumes were significantly smaller in patients in the low-vs high-impedance groups and were significantly correlated with impedance. Impedance was not significantly different between patients with successful defibrillation using a transvenous lead alone compared with those who required either subcutaneous or epicardial patches. Thus, impedance using a non-thoracotomy lead system with monophasic shocks is significantly correlated with both end-systolic and end-diastolic volumes, but elevated impedance does not predict increased defibrillation energy requirements.

Changes in chest electrode impedance were studied by Lateef *et al.* (2000), a group from Singapore. The objective of this prospective study was to measure the electrode skin impedance (ESI) of patients at 5 Hz and 2 kHz frequencies, and assess its change with time from the application of electrodes, the difference between the ESI at two different sets of electrode placement positions, and correlation with patient factors. Patients who were 25 years or older and not critically ill had their ESI measured with a modified Heart-Save 911 defibrillator, using signal frequencies at 5 Hz and 2 kHz, at 10 s, 1 and 2 min after electrodes application. Two sets of positions were used; position 1 where an electrode is placed in the right sub-clavicular region and another just lateral to the apex beat on the left and position 2, which represents the mirror-image of position 1. Thirty-six each of men and women patients were studied. The mean age and weight were $59.9 \pm 13.5$ years and $56.8 \pm 24.1$ kg, respectively. There was no significant correlation between the ESI and patients' body weight or sex. However, there was a significant decrease in the ESI with time from application of electrodes at both positions with the two different frequencies. The ESI was lower when measured at lower frequencies and higher when taken at higher frequencies, but no statistical difference between the two mirror-image positions was found.

Many times, more than one shock is required to bring the ventricles back into normal rhythm. By and large, a secondary effect is a decrease in impedance with repeated discharges, either transthoracic (Dahl *et al.*, 1976) or transventricular (Savino *et al.*, 1986). How important this fact is from a clinical-emergency point of view appears as a matter of speculation; theoretically, such decrease should help in the efficiency of subsequent discharges.

From all of the above, it can be stated that the biological impedance faced by the defibrillator in any case, be it transventricular, intraventricular or transthoracic, lies within the range of 20–120 ohms, the latter value considered as already too high and obviously not recommendable. Typical figures are 25 and 50 ohms, for the myocardium and for the thorax, respectively.

## Is there an inductive element in the TTI?

Guan *et al.* (2000) posed this interesting and rather provocative question proposing a new equivalent circuit model to quantify the defibrillation impedance for short pulses. These authors used six experimental male guinea pigs to validate the model and defibrillated the ventricles delivering square voltage pulses (200 V). Three electrode placements were tested randomly: normal, abdominal, and subcutaneous. The equivalent circuit model was determined according to the best fitting curves of current waveforms in the first 3 ms. An inductor was included in the model to account for the rising current waveforms. The inductors were $213 \pm 57$ mH, $40 \pm 10$ mH, and $236 \pm 39$ mH for the normal, subcutaneous, and abdominal placements, respectively. The skin to the electrodes appears to be the major source of the inductance; the heart and lungs do not make substantial contributions. The mechanism of the inductance could be electroporation of the stratum corneum and cell membranes. This inductive model seems to better predict defibrillation impedance for short waveforms.

Obviously following a similar line of thought, the same group of authors (Malkin *et al.*, 2006) studied electroporation and its effects on defibrillation optimization. They determined impedance changes during defibrillation, thereafter, used that information to derive the optimum defibrillation waveform. Twelve guinea pigs and six swine were the animals employed, measuring current waveform for square voltage pulses of a strength which would defibrillate about 50% of the time, that is, a threshold value. In guinea pigs, electrodes were placed thoracically, abdominally, and subcutaneously using two electrode materials (zinc and steel) and two electrode pastes (Core-gel and metallic paste). The measured current waveform indicated an exponentially increasing conductance over the first 3 ms, consistent with enhanced electroporation or another mechanism of time-dependent conductance. This current was fit with a parallel conductance composed of a time-independent component and a time-dependent component, all these in guinea pigs. Different electrode placements and materials had no significant effect. The stimulating waveform would theoretically charge the myocardial membrane to a given threshold using the least energy from the defibrillator. The solution was a very short, high voltage pulse followed immediately by a truncated ascending exponential tail. Besides, the optimized waveforms and similar non-optimized waveforms were tested for efficacy in 25 additional guinea pigs and six additional swine. Optimized waveforms were significantly more efficacious than similar non-optimized waveforms. In swine, a waveform with the short pulse was 41% effective while the same waveform without the short pulse was 8.3% effective despite there being only a small difference in energy (111 J vs 116 J). The conclusion was that a short pulse preceding a defibrillation pulse significantly improves efficacy, perhaps by enhancing electroporation.

It should be added to clarify ideas that electroporation is used to introduce polar molecules into a host cell through the cell membrane. A large electric pulse temporarily disturbs the phospholipid bilayer, allowing molecules (like DNA) to go into the cell. Electroporation capitalizes on the relatively weak nature of the phospholipid bilayer hydrophobic/hydrophilic interactions and its ability to spontaneously reassemble after disturbance. Thus, a voltage shock may disrupt areas of the membrane temporarily, allowing polar molecules to pass; the membrane reseals quickly leaving the cell intact (for more details see the following website bio.davidson.edu/Courses/Molbio/MolStudents/ spring2003/McCord/electroporation.htm).

*Quick overview recalling the methods to measure TTI*

*Apparent impedance*, either transthoracic or ventricular, is a concept that appeared after a *de facto* measuring technique, fully weird to the eyes of a physicist or an electrical engineer because it boldly makes the ratio of applied peak voltage to measured peak current traversing the load, against all traditional definitions based on pure sinusoidal waveforms. It is found in the literature as early as 1976, and perhaps introduced for the first time by Geddes *et al.* (1976). Other authors applied the idea, as Machin (1978), Lerman *et al.* (1987), Kerber *et al.* (1988), and again Geddes (1994). Sometimes the real or practical world imposes customs opposite to accepted standards. One appropriate analogy taken from linguistics amounts to the way new words enter into the daily language, often as slang or jargon that, with enough time, end up to being recognized by the respective language academies.

Al Hatib *et al.* (2000) reassessed the biological load impedance idea and the corresponding measurement methods with the main purpose of studying the variations of TTI by a continuous measurement technique during the defibrillation shock and comparing the data with results obtained by modeling. Voltage and current impulse waveforms were acquired during cardioversion of patients with atrial fibrillation or flutter. The same type of defibrillation pulse was taken from dogs after induction of fibrillation. The electrodes were located in the anterior position, for both the patients and animals. The *apparent impedance* was used, presenting it as a function of time and as a function of the applied voltage. The skin–electrode interface could be considered in connection with non-linearity, for example, the dependence of its Warburg and Faradic components on current density. Modeling of the thoracic resistance waveform revealed that at least three exponents were needed to reproduce its shape with acceptable accuracy. Therefore, computing the resistance from the tilt of a monoexponent will include an error. They contend that this fact should be considered when optimal voltage and/or current waveforms for efficient defibrillation are searched. Higher transthoracic resistance was observed in the initial parts of both phases of the truncated exponential shock pulse, in spite of the virtually instantaneous rising of both voltage and current to high values. This effect would need further investigation and eventual explanation. The transthoracic resistance variance should be taken into consideration in studying correlation with pre-shock measurement of impedance by high frequency–low amplitude signal. With biphasic pulses, the negative phase in animal experiments met either lower or higher resistances. Therefore, the hypothesis that biphasic pulse efficiency was due to lower impedance during the second phase could not be supported. An example of the recordings of voltage and current waveforms in cardioversion of a patient is shown in Fig. 5.3(a) (first and second trace, respectively). The apparent impedance time course (third trace) was computed and plotted using the ratio of the peak values for each sample. The same type of recording of a dog defibrillated with biphasic pulses is shown in Fig. 5.3(b). Here the fluctuations of $Z_a$ appearing at the end of the first pulse correspond to slight changes in current with its decay to lower values. At the fourth millisecond the pulse switches polarity, with voltage and current reaching the zero level, which results in indeterminate values of the apparent impedance. The dependence of the apparent impedance on the applied voltage during the positive phase of the defibrillation shock is shown in Fig. 5.4, where similar trends were observed in all cases (patients and dogs). An example of the load impedance $Z_L$ measurement by coinciding modeled, computed, and measured voltage waveforms is shown in Fig. 5.5, where the damped sinusoid waveform was obtained from a patient and the truncated exponential waveform from a dog. Note that due to the

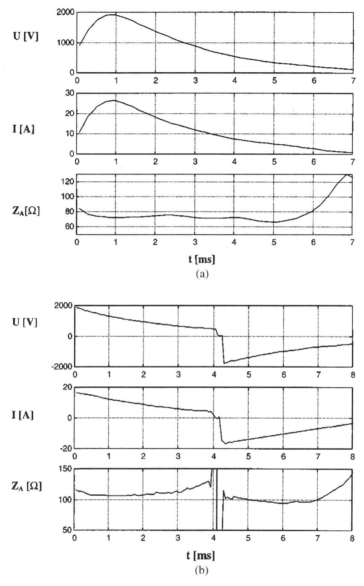

Fig. 5.3. Apparent Impedance. Recorded voltage and current during defibrillating shock. Top set of three records: voltage (volts), current (amps) and apparent impedance (ohms). From a patient, using standard monophasic damped sine waveform. Bottom set, same as above. From a dog, using biphasic truncated exponential waveform. The third signal of each example shows the apparent impedance during the shock. Time in ms. After Al Hatib, Trendafilova and Daskalov (2000), with permission.

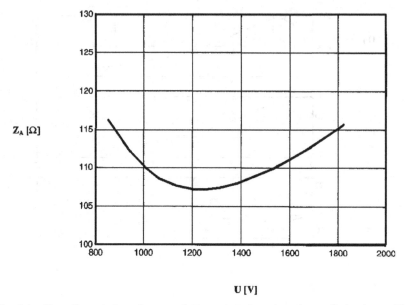

**U [V]**

Fig. 5.4. Transthoracic impedance variations plotted against the applied voltage. The case of Figure 5.3 (bottom set) is taken as an example. After Al Hatib, Trendafilova and Daskalov (2000), with permission.

impedance variations, the measured and the modeled waveforms do not coincide in all time intervals during the shock.

The low constant sinusoidal current of high frequency, as mentioned above, has been the traditional method and, so far, should be considered as the most reliable one, even considered as some kind of golden standard. Older types of defibrillators, using capacitor discharge, allow indirect computation of the load resistance from the time constant of the exponent (Savino *et al.*, 1983). Bridges are also conceivable and references are available in the literature, however, we should not invest time and space in them because they are impractical and rather cumbersome.

### 5.3. Electrode Types

Electrodes can generally be classified into three groups, i.e.:

1. *non-invasive*, or those that are applied to skin surfaces, such as conventional ECG limb electrodes or EEG scalp electrodes;
2. *semi-invasive*, such as nasopharyngeal and tympanic electrodes or EMG acupuncture needle-type electrodes; and

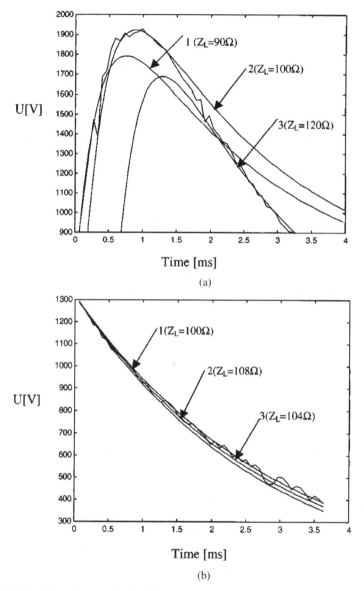

Fig. 5.5. Load impedance obtained by parametric modelling compared to real values through matching experimental and modelled voltage waveforms. (A) For a patient using a standard monophasic damped sine waveform and (B) For a dog using truncated exponential waveforms. After Al Hatib, Trendafilova and Daskalov (2000), with permission.

3. *invasive*, which include needles and grids, and of the catheter type, the
latter to be inserted into an organ.

Defibrillating electrodes fall either into Group 1 or Group 3, the former
for the transthoracic situation and the latter for the direct case or for
implanted units.

Paddles and pads are the typical electrodes applied to the thorax
surface. In 1993, the *Association for the Advancement of Medical
Instrumentation* recommended a minimum electrode size of 50 cm² for
individual electrodes. For adult defibrillation, both hand-held paddle
electrodes and self-adhesive pad electrodes of 8–12 cm in diameter perform
well, although defibrillation success may be higher with electrodes 12 cm
in diameter rather than with those 8 cm in diameter. Small electrodes
(4.3 cm) may be harmful and may cause myocardial necrosis. When using
hand-held paddles and gel or pads, rescuers must ensure that the paddle
is in full contact with the skin (remember the contact resistance). Even
smaller pads have been found to be effective in ventricular fibrillation (VF)
of brief duration. Use of smaller (pediatric) pads, however, can result in
unacceptably high TTI in larger children. It is best to choose larger pads
that can fit on the chest without overlap (see website of *American Heart
Association Guidelines for Cardiopulmonary Resuscitation and Emergency
Cardiovascular Care*, 2005). Rescuers should place AED electrode pads on
the victim's bare chest in the conventional sternal–apical (anterolateral)
position. The right (sternal) chest pad is placed on the victim's right
superior–anterior (infraclavicular) chest and the apical (left) pad is placed
on the victim's inferior–lateral left chest, lateral to the left breast. Other
acceptable pad positions are placement on the lateral chest wall on the right
and left sides (biaxillary) or the left pad in the standard apical position
and the other pad on the right or left upper back. A conductive gel, as
those currently used in ECG recording, spread over the electrode surface is
always recommendable in order to decrease the contact resistance (see text
above), however, care must be taken with the amount because, if too much,
it may run down the skin and eventually make short-circuit with the other
electrode.

TTI is similar when either pads or paddles are used, however, applied
force must be considered because lower TTI has been reported when paddles
were applied at an optimal force of 8 kg compared with pads. Perhaps,
pressure should be better used as evaluating parameter instead of force.
Chronic auricular fibrillation produced similar effectiveness for self-adhesive

pads and manual paddles when monophasic damped sinusoidal or biphasic waveforms were evaluated separately. Several studies showed the practical benefits of pads over paddles in several situations. Apparently, self-adhesive defibrillation pads are safe and effective and are an acceptable alternative to standard defibrillation paddles.

For direct ventricular defibrillation, naked spoon electrodes are of the standard type. They must embrace tightly the myocardium without squeezing it to prevent damage but ensuring an impedance not higher than about 30 ohms. Cardiac surgeons and the associated team have good experience in this procedure.

Several authors have made significant contributions to the subject making it clear, as one reads the papers, that electrode impedance, electrode size, pastes, and operational aspects (such as pressure applied with the hand-held electrodes) are closely interwoven so that it is not easy to separate out their respective effects. Connell *et al.* (1973), Thomas *et al.* (1977), for example, studied the role of paddle size. They belonged to Ewy's group, which has made several contributions in this subject over the years.

Atkins *et al.* (1988), from Kerber's group in Iowa University, found that TTI is a major determinant of successful defibrillation or cardioversion, but no data were available concerning the range and determinants of this parameter in children. Thus, it was measured in 10 ambulatory infants, 6 weeks to 9 months of age, and 37 children, 1.5–15 years of age, using a previously validated "test-pulse" technique that measures TTI without actually delivering a shock. They used hand-held "pediatric" ($21 \, cm^2$) and "adult" ($83 \, cm^2$) electrode paddles coated with either Redux paste or Redux crème finding impedances in children of $108 \pm 24$ ohms (range 61–212) using pediatric paddles. Using adult paddles lowered the resistance by 47% to $57 \pm 11$ ohms (range 29–101 ohms). In infants, TTI (measured only with pediatric paddles) was $94 \pm 17$ ohms (range 74–124 ohms). Using Redux paste as the coupling agent reduced significantly that value by 13%. TTI was significantly but poorly related to body weight and body surface areas, but the correlations were not sufficiently high to be clinically useful. These data indicate that the larger adult electrode paddles will minimize TTI and should be used when the child's thorax is large enough to permit electrode to chest contact over the entire paddle surface. This transition occurred at an approximate weight of 10 kg.

Ewy *et al.* (1977) reported unfavorably on disposable defibrillator electrodes. The TTI to direct-current defibrillation discharge of the half-sinusoidal waveform was compared using disposable defibrillator electrode pads (SAF-D-FIB and DEFIB-PADS) with electrode paste as the interfaces between the defibrillator paddle and chest wall. Twenty-four mongrel dogs with an average weight of 17.3 kg were used. Half were shocked with the defibrillator meter setting at 100 W-S (mean delivered energy, 59 W-S) and half at 400 W-S (mean delivered energy, 205 W-S). Each animal received six shocks with both paste and one of the sets of disposable pads. The sequence of shocks was changed in alternate animals. At a meter setting of 100 W-S, the mean impedance using SAF-D-FIB was (59 ± 6 ohms) compared to (46 ± 6 ohms) with paste, while that encountered with DEFIB-PADS was (57 ± 5 ohms) compared to (50 ± 5 ohms) with paste. At settings of 400 W-S, the impedances encountered were also significantly higher with the disposable electrode. The output of many defibrillators is probably inadequate for consistent defibrillation of adult patients weighing more than 50–80 kg. Since a minimal peak current per unit of body weight is required for ventricular defibrillation and since a higher TTI results in a lower delivered peak current, one should use the paddle electrode–chest wall interface that results in the lowest impedance to defibrillator discharge. The impedance encountered with disposable electrodes is significantly higher than that encountered with electrode paste. Therefore, disposable electrodes for defibrillation or elective cardioversion do not seem as adequate.

Implantable defibrillators nowadays mostly make use of catheters of different types arranged in specific lead systems tending to minimize the myocardial resistance in between. By and large, they are trademarks protected by patents.

Santel *et al.* (1985) reviewed electrode systems for implantable defibrillators. In the beginning, several types have been used, such as metal disks, endocardial catheters, and epicardial patches. These early efforts demonstrated the feasibility of low-energy reversion of ventricular tachyarrhythmias and also provided some insight into the mechanisms of fibrillation and defibrillation. This review describes the evolution of implantable defibrillator electrode systems. Early investigators attempted defibrillation with submuscularly implanted metal disks or a disk electrode paired with an endocardial catheter electrode. Electrode design emphasis turned to transvenous catheter systems with electrodes placed in the right ventricle and right atrium. A more successful configuration placed the proximal electrode in the superior vena cava. In an effort to ensure proper placement of the distal electrode in humans, the catheter was replaced with an epicardial patch. A combination of electrodes and multiple pulses has substantially reduced the energy required to defibrillate.

No doubt, effective electrode systems requiring a minimum of defibrillating energy are constantly evolving. For example, Ideker *et al.* (1987) describe in a patent a pair of defibrillation patch electrodes which is adapted for close fitting placement over the ventricles, either epicardially or pericardially. One of the patches is contoured to fit over the right ventricle, and the other is contoured to fit over the left ventricle in spaced relationship to the first patch to form a substantially uniform gap between confronting borders of the two. The gap is sufficiently wide to avoid the shunting of current between edges of the patches upon delivery of defibrillation shocks, as well as to accommodate the ventricular septum and the major coronary arteries therein. The size and shape of the patches are such that they encompass most of the ventricular myocardium within and between their borders, to establish a nearly uniform potential gradient field throughout the entire ventricular mass when a defibrillation shock is delivered. Flat versions of the two electrodes provide ease of manufacture. In turn, and more recent, Fogarty and Howell (1995), in another patent, disclosed improved implantable defibrillator electrodes and methods of implanting them. One embodiment of the defibrillator electrodes includes a flexible conductive mesh and non-conductive mesh. Another embodiment of the electrodes includes a flexible conductive mesh, a non-conductive mesh and an insulator in-between. A third embodiment of the defibrillator electrode compensates for the shape of a human heart. Methods for implanting the electrodes include rolling an electrode and inserting the rolled electrode into a sub-xiphoid opening while thoracoscopically observing the insertion and manipulation of the defibrillator electrode.

## 5.4. Pastes

At this point, it becomes clear to the reader how difficult it is to independently discuss impedance, electrodes, and pastes, as they are so closely related. Mention of gels and pastes has already been made before in the text as inseparable component parts of the electric path. They are electrolytic materials, spread over the electrode surface area, so acting as conductive bridges to reduce the resistance offered to the passage of current. Ewy (1992) stated clearly that electrode composition and the interface between the electrodes and skin of the chest wall are important elements to take into account. Some care is needed when choosing a particular one because not all show the same properties; for example, electrode gels in disposable units have higher impedance while gels used for echocardiography are not recommendable, as they conduct electricity very poorly.

Studies abound and manufacturers always offer a list specifying their characteristics, including the abrasiveness degree. Aylward *et al.* (1985) determined if the difference in TTI produced by different coupling agents (electrolytic bridges) affects the success of shocks for defibrillation. Three different coupling agents, Harco pads (Hewlett-Packard), Littman pads (3M), and Redux paste (Hewlett-Packard), were assessed in 10 anesthetized dogs in which VF was induced by electrical stimulation of the right ventricle. Defibrillation was attempted 15 s later, using 50, 100 and 150 J. Actual delivered energy, current, impedance, and the percent of the shocks that achieved defibrillation were determined for the three coupling agents. Redux paste gave significantly lower impedance and higher current than the two disposable pads tested. Despite this, there were no significant differences in shock success among the three coupling agents. Thus, in this experimental model, over a threefold energy range, disposable coupling pads were as effective as electrode paste for defibrillation despite the slightly higher impedance of the pads. One might add that canine skin texture is different, coarser, than human epidermis is, and this may affect paste effectivity.

## 5.5. Failures

As any other technological system, emergency defibrillation may show failures; thus, important and significant efforts are spent in developing different procedures, both in hardware and software, for reducing their incidence and aiming always at full safety. Many people focused their studies in this direction.

Cummins *et al.* (1990), at the University of Washington and as part of the so-called Defibrillator Working Group of the Food and Drug Administration (FDA), reviewed a large amount of data regarding the problem of failures in these kinds of equipment. It was concluded that the frequency of defibrillator failures during clinical use may be unacceptably high. Some failures are attributable to component malfunctions, however, evidence suggests that errors in operator use and errors in defibrillator care and maintenance account for a high proportion of malfunctions. Inadequate training increases the chances of errors while lack of running daily checks lead to poor familiarity with the equipment and failure to identify component damages. Many defibrillators and batteries are kept in service beyond their expected lives. In smaller hospitals, periodic maintenance responsibilities are not always appropriately delegated to qualified personnel.

Goyal *et al.* (1996), in turn, analyzed the incidence of lead system malfunction detected during implantable cardioverter defibrillator (ICD) generator replacement. They intended to prospectively determine the frequency of lead system malfunction at the time of device replacement in 55 patients. Forty-nine patients had an epicardial lead system while six patients had a non-thoracotomy lead system. Four (7%) of these fifty-five patients were noted to have previously undetected lead system failure requiring revision. The leads that failed were between 33 and 49 months old. That is, during ICD generator replacement, previously undetected problems with sensing or defibrillation may be identified in approximately 10% of patients. Therefore, a comprehensive evaluation of the sensing and the defibrillation functions should be an essential component of the ICD generator replacement procedure.

Nielsen, Kottkamp, Zabel *et al.* (2008), much more recently, and motivated by reports of unexpected ICD failures, proposed home monitoring (HM) to decrease follow-up workload and increase patient safety. Home monitoring implantable cardioverter defibrillators offer wireless, everyday transfer of ICD status and therapy data to a central HM Service Center, which notifies the attending physician of relevant events. These authors evaluated functionality and safety of HM ICDs in 260 patients for a mean of $10 \pm 5$ months. Times to HM events (ventricular tachycardia or fibrillation and ICD integrity) since implantation and since the latest in-clinic follow-up were analyzed. Mean number of HM events per 100 patients per day was calculated, without and with a 2-day blanking period for re-notifying the same type of event. About 41.2% of the patients had HM events (38.1% medical, 0.8% technical, and 2.3% both types). Probability of any HM event after 1.5 years was 0.50 (95%, confidence interval: 0.42–0.58). More than 60% of new HM event types occurred within the first month after follow-up. A mean of 0.86 event notifications was received per 100 patients per day.

Failures in the overall system are possible and they show a finite probability which tends to decrease as technology is improved. Arnsdorf and Bradley (2008, see http://www.uptodate.com/patients/content/topic.do? topicKey=~vYXPq0f2CRDHW) describe several types of complications dividing them into those that can occur during surgery and those that may show up well after surgery.

In the first category, they list collapse of the lung (pneumothorax), with an incidence of about 1% of cases. Perforation of the heart, causing a collection of blood within the pericardium and, eventually, leading to tamponade. This occurs in less than 1% of cases. Bleeding under the skin, around the defibrillator, is another possibility that requires drainage, with a risk higher in patients who take anticoagulants. The defibrillator is a foreign piece that may bring infection (about 1% incidence). Removal of the whole system becomes a must and is relatively easy to carry out if the device was recently implanted; however, if infection appears after a long time (months or even years, although less likely), risk is significant because the leads can become scarred to the tissues. Lead movement occurs in about 1% of patients and is usually managed by repositioning the lead within the heart. The risk of death from implantation of a modern defibrillator is less than 1 in 500.

In the second category, or long-term risks, Arnsdorf and Bradley mention infection or erosion of the device, which in most cases, calls for removal of the whole system. Lead failure represents the weakest link in the ICD chain so that mechanical stresses may produce breakage of the wires or of the insulation surrounding the leads. Inappropriate detection and subsequent delivery of a shock, which produces intense pain, often described as a "strong kick in the back". Another possibility is battery depletion or device failure, even though ICDs are extremely reliable, but not full proof and in some cases the device must be recalled and replaced. The primary risk of replacement is infection. The decision to replace the device depends on many factors, including the type and likelihood of device failure, the risk to the individual patient if failure were to occur, the risk of replacement, and the patient's preference. Manufacturers, physician groups, and the federal government are paying increased attention to the surveillance of ICDs after implantation. For that matter, patients with ICDs require regular monitoring, typically every 3–6 months throughout their lifetime. Modern ICDs are able to continuously record the electrical activity of heart muscle and record the date and time of each episode. Even technologies are being developed to allow patients to have ICD evaluation from their home using a telephone.

## 5.6. Conclusions and Review Questions

Good contact to reduce resistance to the electrical current flow is an essential condition that must be met in any defibrillatory act, be it transventricular, intraventricular, or transthoracic. Any factor modifying this parameter, such as type of electrode, electrode size, contact surface area, applied pressure, and electrolytic bridges, needs to be considered in order to meet the requirement so that the biological impedance is left as the main current limiting factor. In the case of the ventricles, the defibrillating paddles should see not more than 25–30 ohms, and in the case of the transthoracic procedure an acceptable range would be 50–70 ohms. Endocardial leads, usually much smaller in size, may face in the order of 40–100 ohms. To close this section, even though electrodes and leads represent a bottleneck, defibrillator failures recognize multiple and different origins and many times the human factor sticks out too much.

*Review questions* (T = True; F = False)

1. A defibrillator is a high-energy stimulator.      T      F
2. There is always some hindrance to the current flow termed the *electrode–electrolyte interface impedance.*      T      F
3. The electrode–electrolyte interface impedance plays an essential role in the defibrillation process.      T      F
4. An interface is formed spontaneously the very moment an electrode is immersed in an electrolytic solution.      T      F
5. An array of parallel RC circuits that are usually lumped into one RC network is frequently used to model the electrode–electrolyte interface.      T      F
6. The contact electrode resistance is neither significant nor important in the defibrillation procedure.      T      F
7. Transventricular resistance is usually in the order of (select one value)
         25 ohms      50 ohms      90 ohms      120 ohms
8. Transthoracic resistance is usually in the order of (select one value)
         50 ohms      120 ohms      150 ohms      190 ohms
9. Does sternotomy have a post-surgery effect on chest impedance?
         YES              NO
10. Can electroporation modify chest impedance?
         YES              NO
11. Apparent impedance is defined as (select one answer)
    (A) ratio of mean applied voltage to mean current flow.
    (B) ratio of applied peak voltage to peak current flow.

(C) ratio of root mean square (RMS) voltage to RMS current flow.

(D) none of the above.

12. Paddle electrodes are typical for transchest defibrillation.                                                    T          F

13. An electrolytic bridge is not needed for transchest defibrillation.                                                    T          F

14. Inappropriate detection of fibrillation and subsequent delivery of a shock in ICD may occur.                     T          F

15. Modern ICDs are able to continuously record the electrical activity of heart muscle and record the date and time of each episode.                               T          F

# Chapter 6

# SAFETY AND EFFICACY

*Primum non nocere ... or, first, do not harm ... says an old medical motto ...*

This chapter tackles the problems faced by the defibrillation procedure regarding its safety and efficacy. First, safety — defined as the set of measures to prevent damage or injury of any kind — is introduced in its three levels of importance: the **patient**, the **operator(s)**, and the **equipment** involved, the latter enclosed within a given environment. For that matter, electric isolation appears as an essential condition that must be met by the unit in order to minimize unwanted electrical connections or leaks. Thereafter, sources of electromagnetic interference have to be identified, as they can elicit malfunction. Another aspect refers to the standards regulating design, construction, and operation; however, this book is not intended to describe them, at most and after briefly mentioning them, it may discuss a few particular subjects. Accordingly, herein it merely gives the essential information that the clinical engineer, technician, or manufacturer can take as a beginning. One very peculiar, transient, and obviously undesired effect encompassed by the concept of safety refers to any pain or discomfort the electrical discharge may elicit. The phenomenon has been amply demonstrated and it can be traced back to improper defibrillator discharge, or to such an early ventricular fibrillation or tachyarrhythmia detection and shock delivery that the latter catches the subject still conscious or, in the case of cardioversion, which always captures him/her awake. Possible measures are described among the several proposed in the literature, such as injection of an anesthetic agent or neural inhibiting stimulation, always applied before the shock, or reduction of the energy level. Finally, the concept of efficacy is developed, which is defined as the power, capacity, or ability to produce the sought effect, that is, to successfully defibrillate. It recognizes several factors, all complex and still somewhat under discussion: lead system, pulse waveform (monophasic or polyphasic), pulse duration, and safety margin (in terms of energy or current). The latter tries to determine how much more energy or current is recommended above the minimum required value or threshold, always keeping in mind that a safety margin too large for the sake of efficacy may cause injury to the patient. Thus, an acceptable compromise must be reached.

## 6.1. Introduction

Any medical procedure obviously intends to restore, prevent, or even improve the health condition of an individual. Behind this basic concept, there is always the risk of producing overt damage or the possibility of total or partial failure or even lack of success. The first case is encompassed under the overall name of *safety* and the second enters into the field of *efficacy*. Both words try to offer a responsible, sensible, and highly sensitive answer to the questions very often asked by patients, *what the risks of the procedure are and how well I will feel after it*, questions that in shorter and more professional language amount to how safe and efficacious the procedure is. This is precisely the objective of this chapter: to offer an introduction and to give guiding principles in these two general subjects. The reader, perhaps a clinical engineer or a nurse or an emergency physician or a cardiologist, will need to probe deeper, especially if he or she wants to keep updated with recommendations and standards. As it happens frequently in defibrillation, several aspects overlap leading to repetitions that give the impression of poor organization of the text. In the end, since the approach to a particular subject is always different, the result tends to improve clarity and understanding, at least this is what we hope.

As the text is being developed specific references are given, such as Geddes and Roeder (1995) and Fish and Geddes (2003), to start with, however, more general information can be found in the American Heart Association (AHA) website, where the subject matter of this chapter is carefully detailed and updated every year. Besides, other sites can be mentioned, as **http://www.fda.gov/OHRMS/DOCKETS/dockets/ 94n0418/94n-0418-c000017-01-vol23.pdf** or **http://ucd.webdirect. ie/standards.html**, the latter dealing with defibrillator standards in Ireland, or http://www.jointcommission.org/PatientSafety/NationalPati-entSafetyGoals/. Another good source is ECRI Institute (5200 Butler Pike, Plymouth Meeting, PA 19462-1298, USA; tel +1 (610) 825-6000, fax +1 (610) 834-1275, web **www.ecri.org**, e-mail **hpcs@ecri.org**); it was published in 2007, Defibrillators: External, Automated, Semiautomated, 38 pp., which is a comprehensive compilation including risks, advices, and standards.

Safety and efficacy evolve constantly and concern medical authorities, industry, and professionals alike. A search in a database using the words *defibrillation safety* very quickly retrieved over 1,000 references, looking at the subject from several different viewpoints.

## 6.2. Safety Levels: Patient, Operator, and Equipment

The electric shock delivered during defibrillation, even though is short (not longer than a few milliseconds), means a substantial amount of energy involving tens to hundreds of volts which sustain several amperes of peak current. Thus, there is always a potential risk and, in this respect, three main levels of safety should be considered:

— First, the patient;
— Second, the operator and his/her assistants; and
— Third, the equipment and the environment.

Measures must be implemented to prevent injury to any of these subjects or objects, from the very design stage, where electronic circuits request top quality components, up to the protocol guiding the procedure, when strict steps must be carefully followed. Let us discuss specific points.

## 6.3. Isolation

External defibrillators are mostly powered from the public line. Faulty or poor isolation from such power supply (usually $110\,\text{V}/60\,\text{Hz}$ or $220\,\text{V}/50\,\text{Hz}$) may lead to accidental macroshock either to the patient or to the personnel (Fig. 6.1) because of leak, say, to the cabinet. Can you imagine, the patient in ventricular fibrillation, supposed to be defibrillated, receiving

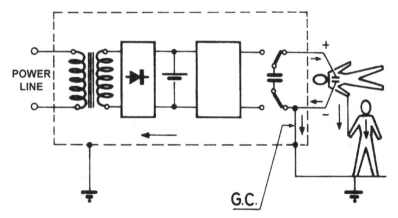

Fig. 6.1. Defibrillator with a single cabinet and a faulty connection providing a current leak. The operator may also get the defibrillating shock. Another situation would be a faulty wire from the transformer primary to the cabinet. GC: faulty ground connection.

a totally uncontrolled shock! The figure depicts one of the paddle wires
making contact to the cabinet. In such case, the operator may receive the
defibrillating discharge if by chance he/she happens to touch the patient and
also depending on the electrical insulation provided by the shoes and the
humidity conditions of the floor (some sort of unwanted Russian roulette).
Another risky possibility is a leak between one of the transformer primary
wires, especially if it is the hot side, and the cabinet. That would endanger
both, the patient and the operator, and the shock would come directly from
the *ac* line.

The solution to the above-mentioned cases is double isolation, i.e. an
internal cabinet, well grounded, enclosed by a second external cabinet built
with a good non-conductive plastic material (Fig. 6.2). Often, an isolation
monitor is included to trigger an alarm if a leak is detected. Leak currents
should not ever be higher than $10\,\mu$A rms. Besides, switches and relays,
when handling large voltages and/or currents, are prone to produce sparks
which may trigger explosions in environments where there is oxygen or
nitrous oxide (such as surgery rooms or coronary units).

Figure 6.3 depicts another situation where the culprit leak is provided
via stray capacitances between the transformer primary coil and the cabinet
or between the former and one of the defibrillating electrodes. The problem
is more difficult than in the previous case, however, a double cabinet
appears as the best answer along with special care in the construction of
the transformer tending to minimize those parasitic capacitances.

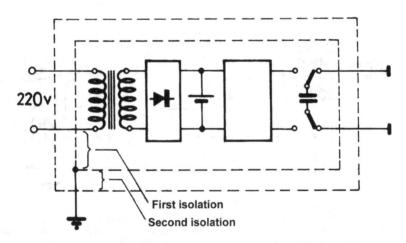

Fig. 6.2.   Equipment with double cabinet and double isolation.

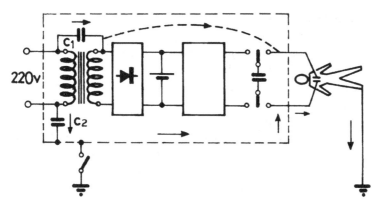

Fig. 6.3.   Capacitive pathway leak that could produce an accidental shock to the patient.

## 6.4. Electromagnetic Interference (EMI)

Even though this perturbation on medical equipment, at large, and on defibrillators or cardiac pacemakers, in particular, has not been fully proved to have had a real and significant deleterious action, the possibility exists and some cases have been reported in the literature. In 1995, the *Radiofrequency/Ultrasound Program of the U.S. Army Center for Health Promotion and Preventive Medicine* (Aberdeen Proving Ground, MD 21010-5422, DSN 584-3353 or Commercial 410-671-3353; email: mchbdsr@aehal.apgea.army.mil) came out with a brochure, available in the WEB, where concerns among health providers is discussed regarding potential deleterious effects on electronic medical devices by electromagnetic energy as well as electrostatic discharges. Problems associated with either one include device failure, loss of control, and erratic operation. They could circumstantially threaten someone's life. Electronic medical devices are increasingly subjected to electromagnetic emissions from sources brought into the hospital environment such as cellular telephones, radios, some paging systems, and security checking machines in airports and governmental buildings. Even the street is contaminated by EMI of different origins (Bostrum, 1991; Silberger, 1993). The American Society for Hospital Engineering (1994) has published several suggestions for reducing the risk of EMI problems associated with electronic medical equipment.

Barbaro *et al.* (1999), in Italy, examined the potential electromagnetic interference (EMI) effects induced by cellular telephones on ICDs. These investigators developed protocols to conduct both, *in vitro* and *in vivo* tests, on several ICD available on the market. From their paper, they conducted trials with three types of cellular phones. A human trunk simulator was used to carry out *in vitro* observations on six ICDs from five manufacturers while *in vivo* tests were conducted on 13 informed patients with eight different ICD models. During the trials in air, some of the telephones induced interference effects on four out of the six cardioverter defibrillators tested. Results were interesting and really raised a cautionary flag: pulse inhibition, reprogramming, false ventricular fibrillation, and ventricular tachycardia detections occurred, which would have entailed inappropriate therapy delivery had this been activated. Effects were circumscribed to the area closely surrounding the connectors. When the ICD was immersed in saline solution, no effects were observed. Three cases of just ventricular triggering with the interfering signal were observed *in vivo*.

Hanada *et al.* (2000) mentioned that there have been a number of reports of EMI on electronic medical equipment caused by mobile telecommunication systems. In Japan, the use of the personal handy-phone system (PHS) has greatly expanded. These handsets transmit signals at a frequency of 1.9 GHz and have a peak radiated power of 80 mW, which is lower than that of other mobile systems. Two parts were carried out: one tried to determine whether these pieces interfere with electronic medical equipment in hospitals while the second study was to observe EMI from 1.9-GHz signals at several radiation power levels. For the former, these authors observed no EMI on electronic medical equipment when the PHS handset was in either the speaking mode or on standby; for the latter, although EMI was not observed at the radiated peak power, EMI on some of the tested equipment was seen when the radiated power was 10 or more times higher than that of the transmitting units.

Interference on cardiac pacemakers is also valid for ICDs. Some clinicians claimed interference from iPods on pacemakers and advised that warning labels may be needed. However, the conclusion reached by Bassen (2008) after an *in vitro* study to evaluate these claims were opposite. Let us scan what he says:

*"We performed in-vitro evaluations of the low frequency magnetic field emissions from various models of iPod music players measuring magnetic field emissions with a 3-coil sensor. Highly localized fields were observed within one square cm area). Also induced voltages were measured inside an 'instrumented-can' pacemaker with two standard unipolar leads. Each iPod was placed in the air, 2.7 cm above the pacemaker case. Case and leads were placed in a saline filled torso simulator per pacemaker electromagnetic compatibility standard ANSI/AAMI PC69:2000. Voltages inside the can*

*were measured. Emissions were strongest ($\approx 0.2\,\mu T$ pp) near a few localized points on the cases of the two iPods with hard drives. Emissions consisted of 100 kHz sinusoidal signal with lower frequency (20 msec wide) pulsed amplitude modulation. Voltages induced in the iPods were below the noise level of our instruments (0.5 mV pp in the 0–1 kHz band or 2 mV pp in the 0–5 MHz bandwidth. Levels of less than $0.2\,\mu T$ exist very close (1 cm) from the case. The measured voltages induced inside an 'instrumented-can' pacemaker were below the noise level of our instruments. Based on the observations of this in-vitro study, it was concluded that no interference effects can occur in pacemakers exposed to the iPod tested".*

> The acronym *iPod* has several and all different definitions, as a quick INTERNET search shows, bringing considerable confusion so that perhaps few people really know what it actually means; one of them reads *Interface Protocol Option Devices*, which in fact does not say much. Introduced in 2001, it is a palm-sized electronic device primarily created to play music. Unlike other traditional players, the *iPod* can store a large number of tracks.

As expected, the low-frequency voltages that could be induced in the pacemaker's (or implantable defibrillation's leads) and inside the case obey classical electromagnetic field theory (Faraday's Law) described by the classical equation,

$$V_\mathrm{b} = \oint E \cdot dl = \frac{d}{dt} \int B \cdot dA,$$

where $V_\mathrm{b}$ = voltage induced between the can and lead tip; $E$ = electric field; $dl$ = unit element of a closed loop; $d/dt$ = the rate of change with respect to time; $B$ = magnetic flux density; and $dA$ = unit element of the surrounded surface area $A$.

On November 16, 2005, the Food and Drug Administration (FDA) issued a public health notification, encouraging its free use, on the *Risk of EMI with Medical Telemetry Systems Operating in the 460–470 MHz Frequency Bands* (all of the FDA medical device Public Health Notifications are available on the Internet at http://www.fda.gov/cdrh/safety.html). A selected verbatim quotation from this report is pertinent:

*In 2000, the Federal Communications Commission (FCC) dedicated a portion of the radio spectrum for wireless medical telemetry. This part of the spectrum is known as the Wireless Medical Telemetry Service (WMTS). The WMTS bands include 608–614 MHz, 1395–1400 MHz, and 1427–1432 MHz. With spectrum dedicated for medical telemetry use, the FCC's intent for the past several years has been to grant new licenses to higher power mobile radio users in the 460–470 MHz band. However, because of the potential for serious interference with existing medical telemetry systems, the FCC has delayed implementing this change in order to allow time for medical facilities to migrate out of the 460–470 MHz band.* **This freeze on new land mobile licenses in the 460–470 MHz band expired on December 31, 2005.**

*After December 31, 2005, the FCC began granting a many licenses for mobile radio transmitters that use new channels in the 460–470 MHz band. The new licenses are for transmitters of 2 Watts or higher. Most of the radio users in this band include hand-held and other mobile transmitters, such as those operated by police, fire and rescue officers, taxis and commercial trucks.*

*Wireless medical telemetry equipment still using channels in the 460–470 MHz band after December 31, 2005, could be adversely affected by mobile radios operating under the new FCC licenses. According to tests conducted by the FDA, the transmitters operating under new licenses in this frequency band can interfere with medical telemetry systems. This could lead to lapses in patient monitoring and missed alarm events, putting patients at risk. The anticipated interference is not limited to urban areas. Any medical facility in the vicinity of a mobile radio could be affected.*

Following the above paragraph, the report recommends,

- *Determine if your current wireless medical telemetry systems are operating in the 460–470 MHz frequency band.*
- *Migrate out of the 460–470 MHz band if you are operating wireless medical telemetry equipment in that band.*
- *Register any WMTS equipment with the frequency coordinator for WMTS — the American Society for Healthcare Engineering (ASHE) of the American Hospital Association (AHA). Registration of WMTS equipment is required by the FCC.*
- *Assess and manage the risks for* **all** *medical telemetry. Medical telemetry still operating in the TV channels 7–13 (174–216 MHz), 14–36 (470–608 MHz), and 38–46 (614–668 MHz) are particularly at risk. This is because in July 2005, the FCC ordered most major commercial broadcasters in the top 100 markets to operate their Digital TV (DTV) transmitters at their maximum licensed power. All others broadcasters were required to do so by July 2006.*
- *Establish lines of communication or meet regularly with local broadcasters so that you can be aware of local changes in the high-power broadcast use of the RF spectrum.*

Additional and background information from FDA on WMTS can be found at http://www.fda.gov/cdrh/safety/emimts.html.

## 6.5. Standards

This book is not intended to describe defibrillators' standards, at most and after briefly mentioning them, it discusses a few particular subjects. Accordingly, herein we merely give the essential information that the clinical engineer, technician, or manufacturer can take as a beginning.

*The primary international standard for external defibrillators is the* **International Electrotechnical Commission** *(IEC) document 60601-2-4, Medical Electrical Equipment, Part 2–4, Particular requirements for the safety of cardiac defibrillators. The second edition of this standard was published in 2002. This standard amends and supplements IEC 60601-1 (second edition, 1988): Medical electrical equipment — Part 1: General requirements for safety, which is an FDA-recognized standard. Improvements from the first edition include new and improved safety requirements for AEDs. Recently, the Defibrillator Standard Committee of the Association for the Advancement of Medical Instrumentation (AAMI) approved the adoption of IEC 60601-2-4 as the new American Standard for external defibrillators. The new standard, AAMI DF80, maintains the full content of IEC 60601-2-4:2002 and also includes additional requirements that the AAMI Defibrillator Committee deemed important for standardization for self-adhesive defibrillation electrodes and external pacemakers. The new standard replaces the previous AAMI standards, ANSYAAMI DF2: 1996 for manually operated external defibrillators and ANWAAMI DF39: 1993 for automated external defibrillators (AED's) Safety Risk Management Standards. The international standard for Safety Risk Management, ISO 14971:2000, Medical Devices — Application of Risk Management to Medical Devices, establishes the requirements for a comprehensive safety risk management approach to the development of medical devices. It is being adapted into the third edition of IEC 60601-1 and should be followed by all AED manufacturers* (selectively downloaded from **www.fda.gov/OHRMS/DOCKETS/dockets/94n0418/94n-0418-c000017-01-vol23.pdf**). The latter is a freely available website.

It is mandatory and ethical duty of design biomedical engineers, manufacturers, clinical engineers, technicians, hospital administrators, physicians, and nurses alike to be aware of these norms, especially if their respective practices involve coronary and intensive care units and medical emergency systems and, very important, to keep updated. Hence, we underline the importance of refreshing short training courses.

## 6.6. Pain

### 6.6.1. *Evidence of the Sensation*

Many people, if not everybody, have received a minor accidental electric discharge when inadvertently placed a hand or finger on a hot conductor. Some had worse experiences because the shock produced burns, loss of conscience, respiratory arrest, or even death in extreme cases due to ventricular fibrillation or respiratory arrest or both. This author, when he was a 23-year-old electrical engineering student working in a large telecommunications transmitting station, received a 2,400-V dc shock while making adjustments on the final power amplifying stage of a 27-MHz transmitter. A combination of several factors, all the odds against, led to the mishap. The result was respiratory standstill for 45 min, which was reverted by quick and skillful manual artificial respiration instituted by local personnel, fortunately with no apparent cardiac arrhythmia. Passing out and severe burns in one hand and arm took place. Skin scars are still there and, yes, there was pain, intense pain; for several months nightmares brought back the shock. Thus, all who went through the experience, from the very mild discharge to the very serious, and survived, know how nasty, unbearable, and unforgettable the sensation is. Imagine what death penalty by electrocution implies! From the above, we see that if the current sustained by the applied voltage traverses the respiratory center located at the level of the medulla, it may inhibit the pacemaking activity that controls the respiratory muscles without triggering cardiac fibrillation (neither atrial nor ventricular). If the center is not too seriously damaged, it recovers with enough time, but artificial respiration must be instituted.

A defibrillator delivers an electric shock, as several times described along this text, a short, well-controlled shock **only** when the heart is in fibrillation, not before and not after the rhythm is restored. In the case of AEDs or ICDs, the mechanism of arrhythmia detection is responsible for triggering the shock. Failure of the system may lead to improper discharge (that is, when the shock is not needed); or external interference may trigger the system, also when not required. Usually, the subject loses conscience during ventricular fibrillation, so that any pain due to the discharge is not felt, but improper shock surprises the subject fully awake and, certainly, he or she would not like it at all. In the case of atrial defibrillation, the patient is always awake, so that electric pain appears as a secondary drawback to take care of. However, even with a normally operating ICD, if detection of fibrillation is too fast, so fast that there is no time for the patient to pass out, the discharge is delivered and the subject feels a strong "kick in the back", as it was described by these kinds of victims. The pain is so unbearable that more than one patient requested removal of the unit, even when they were warned about the risks involved (death because of the arrhythmia).

Defibrillation pain has been well documented beyond any doubt or any hearsaying. Minnesota has an old good tradition in pacemakers and defibrillators. Stationed in this area, Steinhaus *et al.* (2002) recognized the problem specifically during cardioversion. They aimed at evaluating pain perception with low energy internal discharges on 18 patients with ICD devices for malignant ventricular arrhythmias. In the non-sedated state, these patients were to receive shocks of 0.4 and 2 J. Discharges were delivered in a blinded, random order and questionnaires were used to determine discomfort levels and tolerability. Patients perceived discharges at these energies as relatively uncomfortable, averaging a score of 7.3 on a discomfort scale of 0–10, and could not distinguish 0.4 J shocks from 2 J shocks. Second shocks were perceived as more uncomfortable than initial discharges, regardless of the order in which the shocks were delivered. Despite the perceived discomfort, 83% of patients stated that they would tolerate discharges of this magnitude once per month, and 44% would tolerate weekly discharges. The results suggest that ICD systems developed to treat atrial tachyarrhythmias should minimize the number of shocks (last paragraph reproduced from the above-mentioned paper).

In classical physiology, pain has long been recognized as a complex mechanism with neurophysiologic and psychological components not easy to separate out, even in mammalian species (as dogs and horses). Reference to Baumert *et al.*'s (2006) paper, from Germany, appears appropriate. Its objective was to examine whether the strength of perceived shock pain due to ICD activity is influenced by affective and psychophysiologic parameters. "Out of 204 ICD patients, 95 (46.6%) experienced one or more shock. Pain perception was measured by a visual analog scale ranging from 0 to 100. Psychophysiologic arousal (stress estimator) was assessed with skin conductance response (SCR) and electromyogram amplitude (EMG). Classification and regression tree (CART) analysis was applied to assess the effects of psychodiagnostic and psychophysiologic parameters of pain perception. Pain intensity was highly associated with shock discomfort but was largely uninfluenced by clinical and socio-demographic factors.

CART analysis revealed patients with one shock and low EMG magnitude as a subclass with the lowest mean pain perception, whereas patients with more than one shock experience expressed the highest mean pain perception. It was concluded that augmented pain perception of ICD shocks is predominantly associated with the number of perceived shocks, post-shock anxiety, and accompanied by heightened levels of EMG magnitude and impaired EMG habituation, which points to sensitization of central neural structures."

### 6.6.2. *Causes*

Accurate sensing is an essential requirement for appropriate functioning of implantable cardioverter defibrillators (ICDs). Muscular electrical stimulation is becoming very popular, for rehabilitation (say, after surgery), cosmetic (muscle build up), or even massage purposes (simple wellbeing feeling). Chung-Wah Siu *et al.* (2005), in Hong Kong, reported an unusual case of inappropriate ICD discharge in a patient who was using transcutaneous neuromuscle stimulation from a commercially available device.

Alizadeh *et al.* (2006), in Iran, stated that $T$-wave oversensing remains as an annoying problem in currently available ICDs. The Brugada syndrome with its inherent dynamic variations in electrophysiologic phenomena may complicate ICD therapy. These authors report a patient suffering such syndrome who presented with frequent inappropriate therapy due to intermittent $T$-wave oversensing. This problem could not be eliminated by device reprogramming and necessitated implantation of a new sense/pace lead. However, the report does not mention pain sensation even though we think the patient must have felt it.

> Brugada syndrome is a genetic $Na^+$ channel pathology characterized by right bundle branch block (RBBB) and ST segment elevation in the right precordial leads of the electrocardiogram (ECG) without any apparent structural abnormality in the heart, associated with syncope and eventual sudden death (Figs. 6.4 and 6.5). It was in 1992 that the Brugada brothers recognized it as a distinct clinical entity prone to lead to ventricular fibrillation (http://www.brugada.org/).

Atrial defibrillation finds the patient always awake so that he/she is obviously bound to feel pain. In their 2007 study, Dosdall and Ideker, from the University of Alabama at Birmingham, addressed this problem. In their words: "An important factor influencing the outcome of the shock

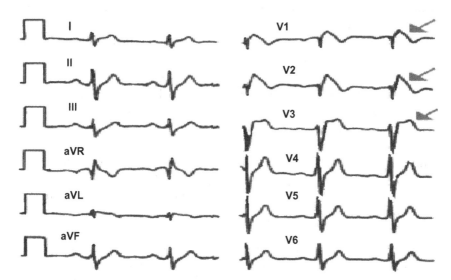

Fig. 6.4. Brugada syndrome. ECG's resembling a right bundle branch block. P–R prolongation and ST elevation in leads V1–V3 (arrows). Downloaded from http://www.brugada.org/about/disease-definition.html; supported by Mapfre Medicine Foundation. With kind permission from Ramon Brugada.

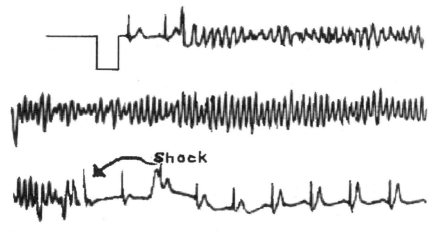

Fig. 6.5. Spontaneous ventricular tachycardia in a patient with Brugada syndrome. The episodes are caused by fast polymorphic tachycardias or fibrillation that appear with no warning. As shown in the third row, defibrillation is required. Downloaded from http://www.brugada.org/about/disease-definition.html; supported by Mapfre Medicine Foundation. With kind permission from Ramón Brugada.

is the potential gradient field created throughout the ventricles or the atria by the shock. A minimum potential gradient is required throughout the ventricles and probably the atria in order to defibrillate. The value of this minimum potential gradient is affected by several factors, including the duration, tilt, and number of phases of the waveform. For shock strengths near the defibrillation threshold, earliest activation following failed shocks arises in a region in which the potential gradient is low. The defibrillation threshold (DFT) energy can be decreased by adding a third and even a fourth defibrillation electrode in regions where the shock potential gradient is low for the shock field created by the first two defibrillation electrodes and giving two sequential shocks, each through a different set of electrodes. However, the addition of more electrodes and sequential shocks complicates both the device and its implantation. Because patients are conscious when the atrial defibrillation shock is given, they experience pain during the shock, which is one of the main drawbacks of intravascular atrial defibrillation. Unfortunately, the pain threshold for defibrillation shocks is so low that a shock less than 1 J is uncomfortable and is not much less painful than shocks several times stronger. Therefore, even though electrode configurations exist that have lower atrial defibrillation threshold energy requirements than the atrial defibrillation threshold with standard defibrillation electrode configurations used in ICDs for ventricular defibrillation, they are not clinically practical because their shocks are almost as painful as with the standard ICD electrode configurations. Such electrode configurations would make the ICD more complicated, leading to greater difficulty and longer time required for implantation." Thus, their conclusion is disheartening.

### 6.6.3. *Proposed Measures to Prevent it*

Cammilli *et al.* (1998, 2006), in Italy, filed for an interesting patent that seems to take care of the pain problem described above. They described "an implantable defibrillation system for ventricle and atrium that is able to diagnose the type of arrhythmia within a maximum time of 2 seconds from its onset delivering the therapeutic shock by electrodes implanted in the region to be defibrillated no more than 4–5 seconds after the recognition of the arrhythmia, if it is ventricular fibrillation, so that the patient does not loose consciousness; immediately after the onset of the arrhythmia and before the defibrillation shock is delivered, the unit can prevent conduction of neural pain signals by nerve stimulation with a catheter inserted in the spinal column, utilizing the gate effect, or by the perfusion of a drug with analgesic effect by an infusion pump and a catheter positioned in the affected region. This system enables defibrillation or conversion to be carried out with the patient conscious and within a sufficiently short time to be able to use low shock energy and with prevention of the consequent painful shock." We do not know if the unit was ever built and used.

The World Intellectual Property Organization describes an invention, identified as WO/2004/041350, Auxilary Central Nervous System Pre-pulse for Shock Pain Inhibition (http://www.wipo.int/pctdb/en/wo.jsp?WO= 2004041350&IA=WO2004041350&DISPLAY=DESC), without giving the author's name, which (partial verbatim quotation) *relates generally to an implantable device for* **delivering a pain inhibiting stimulation pulse to the central nervous system prior to delivering cardioversion shock** *therapy (as for example disclosed in U.S. Patent No. 6,438, 418, issued to Swerdlow et al.). These high-voltage shocks can be very painful. Some patients have recurring arrhythmias and are subject to repeated shock therapies. Patient anxiety over receiving a painful shock therapy can affect a patient's overall quality of life and their acceptance of ICD use. Another approach for reducing the pain associated with cardioversion shocks is* **to minimize the energy of the shocking pulse***. While this approach may reduce the amount of pain perceived by the patient, it does not eliminate the pain and potentially compromises the effectiveness of the shock therapy. A third possibility approach to alleviating pain is* **to deliver an analgesic drug** *prior to delivering a shock (as disclosed in U.S. Patent No. 5,662, 689, issued to Elsberry et al.).*

Since atrial defib acceptance is limited by shock-related anxiety and discomfort, Ujhelyi *et al.* (2004) made use of nitrous oxide ($N_2O$) as potent sedative-analgesic-anxiolytic agent that may mitigate such sensations. Thus, "patients with more than one ambulatory atrial shock within 12 months were enrolled and grouped by shock method; awake ($n = 9$) or asleep ($n = 4$), when ambulatory defib was delivered. A baseline questionnaire assessed the most recent ambulatory shock ($3 \pm 3$ months). A 65% $N_2O$/35% $O_2$ mixture was inhaled for 4 minutes followed by a test shock ($18 \pm 8$ J). The test shock mimicked the awake shock method. The test shock experience during $N_2O$ was evaluated via questionnaire immediately following and 24 hours after the shock. Shock-related anxiety, intensity, pain, and discomfort were assessed using a ten-point rank scale. Baseline test shock scores were similar between the shock method groups. In the awake shock method group, $N_2O$ greatly reduced pre-shock anxiety by 48%

($6.4\pm2.4$ to $3.3\pm2.0$) and shock-related intensity ($5.9\pm3.1$ to $3.3\pm2.5$), pain ($5.0\pm2.6$ to $2.0\pm2.1$), and discomfort ($5.6\pm2.4$ to $1.3\pm1.4$) from baseline values by 45%, 60%, and 78%, respectively. The asleep shock method group reported no changes in shock-related anxiety, intensity, pain, or discomfort. Atrial shock concern, assessed via a five-point rank scale ($5 =$ extreme concern) was improved by $N_2O$ but only in the awake group ($3.1\pm1.0$ baseline to $1.6\pm0.5$). There were no adverse events with $N_2O$ and patients fully recovered within 5 minutes after $N_2O$. In conclusion, 65% $N_2O$ greatly reduced shock related pain and discomfort, and significantly reduced atrial shock concern but only in the awake shock method group. The benefits of $N_2O$ therapy may expand the use and acceptability of atrial defib."

In short, the possible pain prevention techniques, either for atrial or ventricular defibrillation, can be described as,

(1) CNS inhibition by delivering a pre-shock pulse;
(2) administration of an analgesic drug prior to the shock; and
(3) minimizing the energy of the defibrillation discharge.

In the case of ventricular defibrillation, a fourth possibility would be to slightly delay the shock thus giving time for the patient to fall unconscious. Some people may object the procedure as potentially risky and even unethical.

### 6.7. Efficacy

Even if there is no discomfort or pain, the procedure may not produce the therapeutic effects it intends to, that is, reversion of the arrhythmia, in which case human health is not preserved. This potential risk leads to the concept of efficacy (defined by the Merriam-Webster Dictionary as *the power to produce an effect*). Apparent synonyms are *efficiency* and *effectiveness*; however, a quick search indicated that minute semantic differences might exist in their respective meanings (see below). Since this book does not deal with linguistics, we will stick to the first word, which is the one currently found in the specialized scientific literature.

> The relationship between the resources used in a project and the results obtained is defined sometimes as efficiency (also efficacy); thus, the lower the resources, the higher the efficiency. Effectiveness, instead, refers to the ability to reach an objective irrespective of the used means. When dealing with defibrillation, however, these differences tend to blur.

Efficacy of a defibrillation shock, either atrial or ventricular, recognizes several factors, all complex, eventually overlapping, and still somewhat under discussion because of conflictive results, such as *lead system, pulse waveform* (monophasic or polyphasic), *pulse duration,* and *safety margin* (in terms of energy or current).

### 6.7.1. Leads

It is impossible to review exhaustively the defibrillation leads that have been tested and even more those currently in use, especially for implanted devices, for there are many and still they represent a subject of development. The appearance of the emulators has complicated the picture because such units allow fast testing of different possibilities, including the detecting stage as forerunner of the actual defibrillation attempt.

One of the many contributions in this area is the US Patent #5662696, by Kroll *et al.* (1995); it describes a disposable pulse generator for emulating a subcutaneous ICD having an active housing electrode. The emulator of the invention is for use with an external test system to screen a patient for candidacy for an ICD by determining the patient's minimum defibrillation threshold (DFT) voltage. This emulator has a housing that has substantially the same conductive geometry as the desired implantable pulse generator. Gold *et al.* (1998) tried a single vs a dual-coil active pectoral defibrillation arrangement while de de Jongh, Entcheva, Replogle *et al.* (1999) measured the defibrillation threshold (DFT) associated with different electrode placements using a three-dimensional anatomically realistic finite element model of the human thorax. The DFT's measured at each configuration fell within one standard deviation of the mean DFT's reported in clinical studies using other leads. The relative changes in DFT among electrode configurations also compared favorably. This model allows measurements of DFT or other defibrillation parameters with several arrangements saving time and cost. In another study, KenKnight *et al.* (2000) showed a reduction in the DFT by application of an auxiliary shock to an electrode in the canine left posterior coronary vein.

Mazur *et al.* (2001) hypothesized that electrograms (EGMs) recorded from electrodes on the ICD surface may improve diagnostic capabilities of the device. "The Buttons on Active Can Emulator (BACE), an ICD-sized device containing four button electrodes, was temporarily placed into a subcutaneous or submuscular left pectoral pocket in 16 patients during

ICD implantation. Simultaneous recordings were obtained from the ECG lead II, bipolar EGM's using BACE electrodes, and a bipolar atrial EGM during sinus rhythm (SR), ventricular pacing (VP) at cycle lengths of 500 and 400 ms, and ventricular tachycardia (VT). Visible P waves were present in all patients during SR ($n = 15$), in 5 (33%) of 15 patients during VP, and none of the patients during VT ($n = 4$) using BACE EGM's and lead II. P and QRS amplitudes and the P:QRS ratio during SR in BACE EGM's were significantly lower than those in lead II. BACE EGM's showed prominent changes in QRS morphology and duration during VP and VT compared to SR, and the magnitude of QRS prolongation during VP was similar to that in lead II. In conclusion, EGM's recorded from electrodes embedded on the ICD housing may potentially improve visual discrimination between supraventricular and ventricular arrhythmias. They also may be useful as a surrogate of the ECG for analysis and monitoring of different components of P-QRS-T complex."

Defibrillation thresholds (DFTs) with standard ICD leads in the right ventricle (RV) may be determined by weak shock field intensity in the myocardium of the left ventricle (LV); that was the initial comment of Butter *et al.* (2001). Adding a shocking electrode in a coronary vein on the middle of the LV free wall, that is, using a biventricular defibrillation lead, substantially reduced defibrillation requirements in animals. Thus, these investigators studied the feasibility of this approach in 24 patients receiving an ICD. "The LV lead was inserted through the coronary sinus into a posterior or lateral coronary vein whose location was determined by retrograde venography. Paired DFT testing compared a standard system (RV to superior vena cava plus can emulator [SVC + Can], 60% tilt biphasic shock) to a system including the LV lead. The biventricular system was tested with a dual-shock waveform (20% tilt monophasic shock from LV to → SVC + Can, then 60% tilt biphasic shock from RV to → SVC + Can). Twenty patients completed DFT testing. The biventricular system significantly reduced mean DFT by 45% ($8.9 \pm 1.1$ J vs $4.9 \pm 0.5$ J). Twelve patients (60%) had a standard system DFT $\geq 8$ J, and the biventricular system gave a lower DFT in all patients." They concluded that internal defibrillation using a transvenously inserted LV lead is feasible, produces significantly lower DFTs, and seems safe under the conditions tested. Biventricular defibrillation may be a useful option for reducing DFTs or could be added to an LV pacing lead for heart failure.

Rashba *et al.* (2004), in the case of atrial defibrillation, stated that the optimal configuration is unknown and, thus, established as their objective to compare atrial defibrillation thresholds (DFTs) with three shocking configurations currently available with standard ICD leads. It was a prospective, randomized, paired comparison of leads carried out in 58 patients. The system evaluated was a "transvenous defibrillation lead with coils in the superior vena cava (SVC) and right ventricular apex (RV) and a left pectoral pulse generator emulator (Can). In the first 33 patients, atrial DFT was measured with the ventricular triad (RV → SVC + Can) and unipolar (RV → Can) shocking pathways. In the next 25 patients, atrial DFT was measured with the ventricular triad and the proximal triad (SVC → RV + Can) configurations. Delivered energy at DFT was significantly lower with the ventricular triad compared to the unipolar configuration ($4.7 \pm 3.7$ J vs $10.1 \pm 9.5$ J). Peak voltage and shock impedance also were significantly reduced. There was no significant difference in DFT energy when the ventricular triad and proximal triad shocking configurations were compared ($3.6 \pm 3.0$ J vs $3.4 \pm 2.9$ J for ventricular and proximal triad, respectively). Although shock impedance was reduced by 13% with the proximal triad, this effect was offset by an increased current requirement (10%). In conclusion, the ventricular triad is equivalent or superior to other possible shocking pathways for atrial defibrillation afforded by a dual-coil, active pectoral lead system. Because the ventricular triad is also the most efficacious shocking pathway for ventricular defibrillation, this pathway should be preferred for combined atrial and ventricular defibrillators."

### 6.7.2. *Pulse Waveform (Monophasic or Polyphasic)*

As already described before in the text, defibrillators started with damped sinusoidal pulses; thereafter, biphasic pulses were introduced finding that the energy requirements were lower. The latter, first send energy through the heart in one direction repeating the shock in the opposite direction slightly later. By and large, less energy is required with biphasic discharges. Both, monophasic and biphasic procedures have been approved by the FDA and meet the general guidelines for cardiovascular care. Monophasic waveforms with increasing energy produced better success in some patients, especially in subjects showing higher chest impedances. For example, in the transchest situation, in the order of 350 J at, say, 5,000 peak volts may be needed with a damped monophasic pulse vs 150 J, at about 1,700 peak volts, when biphasic truncated pulses are applied. In fact, this is standard knowledge now, as reported by many authors who started with experimental animals, such as Chapman *et al.* (1988), or as can be easily found in the INTERNET (see http://www.expresshealthcaremgmt. com/20050515/criticare07.shtml; Health Care Management, May 15, 2005). The latter investigators studied pentobarbital-anesthetized dogs to determine the relative efficacy of monophasic and biphasic truncated exponential shocks employing a non-thoracotomy internal defibrillation pathway that consisted of a right ventricular catheter electrode (cathode) and a subcutaneous chest wall patch electrode (anode). "In part 1 of the experiments, six dogs (19.6 ± 1.1 kg) were utilized. Monophasic pulses of 5, 7.5, 10 and 12.5 ms duration were compared with biphasic pulses of the same total duration. The biphasic pulses had an initial positive phase (P1) followed by a terminal negative phase (P2) with the initial voltage equal for each phase. For each biphasic total pulse width, five relative P1 vs P2 durations were tested (50% and 50%, 75% and 25%, 90% and 10%, 25% and 75%, 10% and 90%). Ventricular fibrillation was induced by alternating current and pulse configurations were tested randomly to determine the minimal voltage and energy for defibrillation (threshold). Biphasic shocks with P1 longer than P2 were associated with significantly lower energy thresholds than were monophasic shocks. Additionally, there was no significant relation between pulse width and voltage or energy thresholds. In part 2 of the experiments, six dogs (20.2±1.6 kg) were studied. Monophasic shocks were compared with biphasic shocks with P1 vs P2 durations of 75% and 25% and 90% and 10% for total pulse widths of 7.5, 10 and 12.5 ms. Threshold determinations were performed as in part 1. Subsequently, five initial voltages clustered about threshold were randomly tested four times and dose-response curves constructed for each pulse configuration with the use of stepwise logistic regression. Biphasic shocks resulted in significantly lower energy and voltage requirements than did monophasic shocks."

In 2003, Fado commented that even though biphasic waveforms are routinely used for implantable defibrillators, such technology has been less readily adopted for external defibrillation. For that reason, he intended to evaluate the efficacy and harms of biphasic waveforms over monophasic waveforms for transthoracic defibrillation of patients in ventricular fibrillation (VF) or hemodynamically unstable ventricular tachycardia. "Randomized trials compared monophasic and biphasic external defibrillation for participants with VF or unstable ventricular tachycardia. Seven trials (1,129 patients) were included in the analysis. All trials were conducted during electrophysiology procedures or implantable cardioverter/defibrillator testing. Compared with 200 J monophasic shocks, 200 J biphasic shocks reduced the risk of post-first shock asystole or persistent VF by 81% for the first shock. Reducing the energy of the biphasic waveform to 115–130 J resulted in similar effectiveness compared with the monophasic waveform at 200 J. Low energy biphasic shocks produced less myocardial injury than higher energy monophasic shocks. Their conclusion: Biphasic waveforms defibrillate with similar efficacy at lower energies than standard 200 J monophasic waveforms and greater efficacy than monophasic shocks of the same energy. It is suggested that lower delivered energy and voltage result in less post-shock myocardial injury."

### 6.7.3. *Pulse Duration*

Basic neurophysiology teaches that the shorter the pulse, the lower the probability of inducing pain or discomfort. The chronaxie characteristic of each particular excitable tissue, another classical parameter, is the reference criterion to determine what pulse duration is either long or short (Valentinuzzi, 2004). Since rarely, if ever, a defibrillation shock exceeds 10 ms, it can be stated that this parameter is of not much concern, except that it must guarantee depolarization of a minimum number of cardiac fibers. The previous section also mentions duration in the case of monophasic vs biphasic discharges; thus, this section can be regarded as a continuation of the former.

As early as 1989, in Duje University, Tang *et al.* "tested, in 14 anesthetized open chest dogs with large contoured defibrillation electrodes, the effect on defibrillation efficacy of varying the duration of the two phases of biphasic waveforms. All combinations of 0, 1, 3.5, 6 and 8.5 ms duration were used for both the first and the second phase. The 3.5-2 waveform (3.5 ms first phase and 2 ms second phase) was also tested. All the hearts were defibrillated with less than or equal to 5 J using any of the 25 waveforms. However, biphasic waveforms with the second phase shorter than or equal to the first had significantly lower defibrillation thresholds than did those with the second phase longer than the first or than did monophasic waveforms of approximately the same total duration. A plot of defibrillation threshold current strength vs second phase duration for all biphasic waveforms with a 3.5 ms first phase did not produce a hyperbolic strength-duration curve as seen with monophasic waveforms. To verify these findings, defibrillation dose-response curves were obtained for the 3.5-2, 6-6 and 3.5-8.5 biphasic waveforms in another six dogs. The 50 and 80% successful voltage doses of the 3.5-8.5 waveforms were significantly higher than those of the other two waveforms, which were not different from one another."

### 6.7.4. *Safety Margin (in Terms of Energy or Current)*

Each time an ICD is implanted in a patient, a testing procedure is carried out in order to determine the DFT in terms of the electrical energy required to successfully defibrillate for the particular electrode lead combination installed in that patient. We contend in this book, however, as already discussed before, that current ought to be used instead. The procedure involves inducing ventricular fibrillation and then immediately delivering a countershock of a specified initial energy (for example, 20 J for a monophasic pulse). If defibrillation is successful, a recovery period is provided for the patient and the procedure is sometimes repeated one or more times using successively lower energies until the shock is not successful. If defibrillation is not successful, subsequent discharges are immediately delivered to resuscitate the patient. After a recovery period, the procedure is repeated using a higher initial energy (for example, 25 J). It is also possible that during the recovery period and prior to attempting a higher initial value, the electrophysiologist may attempt to lower the energy for that patient by changing the configuration of the electrodes. Typically, if more than 30 to 35 J are required for successful defibrillation with a monophasic countershock, the patient is not considered to be a good candidate for an ICD. Otherwise, the lowest successful discharge is considered to be the DFT for that patient. The accepted guideline is that the lower the energy, the lower the likelihood of damage to the heart. Usually, the actual value for adjusting the unit is larger than the threshold. The difference between that working value and the threshold is the safety margin.

Gold *et al.* (2002), after trials within the frame of the so-called Low Energy Safety Study (LESS), analyzed the efficacy of ventricular defibrillation. These authors say: "Traditionally, a safety margin of at least 10 J between the maximum output of the pulse generator and the energy needed for ventricular defibrillation has been used because lower values were associated with unacceptably high rates of failure. The Low Energy Safety Study (LESS) was a prospective, randomized assessment of the safety margin requirements for implantable cardioverter-defibrillators. A total of 636 patients undergoing initial ICD implantation with a dual-coil lead and active pulse generator were evaluated. The DFT was measured using a modified step-down protocol. The induced ventricular fibrillation data had conversion success rates of 91.4%, 97.9%, 99.1%, 99.6%, and 99.8% for safety margins of 0, 1, 2, 3, and 4 steps above threshold, respectively. A margin of 4 to 6 J was adequate to maintain high conversion success over time (98.9%). Over a mean follow-up of $24 \pm 13$ months, conversion of spontaneously occurring ventricular tachyarrhythmias ($>200$ bpm) was identical (97.3%), despite a safety margin difference of $5.2 \pm 1.1$ J vs $20.8 \pm 4.2$ J for maximal output. In conclusion, with a rigorous implantation algorithm, a safety margin of about 5 J is adequate for safe implantation of modern ICD's."

Another possibility to determine the safety margin makes use of the upper limit of vulnerability (ULV) using ICD EGMs (Swerdlow, Shehata, Belk *et al.*, 2007). The ULV is the weakest shock that does not induce fibrillation in the vulnerable period. It correlates with the DFT so permitting assessment of ICD safety margins without inducing VF. To determine the ULV, T-wave shocks must time at the most vulnerable intervals (corresponding to the strongest shock that induces VF), which are estimated using multiple ECG leads. To automate the ULV method, these intervals must be identified from an ICD EGM. These authors determined the range of most vulnerable intervals and compared the accuracy of estimating them using timing points based on either ECG or EGM.

Years ago, a "protective zone" near the T-wave region of the ECG was proposed (Verrier *et al.*, 1978); however, not much came out of the concept and, for the time being, it only has a historical interest. Thereafter, and somehow related to that idea, Chen *et al.* (1986) supported the hypothesis that successful defibrillation with epicardial electrodes requires a shock strength that reaches or exceeds the upper limit of ventricular vulnerability and that shocks slightly lower than the DFT fail because they reinitiate ventricular fibrillation by stimulating portions of the myocardium during their vulnerable period. They demonstrated the existence of an upper limit to the shock strength that can induce fibrillation during the vulnerable period of paced rhythm. Is that the "protective zone or effect"?

Strickberger *et al.* (2007) stated that in patients undergoing defibrillator implantation, an appropriate safety margin has been considered to be either 10 J or an energy equal to the defibrillation energy requirement. However, a previous clinical report suggested that a larger safety margin may be required in patients with a low defibrillation energy requirement. Therefore, their purpose was to compare the defibrillation efficacy of the two safety margin techniques in patients with a low defibrillation energy requirement. "Sixty patients who underwent implantation of a defibrillator and who had a low defibrillation energy requirement ($\leq 6$ J) underwent six separate inductions of ventricular fibrillation. For each of the first three inductions of ventricular fibrillation, the first two shocks were equal to either the defibrillation energy requirement plus 10 J ($14.6 \pm 1.0$ J), or to twice the defibrillation energy requirement ($9.9 \pm 2.3$ J). The alternate technique was used for the subsequent three inductions of ventricular fibrillation. For each induction of ventricular fibrillation, the first shock success rate was $99.5\% \pm 4.3\%$ for shocks using the defibrillation energy requirement plus 10 J, compared to $95.0\% \pm 17.2\%$ for shocks at twice the defibrillation energy requirement. The charge time and the total duration of ventricular fibrillation were each approximately 1 second longer with the defibrillation energy requirement plus 10 J technique. It was concluded that in patients with a defibrillation energy requirement $\leq 6$ J, a higher rate of successful defibrillation is achieved with a safety margin of 10 J than with a safety margin equal to the defibrillation energy requirement."

## 6.8. Conclusions and Review Questions

The enormous and even perhaps disproportionate number of contributions (with a concomitant large expenditure of resources) and the variety of approaches and results, some of them even conflicting, indicates that, in spite of the elapsed decades, safety and efficacy are subjects not fully solved yet. Consensus is not at hand, only accepted practice is. Electrical and magnetic isolation obviously is agreed upon and, whenever possible, battery powered units gain rapidly the market, although interferences come from essentially everywhere and only minimization seems to be left as a way out along with strict adherence to international standards. What perhaps should trouble more is the still purely empirical methodology disclosing clearly the lack of a solid theoretical ground. The concept of safety goes beyond the simple fact of an accident due, say, to a broken wire or a current leak; it is indeed closely linked to the efficacy of the procedure, without any discomfort or pain to the patient. If the shock does not have a high probability of success, then the procedure loses safety, too; in principle, it should follow the formula "the higher, the better", but simultaneously accepting that 100% success is an unreachable ideal, limited by the counterpart formula stating that "too high may produce injury". The possible pain prevention techniques, either for atrial or ventricular defibrillation, can be summarized as, central nervous system (CNS) inhibition by delivering a pre-shock pulse, administration of an analgesic drug prior to the shock and minimizing the energy of the defibrillation discharge while efficacy still searches for the best lead system while biphasic pulses seem to have attained consensus. Recommendations for a defibrillator operator can be found in Linda Cook's "Staying current on defibrillator safety", *Nursing*, Nov 2003 (http:// findarticles.com/p/articles/mi_qa3689/is_200311/ai_n9324429). Besides, a quick search in the WEB easily retrieves over 1,000 references on *defibrillation safety and efficiency.*

*Review questions* (T = True; F = false or choose the most appropriate answer)

1. Isolation of a defibrillator intends to
   (A) avoid humidity to get into it
   (B) to prevent an accidental shock because of an electrical hot wire touching, say, the cabinet
   (C) to avoid an unduly temperature increase.
2. Starting of a large electric motor (such as that moving an elevator or a compressor) may trigger a defibrillator.     T     F
3. Cellular phones are totally and absolutely harmless devices from the viewpoint of an implantable cardiac defibrillator.     T     F
4. Coronary Care Units' (CCU) nurses and physicians are not required nor need to be current in standard norms regarding use and maintenance of defibrillators at large.     T     F
5. A defibrillator discharge if improperly applied
   (A) cannot trigger bowel activity
   (B) can produce respiratory arrest
   (C) can produce pain
   (D) it is irrelevant.
6. Defibrillation *efficacy* is defined as
   (A) how well the battery energy is used in each shock
   (B) how high the probability is of reversing the arrhythmia
   (C) how long the unit is expected to operate properly.

7. Select, from the material herein presented, an effective
   lead configuration, first for an automatic external
   defibrillator, and second for an implantable unit. Make
   drawings to better visualize them. Search numbers in
   percent to validate your choices. If necessary, state what
   type of pulse or pulses you would select.
8. Search in the literature what an emulator is. Search and
   better study what an emulator is used for in the field
   of cardiac defibrillation.
9. Biphasic shocks are more efficacious or defibrillation.          T      F
10. Define what *defibrillation safety margin* is. Discuss it
   briefly. Can you increase it as much as you wish? What
   would the limitations be?

# Chapter 7

# THEORETICAL MODELS

*Empirical knowledge is fine, but how much better when it stands on solid grounds...*

Diego L. González, Simone Giannerini, and Max E. Valentinuzzi

This is, no doubt, the most difficult chapter of the book, written mostly by its first author, a specialist in non-linear dynamic systems, and seconded by a statistician that has been working on the connections between Chaos Theory and Statistics; the third co-author, responsible for the whole book, acted mainly as editor, adding, removing, or changing minor pieces. A good deal of exchange occupied considerable room and time in the cybernetic emailing space making the task enjoyable and fruitful. In the introduction, attention is called to the heart as paradigmatic case of high biological complexity reminding that interaction with several factors contributes often to further complicate its framework. No wonder, then, if complex theories become necessary to tackle pathological cardiac dynamics, in general, and ventricular fibrillation, in particular. Thereafter, the *bottom-up* and the *top-down* strategies are mentioned to start the modeling adventure. The Hodgkin–Huxley equations are presented as example of the first approach from which *dynamic bifurcations* can be derived. Linearization is also discussed as a possible simplification; however, a linear system might not show the same qualitative behavior as that of a non-linear one because it loses information. Alternatively, numerical integration becomes as a way out, but there are many and severe drawbacks. Thus, we expect better contributions from other top-down non-linear dynamic methods; they reduce microscopic bottom-up models to their minimal expression exhibiting also the main features of the complete model. Fibrillation is divided into two functional phases, its onset and as an already developed condition. The former can be considered as a bifurcation from a periodic condition of relatively low dimensionality; the latter, instead, implies rapid and irregular activity of the heart. From a medical point of view, the interest in modeling the onset of fibrillation relates to the possibility of avoiding the arrhythmia and/or diagnosing a propensity of falling into it. The interest in modeling established fibrillation lies in how to best intervene to revert the condition. The three sections after the introduction deal, respectively, with non-linear microscopic models, non-linear dynamics and the onset of fibrillation, and extended models and connection with sustained fibrillation, thus getting deeper into the subject. The relaxation oscillator of van der Pol appears as the starting mark up to more recent authors, as Winfree and others, going through a fascinating series of intermediate contributions. Several include experimental validations. For sustained fibrillation, the ventricular surface may be viewed as a sea of little reentry waves wandering on the ventricles; these waves arise from destabilization of one or a few greater spiral waves formed around an anatomical or dynamical singularity. The induced pathological dynamics can produce new singularities and also two singularities can merge and eventually annihilate or reduce to one. The statistical analysis relies on the reconstruction of the whole state space of the process (say, fibrillation) when just one or few time series components are available. Thereafter, Lyapunov exponents are discussed and followed by the concepts of complexity and entropy, all to better assess the cardiac signal under study. Heavy math is a characteristic of the section ... and there is no other way. As in previous chapters, we end with a discussion, a few review questions and a good list of backing up references.

## 7.1. Introduction

Why does the construction of models appear as a pertinent question? Medical heart care needs to rely on sound understanding of experimental and clinical data for dealing safely and efficiently with pathological rhythms; it is, however, a difficult endeavor because cardiac dynamics represents, in fact, a paradigmatic case of high biological complexity. Moreover, the interaction with drugs, electric stimulation, and other physico-chemical factors, contributes often to further complicate the conceptual framework by altering heart dynamics in not always predictable ways. No wonder, then, if complex theories become necessary to tackle pathological cardiac dynamics, in general, and ventricular fibrillation, in particular, especially when the aim is to obtain the best accuracy in model predictions.

Historically, two main attempts have been used for modeling complex biological systems; they can be called, without loss of generality, the *bottom-up* and the *top-down* strategies. A complex system appears usually as a collection of many interacting elements pertaining to a few discrete classes or categories; for example, coupled excitable, conducting, and auto-oscillating cells in cardiac tissue. Thus, we can try to construct a bottom-up model by representing an organ or tissue as a great number of coupled basic elements (Fig. 7.1). Successively, we define as precisely as we can (from a mathematical point of view) a single cell or element of this model. After that, we choose an appropriate coupling between elements of the tissue (say, physiologically suggested) including also possible excitations (such as natural pacemakers, vagal stimulation, external perturbations or pacing, or others.). This seems to be a natural and simple strategy for having a good mathematical model of the complete organ; however, for a wide range of complex systems, including the cardiovascular one, it leads

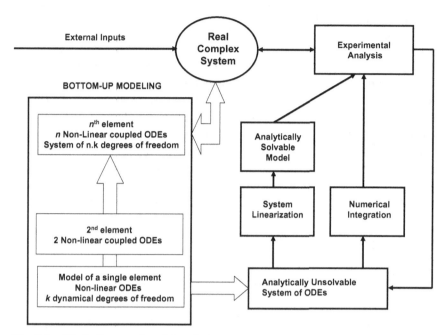

Fig. 7.1. Block diagram describing the bottom-up or microscopic modeling approach. A model is constructed coupling many systems of ODEs that accurately describe, from a mathematical point of view, a single (or microscopic) component of the complex system.

invariably to almost intractable dynamic equations. The main reason is that accurate mathematical models of a complex system single-constitutive element (the microscopic models) are in general non-linear. This means that the superposition of particular elementary solutions is not valid for generating a general solution and, consequently, no general mathematical approach for solving them exists. Two alternatives can be followed in the bottom-up approach, as illustrated in Fig. 7.1,

(i) to linearize the dynamic equations, or
(ii) to numerically integrate them.

> **Top-down** and **bottom-up** are strategies of information processing and knowledge ordering, mostly involving software models, but also other humanistic and scientific theories. They can be seen as a style of thinking and teaching; often *top-down* is used as a synonym of **analysis** and *bottom-up* of **synthesis**. A **top-down** approach is essentially breaking down a system to gain insight into its compositional sub-systems. A **bottom-up** approach, instead, is piecing together systems to give rise to grander systems, thus making the original systems sub-systems of the

emergent system. In a bottom-up approach the individual base elements of the system are first specified in great detail.

As a concrete example of the bottom-up approach, we can start with the Hodgkin–Huxley equations, frequently referred to as H–H equations, for modeling a single excitable cell (Hodgkin and Huxley, 1952); qualitative changes, known as *dynamic bifurcations*, can be derived from it by changing its parameters to obtain other behaviors qualitatively different from the excitable case, such as oscillatory or bi-stable. The Hodgkin–Huxley equations form a system of non-linear ordinary differential equations (ODEs) of the fourth order (if only the dynamics of $K^+$ and $Na^+$ ions are considered). They read,

$$C_m \frac{dV}{dt} = -g_L(V - E_L) - \tilde{g}_{Na} m^3 h (V - E_{Na}) - \tilde{g}_K n^4 (V - E_K)$$

$$\frac{dm}{dt} = \alpha_m(V)(1 - m) - \beta_m(V)m$$

$$\frac{dh}{dt} = \alpha_h(V)(1 - h) - \beta_h(V)h \qquad (7.1)$$

$$\frac{dn}{dt} = \alpha_n(V)(1 - n) - \beta_n(V)n.$$

The H–H system can be understood as a parallel electric circuit with variable conductances for potassium and sodium ions (Fig. 7.2). The first equation describes the current conservation in the system. The left term corresponds to a capacitive current due to voltage variation across the capacitor formed by the cell membrane, i.e. $C_m$ (measured in $\mu F$/unit area), and the right terms stand for the conductive currents due to the flow of sodium ($Na^+$) and potassium ($K^+$) ions plus a leakage term (L) including all other ionic current components with slower dynamics. In the above equations, $g_L = \tilde{g}_L$, $g_{Na} = \tilde{g}_{Na} m^3 h$, and $g_K = \tilde{g}_K n^4$ are the respective ionic conductances; each can be described by the product of a maximal conductance $\tilde{g}_i$ and other dynamic variables depending on the state of some ion gates. Hodgkin and Huxley in their original paper defined them as $m =$ proportion of activating molecules on the inside and $(1-m)$ their proportion on the outside; $h =$ proportion of inactivating molecules on the outside and $(1 - h)$ the proportion on the inside, both for the potassium conduction channels; $n =$ dimensionless variable between 0 and 1, which describes the proportion of activating particles for the sodium conduction channels inside the membrane while $(1 - n)$ is the proportion outside it. Besides,

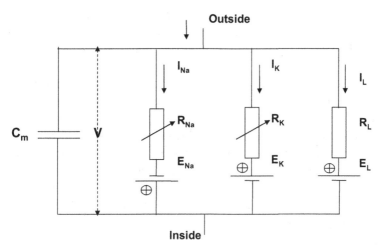

Fig. 7.2. Electric circuit representing the excitable membrane. $R_{\text{Na}} = 1/g_{\text{Na}}$; $R_{\text{K}} = 1/g_{\text{K}}$; $R_{\text{L}} = 1/g_{\text{L}}$. $R_{\text{Na}}$ and $R_{\text{K}}$ vary with time and membrane potential; the other components are constant. This is the famous model proposed by Hodgkin and Huxley in 1952.

$\alpha_{\text{n}}$ determines the rate of transfer from outside to inside and $\beta_{\text{n}}$ does it for the transfer in the opposite direction. By the same token and referring to the activating and inhibiting molecules, $\alpha_{\text{m}}$ or $\beta_{\text{h}}$ and $\beta_{\text{m}}$ or $\alpha_{\text{h}}$ represent the transfer rate constants in the two directions, respectively. Finally, $V$, $E_{\text{Na}}$, $E_{\text{K}}$, and $E_{\text{L}}$ are electric potentials measured as displacements from the resting potential $E_{\text{r}}$.

It is supposed that four identical activators govern the opening of the $K^+$ ion channels and three activators plus one inhibitor do it for the $Na^+$ channels. The parameter $n$ can be seen as the probability of the $K^+$ activator while $n^4$ would describe the conduction state; analogously, $m^3h$ represents the activation of the sodium channels. The three remaining equations describe the dynamics of the probabilities $n$, $m$, and $h$, which is supposed to be of the first order. This fact is well supported by experiments on the giant squid axon and led Hodgkin and Huxley to the uncovering of Eq. (7.1) shown above.

In general, the degrees of freedom of a given dynamic system, like the H–H equations, are defined as the number of coupled first-order differential equations needed to describe it. Thus, one speaks of low-dimensional dynamic systems whenever their degrees of freedom are a relatively small integer. If we construct an excitable tissue model by coupling many of these excitable cells (represented microscopically by the

H–H equations), we need first to choose the type of coupling among them, a difficult and very important aspect of the modeling process, indeed, for it strongly affects the resulting dynamics. Furthermore, the number of elements (cells) in the model requires estimation, preferably based on values obtained from the real tissue; finally, their spatial organization has to be established in order to determine its coupling feasibility.

All of the above amounts to building a very high-dimensional *non-linear* dynamic system of, say $\cong 10^{10}$ degrees of freedom (four first-order differential equations, that is, four dynamic degrees of freedom for **every cell** in the tissue model). As said before, there is no analytical way of solving such a system. Thus, a first attempt may be the linearization of the model, not only the equations characterizing a single element, but also any non-linearity present in the coupling terms. Thus, the coupled system becomes amenable.

> Adler and Costabel (1975), based on the DNA content of 30 human hearts from different age groups and of different weight classes, determined the total number of heart muscle cells. The number of heart muscle cells is $2 \times 10^9$ in normal hearts of children and adults, and may rise to $4 \times 10^9$ in excessively hypertrophied hearts. Thus, considering four equations per cell and the previous range of cell number, the number of degrees of freedom can be acceptably estimated as $10^{10}$.

The main drawback with linearization is that a linear system might not show the same qualitative behavior as exhibited by a non-linear one because it loses information when compared with the complete non-linear system. Paradoxically, the complete *non-linear* equations of a *single* element may show qualitative behaviors that are absolutely absent in a system of *thousands* of coupled linear differential equations. Mainly for this reason, linearization is not a very promising approach for describing complex cardiac dynamics in the bottom-up modeling approach. As an alternative strategy to cope with the loss of essential qualitative behavior, we can try to numerically integrate the original non-linear equations (instead of linearizing them). Even though this strategy offers some advantages, as for example, the possibility of running virtual experiments in a controlled way, it has many and severe drawbacks. Say,

(i) massive computing power is required (numerical integration of a huge number of non-linear differential coupled equations);

(ii) the results of the simulation are not as faithful as the data arising from the real system itself; and

(iii) simulation results are often as difficult to interpret as the real data themselves (enormous quantities of data simulating real physiological signals).

Thus, also in the case of numerical integration of the original complex ODE's system, we expect a more significant contribution from alternative top-down methods. Out of the different approaches so far available, let us refer only to the dynamic systems-based viewpoint because we consider it is the best suited for cardiac (and also neural) modeling. Dynamic systems modeling also offer a good opportunity for reducing microscopic bottom-up models to their minimal expression exhibiting simultaneously the main features of the complete model. Hence, it represents some kind of minimal modeling. It is based on three concurrent characteristics of the non-linear dynamical systems behavior, i.e.:

(i) dynamic dimensionality reduction;
(ii) complex or chaotic behavior of low-dimensional systems; and
(iii) qualitative and, to some extent, quantitative universality of the observed behavior (Gonzalez, 1987; Gonzalez and Rosso, 1997; Cartwright *et al.*, 1999a, 1999b).

In fact, a microscopic bottom-up model is characterized by a very high dimensionality. With qualitative modeling, instead (Fig. 7.3), the significant qualitative features of the complex system are described by models with only a few degrees of freedom; thus, in order to implement top-down modeling, we need usually an enormous dimensionality reduction. However, such reduction is really a natural property of non-linear dynamic systems. In a few words, one or a few dynamic modes slave a myriad of subsidiary modes, which, as a consequence of their slavery, are not relevant for the resulting dynamics. This is the so-called **dynamic dimensionality reduction property**. On the other hand, if we intend to describe complex behavior with low dimensional systems, it is required that these systems, although low dimensional, exhibit complex behavior; this is the case, indeed, in the so-called chaotic deterministic systems. Finally, the search of a qualitative model in-between the category of low dimensional dynamic systems will be an impossible task without the aid of qualitative (and to some extent quantitative) universality. Qualitative universality ensures that the relevant properties of the dynamics do not depend on the details of the system model; in other words, small perturbations of the system parameters should not break its qualitative behavior. The latter property is known

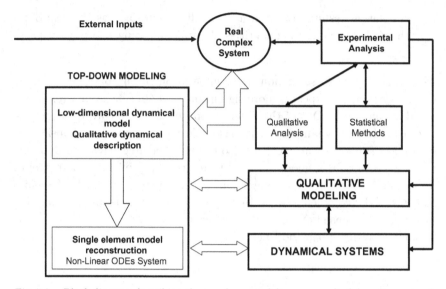

Fig. 7.3. Block diagram describing the top-down modeling approach. A low-dimensional dynamical model describing the qualitative dynamics is constructed. The main idea is to describe the relevant dynamics with a minimal model. Successively, a microscopic faithful model can also be identified. This model can serve as input for improved qualitative modeling including also bottom-up strategies.

as the *structural stability* of a system model. It is equivalent to say that large classes or categories of systems share the same qualitative dynamics. Moreover, qualitative universality is observable in real complex systems. This is because stable responses known as *dynamic attractors* exist on open regions of the parameter's space and, thus, we have a finite probability of observing them in measuring a real complex system around a neighboring parameter's space region.

Application of the above-mentioned concepts to cardiac arrhythmias such as fibrillation requires, first, to distinguish two aspects of the problem,

(i) the onset of fibrillation, and
(ii) fibrillation as an already developed condition.

Fibrillation is a condition in which control of the normal heart rhythm from the natural sinus node was lost; its onset refers to the different scenarios in which the heart loses such synchronism with the sinus node. It can be considered as a bifurcation from a periodic or almost-periodic condition and, thus, it is a phenomenon of relatively low dimensionality (for the description of a sustained oscillation a minimum of two dynamic degrees of freedom are required); sustained fibrillation, instead, implies rapid and irregular activity of the heart, when different tissue regions act apparently on their own or in uncoordinated way. It is a dynamics analogous to developed turbulence in fluids. From a medical point of view, the interest of modeling the onset of fibrillation is related to both aspects, the possibility of avoiding the arrhythmia and/or the diagnosis of a propensity of falling into it. The interest in modeling established fibrillation is exactly the inverse, that is, how to best intervene in order to revert the condition. From a dynamic point of view, the onset of fibrillation is simpler than the developed fibrillation because it can be described with fewer variables. Steady fibrillation, instead, can be thought of as a process of growth into effective dimensionality and, consequently, as getting into higher complexity.

## 7.2. Non-linear Microscopic Models of Cardiac Dynamics

Probably, the first research describing in a mechanistic way the dynamics of the heart is represented by the contribution of B. van der Pol and J. van der Mark (1928, 1929), both investigators from the Philips Physical Laboratory in The Netherlands, using electronic oscillators as analog dynamic systems. Curiously, the equation of a triode oscillator discovered by these authors became the paradigm of non-linear auto-oscillations being known today as the *van der Pol oscillator*. Such device is one of the simplest non-linear systems able to show sustained oscillations; in fact, the dynamic equation is a second-order non-linear differential equation. Notwithstanding its simplicity, several non-linear behaviors can be tested and modeled with this basic equation (or with an enlarged system of forced or coupled van der Pol oscillators). The equation reads,

$$\frac{d^2x}{dt^2} - \mu(1 - x^2)\frac{dx}{dt} + x = 0, \tag{7.2}$$

which is equivalent to a system of two coupled first-order differential equations, i.e.:

$$\frac{dx}{dt} = y$$

$$\frac{dy}{dt} = \mu(1 - x^2)\frac{dx}{dt} - x. \tag{7.3}$$

Putting the van der Pol equation in this form shows explicitly that there are two dynamic degrees of freedom corresponding to the variables $x$ and $y$. Years later, Bonhoeffer (1948, 1953), in Germany, using these equations came up with an iron model of a neuron. These equations, in the final form given by FitzHugh (1961), are also called the Bonhoeffer–van der Pol oscillator.

The main difference between a linear and a non-linear oscillator is related to the stability of the oscillations. A linear oscillator is marginally stable, meaning that the amplitude of the oscillator is undefined: any perturbation alters the oscillation amplitude. On the contrary, a non-linear auto-oscillator shows one or more stable solutions defining oscillations with definite amplitude. Such solutions are termed in the Poincaré terminology *limit cycles*, that is, stable trajectories reached by the temporal evolution as an asymptotic limit.

If the parameter $\mu$ in the van der Pol equation is very low, the oscillations are nearly linear; they resemble a sinusoidal function (actually, it is slightly deformed because of the presence of weak harmonics). When this parameter grows, the non-linearity increases, too, and the waveform becomes more and more deformed and tends to what is called a *relaxation oscillation*. A distinct characteristic of this kind of oscillations is that they remain almost constant for a long period and, suddenly, go onto a different state, and thus the cycle restart. There are many examples of this behavior in the real world, as the case of the cover of a boiling water pot, which maintains a pulsated periodic steam leak.

In Fig. 7.4 we can see the temporal evolution of the van der Pol oscillator $x$ and its derivative $y$ for a value of the equation's parameter $\mu = 1$. The variable $x$ can be thought of as the position of the oscillator and $y$ as its velocity at a given instant. More insight can be gained if we represent the oscillation in a plane called the *phase plane* (this is part of the geometrical methods developed by Henry Poincaré for studying systems of non-linear ODEs at the end of the nineteenth century). Such plane is defined by the dynamic variables, in our case, the variables defining the van der Pol oscillator, i.e. $x, y$, the position and the velocity of the oscillator, both represented on the horizontal and vertical axes, respectively. Figure 7.5 displays a phase plane representation of the van der Pol oscillator evolution. Interesting aspects appear as outstanding characteristics: irrespective of the initial condition, the point describing the solution of the oscillator tends to a fixed curve that describes the stable auto-oscillations (the limit cycle, consisting of the points in the figure most elongated from the origin and forming a closed curve). Moreover, initial conditions near the origin tend to evolve away from this point (following the arrows in Fig. 7.5); thus, the origin is an unstable point or focus because all trajectories revolve around it.

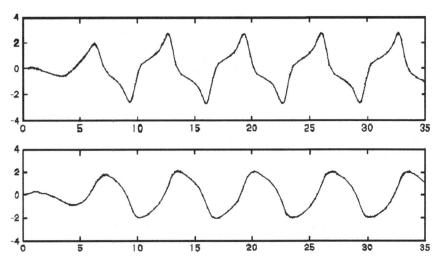

Fig. 7.4. Temporal evolution of the solutions of the van der Pol oscillator (the abscissae represent time, $t$). Upper trace: Ordinate position ($x$ variable). Lower trace: Velocity or position derivative, $y$. The parameter $\mu$ controls the non-linearity. Both plots correspond to $\mu = 1$; smaller values lead to more linear oscillations (not represented) and at the limit 0, the oscillation becomes a pure sinusoid. Larger values produce non-linear oscillations quite similar to a square waveform.

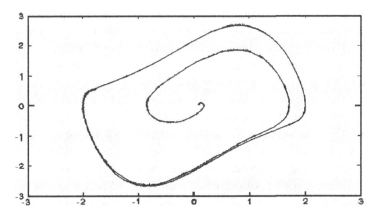

Fig. 7.5. Phase-plane representation of the van der Pol oscillator. Same parameters as in Figure 7.4 with an initial condition very close to the origin $(0,0)$. Coordinates correspond to $x$ and its derivative $y$ and, thus, can be interpreted as the position and the velocity of the oscillator, respectively, at a given instant (Eq. (7.3)). The trajectory converges to a closed curve or limit cycle, i.e., a stable oscillatory solution with definite amplitude, typical behavior of auto-oscillatory nonlinear systems.

   The observation of the qualitative behavior of a forced non-linear oscillator with an unstable focus led to one of the first predictions for heart dynamics (Winfree, 1983). This investigator first analyzed the phase evolution of non-linear oscillators by means of a map or recurrence where the old phase is written as a function of the new phase attained after the application of a suited perturbation. In fact, if we launch two non-linear oscillators and an impulsive excitation is applied to one of them, after a transient the two oscillators attain the cycle limit oscillation but the perturbed one has a different oscillation phase. Following the strength of the perturbation, the phase map shows topological changes: The phase may vary slightly with respect to the unperturbed oscillation and, thus, shows a complete excursion around all its possible values. This defines a Type 1 phase map that can be considered as a perturbation from the identity, i.e. new phase = old phase; or it may remain confined to a phase interval without completing a circle over the phase of the unperturbed oscillator. This defines a Type 0 phase map (0 turns of the new phase for a complete oscillator cycle). This topological change of the phase map implies that there exists an appropriate stimulus which leads the oscillator to an undefined phase (a singularity or singular point). Winfree performed experiments for determining phase maps in real biological systems, but all these observations have their counterpart in the dynamics of non-linear oscillators. Usually, if we perturb a non-linear oscillator (as the van der Pol) with a periodic impulsive force, the associated phase map is of topological Type 1 for small amplitudes of the perturbation, and of Type 0 for high amplitudes. If a perturbation with an amplitude equal to the oscillation amplitude (in-between the former two cases) is applied just when the oscillator traverses the position $x = 0$ (the so-called vulnerable phase), the forcing leads the oscillator into the unstable focus producing a temporary death of the oscillation and, consequently, an ambiguity of the phase. Indeed, Winfree demonstrated the existence of the vulnerable phase in an experimental biological system, i.e. the circadian rhythms of a population of flies (Winfree, 1970). Interpreting oscillation silencing as the onset of conditions for triggering fibrillation, Winfree advanced on this basis the idea for an explanation of the Sudden Death Syndrome, notwithstanding any drawback or controversial opinions it might carry. In fact, a simple electrical stimulus of the right strength at just the right time (phase) could produce a pair of singularities, similar to those described above, around which two counter-rotating spiral waves can form; in turn, these spiral waves can destabilize dramatically the normal cardiac dynamics and lead to complex cardiac functional derangements. Hence, there is an attractive and intrinsic conceptual power arising from the qualitative analysis of non-linear differential equations. In fact, the study of phase maps (related to the concepts of phase resetting and transition) has inspired many key studies (Jalife and Antzelevich, 1979; Guevara *et al.*, 1981; Glass and Perez, 1982; Glass *et al.*, 1984; Gonzalez and Piro, 1984) and continue to be a source of insight in heart complex dynamics (Glass *et al.*, 2002; Croisier *et al.*, 2009).

**Jules Henri Poincaré** (1854–1912) was a French mathematician and theoretical physicist. He made several fundamental contributions, as for example, the concept of chaotic deterministic system, so laying the foundations of modern chaos theory. Besides, Poincaré introduced the principle of relativity and was the first to present the Lorentz transformation in its symmetrical form, as preliminary essential step in the formulation of the current theory of special relativity.

**Balthasar van der Pol** (1889–1959), Dutch, studied physics in Utrecht. Besides, he was also a student of John Ambrose Fleming and Sir J.J. Thomson in England, joining Philips Research Labs in 1921, where he worked until his retirement in 1949. His main interests were radio wave propagation, theory of electrical circuits, and mathematical physics. He was awarded the Institute of Radio Engineers (IRE, now IEEE) Medal of Honor in 1935.

**Karl Friedrich Bonhoeffer** (1899–1957) studied with Walther Nernst. He was successively professor of physical chemistry at the Universities of Berlin, Frankfurt, and Leipzig, returning to Berlin in 1947. In 1949, he was appointed director of the Max Planck Institute for Physical Chemistry in Goettingen. The institute was restructured long after his death in 1971 and is now named after him. In 1929 Bonhoeffer, together with Paul Harteck, discovered orthohydrogen and parahydrogen. Bernhardt Hassenstein was also one of his collaborators working out the properties of insect motion detection. Karl was an older brother of the martyred theologian Dietrich Bonhoeffer (1906–1945), who participated in the resistance against Nazism (http://es.wikipedia.org/wiki/Dietrich_Bonhoeffer). The author of this book, MEV, when a young engineering student met personally Dr. Hassenstein during a visit to Argentina after an invitation of Drs. Josué Núñez, a behavioral biologist, and Máximo Valentinuzzi, a biophysicist and MEV's father.

**Arthur Taylor Winfree** (1942–2002) was a theoretical biologist who produced significant mathematical modeling of biological phenomena. He became interested in the spontaneous synchronization of populations of biological oscillators. For example, the pacemaker region of the heart with its thousands of cells that produce a regular, collective rhythm of electrical signals. In some species of fireflies, males congregate in a tree and flash in synchrony to the presumed delight of their lady friends. Thousands of slime mould cells secrete synchronous pulses of cyclic AMP, a molecular signal that calls them to forego their solitary existence and adopt a communal lifestyle. For all this and more, he shared the 2000 Norbert Wiener Prize with Alexandre Chorin, among other distinctions (Tyson and Glass, 2004).

Interestingly enough, a slight modification of the van der Pol oscillator leads to a simplified model of the Hodgkin–Huxley equations. In fact, canceling the non-linear term in the dissipation, i.e. $(x^2 dx/dt)$, and adding a non-linear term in the restoring force, i.e. $V^3/3$, the well-known system of FitzHugh–Nagumo (FHN) equations is obtained (FitzHugh, 1961; Nagumo *et al.*, 1962),

$$\dot{V} = V - \frac{V^3}{3} - W + I$$

$$\dot{W} = \varepsilon(aV - bW + c). \tag{7.4}$$

The FHN equation is a new interpretation of the H–H equations, which started with the Bonhoeffer equation mentioned previously; thus, perhaps they ought to be better abbreviated as BVDP-FHN. As a simplified (two-dimensional) version of the H–H equations, $V$ represents the membrane potential, $W$ can be associated to a recovery variable, whereas $I$ represents the external driving current and $\varepsilon$, $a$, $b$, and $c$ are the model parameters. From a dynamic point of view, the BVDP-FHN equations allow the separation of the responses in two different paths, a slow one, and a fast one, typical of relaxation oscillators. Doing so, it is possible to study geometrically the effect of the excitation and separate it from the successive evolution of the equations. Figure 7.6 displays the possible responses as a function of the system parameters and stimulus amplitude. This example, extensively used in cardiac modeling, shows the usefulness of the Qualitative Theory of the ODEs of Poincaré at work. First, as previously shown in the case of the van der Pol equations, the phase plane representation is used. By and large, we have an $n$-dimensional phase space, but in this case the BVDP-FHN equations have two dynamic degrees of freedom and, thus, two variables (a plane) suffice for describing the evolution. The intersection of the curves determines the position of the fixed point. This is because the two curves simply represent the geometrical locus where derivatives in Eq. (7.4) are null, i.e. the fixed point resolves simultaneously the two equations,

$$W = V - V/3 + I$$

$$W = (a/b)V + (c/b). \tag{7.5}$$

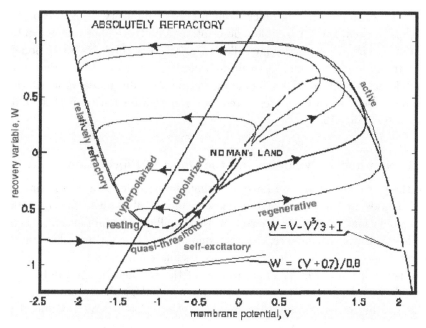

Fig. 7.6.   Phase-space representation of the possible trajectories of the Bonhoeffer-van der Pol–FitzHugh–Nagumo equations, for $e$ or epsilon = 0.08, $a = 1, b = 0.8, c = 0.7$.

As the derivatives indicate the rate of change of the respective variables, this fixed point, where all derivatives cancel, is necessarily a resting point (without some perturbation the system cannot exit from such point). Moreover, we can complicate a little more the picture by taking into account the effect of the stimulus current (fixed or impulsive, as typical in physiological experiments). The effect of a constant current can be interpreted as a vertical translation of the second null curve with the N shape (observe the first of Eqs. (7.5)). As the stability of the fixed point depends on the location along this curve, the excitation can change the stability of that point and consequently the associated dynamics. When the fixed point is on the middle branch of the N-shaped curve (No Man's Land in Fig. 7.6), the singularity is unstable and thus the trajectories go necessarily away from this region determining autonomous oscillations. In this way, we can explain the transition between excitable and auto-oscillatory regimes produced by current injection (displacement of the fixed point from the No Man's Land region to one of the branches of the N-shaped region), and many stationary and transient phenomena which are typical of physiological experiments on excitable cells; for example, spiking block at high current intensity or excitation by impulsive excitation. A complete description of all these phenomena can be found at http://www.scholarpedia.org/article/FitzHugh-Nagumo_model. The transition from excitable to auto-oscillating states has also been studied in different models of ODEs, including an exact solvable model in which the current injection can be interpreted as a renormalization term (Feingold, Gonzalez *et al.*, 1988).

### 7.3. Non-linear Dynamics and the Onset of Fibrillation

In the previous section, we have seen that the presence of a singularity — i.e. a node in the origin of the phase plane — allows the phenomenon of oscillation death. Of course, if the oscillation annihilation affects a key natural pacemaker, as the sino-auricular one, the absence of excitation can free the heart tissue to assume complex behaviors, which are normally initiated by amplification of the residual background noise. Oscillation disappearance is caused by a topological characteristic of the non-linear oscillation that manifests the existence of a vulnerable phase (corresponding also to a defined magnitude excitation). Oscillation death has been experimentally observed by stimulating the sinus node (Jalife and Antzelevich, 1979; Guevara *et al.*, 1981) and also in self-oscillating squid axons (Guttman *et al.*, 1980). The same dynamics has been observed also in auto-oscillating Purkinje fibers (Jalife and Antzelevich, 1979) notwithstanding the very different characteristics of this kind of tissue. Oscillation annihilation can be found, too, on a single H–H cell model and represents a universal behavior of impulsively forced hard-oscillators (Cechi *et al.*, 1993). Moreover, the concept of phase resetting, associated in principle with an auto-oscillator, can be extended to excitable systems, which can be driven dynamically to oscillating states of similar properties (Feingold *et al.*, 1988). However, the probability that in normal circumstances an impulse of the appropriate amplitude hit the natural pacemaker, particularly during the vulnerable phase, is indeed very low (excluding the possibility of an external random excitation applied over a long time or a controlled electrical shock for obtaining such result). Moreover, this mechanism is in some sense static, that is, it does not involve in itself a complex dynamic behavior (there are other means to causing oscillation death, for example, asynchronic extinction, which consists of a periodic forcing of very high frequency compared with the natural oscillator frequency). More interesting than the vulnerable phase resetting is the possibility of having truly complex dynamic behavior and to studying the associated bifurcation routes that a system may follow for entering into those states, that is, the different dynamic routes to fibrillation.

As previously noted, established fibrillation is not expected to be well described by a low dimensional model; however, the normal heart dynamics is low dimensional and, thus, we may expect the onset of fibrillation to be associated with the destabilization of such at a lower-dimensional behavior (the breaking of a low-dimensional dynamic attractor). In this sense, many studies of non-linear dynamics have contributed to elucidating the different routes followed by a system to attain complex dynamics. In fact, one of the most important routes is known as the Feigenbaum scenario (Feigenbaum, 1978, 1980) or period-doubling bifurcation route to chaos. This route appeared to be relevant for studying the transition to developed fibrillation in cardiac dynamics. Different clinical studies have revealed that a period-doubling bifurcation in different heart physiological signals is strongly correlated with severe arrhythmia risk and, in fact, it is used as a predictor for sudden death risk (Karma and Gilmour, 2007). The period-doubling bifurcation is also known in cardiology as electrical alternans (Traube, 1872), manifested as a different waveform amplitude from one oscillation to the following one. Alternans can be seen in the T-wave portion of the electrocardiogram and also in the concentration of $Ca^{+2}$ ions. As this period-doubling is a signature of the Feigenbaum route to chaos, it appears sound to ask whether if we are indeed observing the initial state of that route when detecting such physiological signals. In fact, the Feigenbaum route to chaos has been experimentally observed in toad ventricles, as illustrated in Fig. 7.7 (Savino *et al.*, 1989). The electric alternans are clearly observed in Panel A together with the corresponding component at half the pacing frequency in the Fourier spectrum (on the right hand). In the second panel, the next period-doubling response producing a Fourier component at $1/4$ of the pacing frequency is clearly observed. The last panel displays the broadband spectrum typical of noisy or chaotic signals; this corresponds to the transition to chaos after the accumulation of period-doubling bifurcations (see also Giannerini *et al.*, 2007). The Fourier spectrum can give significant information about the onset of ventricular fibrillation as the former case illustrates.

**Electrical alternans and pulsus alternans.** The first term is a broad term that describes alternate-beat variation in any component of the ECG waveforms. It was first recognized by Hearing in 1908–1909 and further characterized by Sir Thomas Lewis in 1910. Kalter and Schwartz first identified electrical alternans on surface ECG in 1948. It must be distinguished from mechanical alternans (pulsus alternans), as

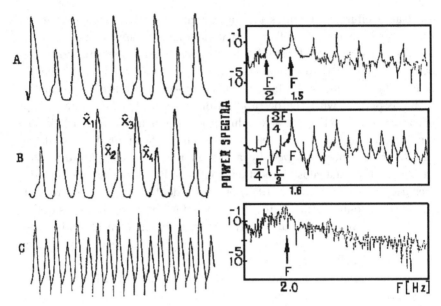

Fig. 7.7. Period doubling in paced toad ventricle. A: Period doubling (electrical alternans) observed in signals obtained from the epicardium by means of a suction electrode. B: A second period doubling bifurcation; amplitudes returned to the original value after four cycles; until the third period doubling bifurcation (Period 8) was observed in this experiment. C: Ventricular fibrillation with aperiodic variation in amplitude. Right hand panels: Fourier power spectra for each case (after Savino *et al.*, 1989, with permission).

originally described by Traube (1872), although both may coexist. Often both terms are loosely used without making the distinction. Electrical alternans may occur without a concomitant pulsus alternans.

However, heart dynamics is very different in mammals than in amphibians. Perfused toad ventricles do not suffer from circulation deficiency when entering in abnormal dynamics because their tissue is able to maintain its metabolic activity by passive particle exchange; conversely, for a mammalian heart, falling into fibrillation affects the coronary circulation and worsens its dysfunction by blood supply tissular deficiency. In toad ventricle, it has been demonstrated, too, that the sustained fibrillation is of relative low dimensionality and could be characterized by a transient state with two positive Lyapunov exponents (Giannerini *et al.*, 2007); it returns spontaneously to normal function after stimulation disruption. In recent mammalian studies, it has been demonstrated, however, that spatial distribution of alternans affects the triggering of fibrillation. In fact, the dangerous pre-fibrillation state is characterized by a spatial heterogeneity regarding the phase of the alternans: some tissular regions display alternans which are inverted with respect to others in somewhat distant regions. In other words, when the oscillation appears with given amplitude in one ventricular region, it may be smaller or bigger in other neighbor area or vice versa. This fact shows that an important spatial cardiac non-homogeneity can be produced as a consequence of the dynamic regime, even in the absence of other pathological causes.

The latter findings and ideas lead to the concept of cardiac dynamic disease and point out to the importance of understanding dynamic instabilities for therapeutic purposes. No doubt, insight can be gained in the understanding of these complex phenomena mainly through the use of appropriate models. Prior to describing how spatial non-homogeneities may trigger complex spatial dynamics and, in particular, sustained fibrillation, we mention that other scenarios different from the period-doubling route to chaos are feasible for entering into a complex situation; all of these imply a number of successive bifurcations from a low-dimensional attractor when one or more key parameters are changed. Among the different routes to chaos, the quasi-periodic one shows up as very important. In such case, new incommensurate frequencies are dynamically added to the fundamental frequency of a non-linear oscillator until the oscillation destabilizes and ends up in a chaotic state. Outstanding in this case, the Newhouse–Ruelle–Takens Theorem (Newhouse *et al.*, 1978), for short NRT, clearly establishes the necessary conditions for this kind of dynamic destabilization. In simple terms, the theorem says that, in addition to the natural oscillation frequency, the generation of other two incommensurate frequencies suffices for destabilizing the system and so ending into chaotic oscillations. In such scenario, the possible behavior of ⋅higher complexity prior to chaos is called a three-frequency resonance (Cartwright *et al.*, 1999a, 1999b), corresponding to a particular case of two-frequency quasi-periodicity: three incommensurate frequencies satisfy a Diophantine relation (a linear combination with integer coefficients). The NRT theorem implies that in a real system we cannot observe truly three-frequency quasi-periodicity (three simultaneous incommensurate frequencies) because infinitesimal perturbations of the system drive it onto a chaotic attractor. Destabilization to a quasi-periodic solution is highlighted in the phase space by the grouping of iterated points around the neighborhood of a torus surface (a tube closed in itself or a doughnut-like shape). In fact, this behavior has been observed in both, experimental and simulation data of ventricular fibrillation (Weiss *et al.*, 1999).

**Incommensurate frequencies.** Two frequencies are commensurate when there are two positive integers, $p$ and $q$, that satisfy the equation $f_2/f_1 = p/q$, or, in other words, when the frequency ratio is rational. If no integers satisfy the above equation, the frequencies are said to be incommensurate or irrational (Hilborn, 2001).

**Diophantine equation** is an indeterminate polynomial that allows the variables to be only integers. Diophantine problems have fewer equations than unknown variables and involve finding integers that work correctly for all equations. The word *Diophantine* refers to the mathematician of the third century, Diophantus of Alexandria, who made a study of such equations (http://en.wikipedia.org/wiki/Diophantine_equation).

We should mention that other scenarios have been studied for the transition to chaos from periodic oscillations in relation to cardiac dynamics, mainly as in the case of intermittency, which consists of bursts of periodic activity followed by irregular silent periods (Pomeau and Manneville, 1980). The most relevant scenarios for fibrillation, however, seem to be the quasi-periodicity chaos route and the Feigenbaum one, the latter preceded by the birth of alternans, either in electrical or chemical cardiac signals. Moreover, the above-mentioned mechanism for creating dynamic spatial non-homogeneities and to destabilize normal heart beating may lead to the creation of spiral waves in the surface of the cardiac tissue. Spiral waves are an extended phenomenon dealt with in the following section and that has been observed in different experiments and corresponding spatial non-linear models. In particular, spiral waves are typical of the well-known chemical reaction called the Belousov–Zabotinsky reaction (Belousov, 1959; Zhabotinsky, 1964), which easily generates also concentric (spherical) waves. Bidimensional spiral waves are produced around a point singularity and can interact with the normal wave mode of the heart or interfere constructively or destructively and create the conditions for fibrillation triggering.

Thus, from a medical point of view, it is of great interest that the research focuses on methods for avoiding the onset of spatial alternans. Actual therapy makes use of electrical and chemical means but, in both cases, there is not a clear understanding of the dynamic consequences of the intervening procedures with the extreme case that the administration of anti-arrhythmic drugs can raise the risk of cardiac sudden death (CAST (1989) and SWORD (1996) trials). From a dynamic point of view, this is part of the theory of control of dynamic systems and some new results are encouraging for controlling electrical alternans; for example, by applying control to a point in a cable of Purkinje fibers we can eliminate the spatial alternance (Karma and Gilmour, 2007).

## 7.4. Extended Models and Connection with Sustained Fibrillation

As we have pointed out in the previous section, electrical alternans seem to be the most probable bifurcation route for the onset of fibrillation. In fact, once spatial alternans have developed, there is an increased probability of ventricular tachycardia (VT) as a state previous to fibrillation. It is generally accepted that these pathological states are maintained by means of wave reentry. Ventricular tissue is excitable and, as such, characterized by an excitation threshold and a refractory period. The excitation threshold represents the minimal amount of excitation needed to triggering the impulse; once excited, the single cell needs a variable time for repolarizing and, thus, becoming ready for another excitation. Repolarization and depolarization are provided mainly by the inward and outward currents of calcium and sodium ions through the cellular membrane. This description is approximate because the form of the excitation and the response depend also on the cell dynamics (mainly due to the polarization state of the cell when reached by the excitation front); in fact, the threshold level is not constant but a function of the repolarizing process (depending also on the influx of other ions, as for example $Ca^{+2}$). In a normal heart cycle, a wave starting in the sinus node propagates, passes through the auricles, and produces a single contraction in the ventricular cells. Once the activation wave has passed, single cells repolarize and remain in an idle state ready for the next excitation. However, in the presence of anatomical or dynamical heterogeneities (ischemia, blocks), the normal single wave can break and generate many new waves (wavelets) that may spread in different directions. The main consequence of such wave breaking is that some re-entering paths can be activated, that is, an anomalous wave following a closed path different from the normal one may be excited. However, certain dynamic conditions need to be met for sustaining the propagation of such reentry waves. First, the front end of the anomalous reentry wave needs to reach regions sufficiently repolarized in the closed path. This possibility depends, in turn, on the relationship between the wave propagation velocity and the reentry path length; the condition for reentry, thus, will be that the travel time along the path, i.e. $\tau_p = c/L$ — where $c$ represents the wave propagation velocity and $L$ the path length — be greater than the refractory period $\tau_R$ (the time needed for repolarization of the cell) (see also Chap. 1). In the normal heart cycle, one excitable cell is excited once in a complete cycle and the time interval comprised between two successive excitations is sufficiently long to ensure complete repolarization, that is, $\tau_R \gg c/L$. However, heterogeneities of physiological and/or dynamical origin may break the former inequality opening the door for the triggering of different arrhythmias and fibrillation. Dynamic causes may be as simple as ectopic excitations, the wrong pulse at the wrong phase. Also tachycardia can produce dynamic instabilities because increase in beat frequency diminishes the time available for repolarization. The induced refractory abnormalities would produce, in turn, breaking of normal waves and the birth of reentry paths. We know that one of the most common behaviors observed in these reentry waves is the genesis of spiral waves. Spiral waves are excitation vortices moving around a singular region, usually an unstable focus. As mentioned before, spiral waves have been observed first in a typical non-linear chemical system, the Belousov–Zabotinsky reaction (1959, 1964) and are also characteristic of the route to fibrillation in heart dynamics. In Fig. 7.8 we can see spiral and concentric waves in the Belousov–Zabotinsky reaction implemented on a Petri dish.

Bidimensional spiral waves in the B–Z reaction have been reported by Winfree in 1972. They are natural in a system as described in Fig. 7.8 because the third dimension often can be neglected. However, Winfree asked himself about the organization of spiral waves in a true three-dimensional case (that is, when the third spatial dimension of the chemical reaction cannot be neglected). In doing this, Winfree (1973) discovered that spiral

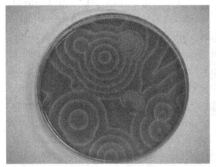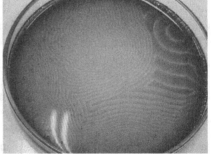

Fig. 7.8. Belusov–Zabotinsky (B–Z) reaction showing concentration fronts shaping up different geometrical patterns. The most common are spiral and concentric waves. (Courtesy of Oreste Piro).

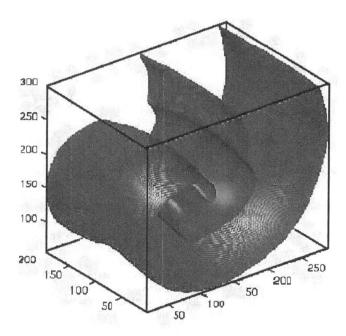

Fig. 7.9. Representation of a scroll wave. Observe the intersection of the scroll wave with the $(x, y)$ surface forming a spiral. The spiral is organized around a singular point, which prolongs in the depth dimension as singular filament (R.H. Keldermann, University of Utrecht, 3D Organization of Ventricular Fibrillation in a Heterogeneous Model of the Human Ventricles, 21-06-2006; http://bioinformatics.bio.uu.nl/rikkert/talks/CLS.pdf; with permission).

waves prolonged in the third dimension forming a three-dimensional "scroll" wave or rotor (Fig. 7.9). Scroll waves are organized around a line or filament of singular points. The appearance of the scroll wave on the reaction surface is such of a spiral wave organized around a singular point; the singular point truly is the end point of the singular filament on the reaction limit surface.

Multiple ectopics can be mainly considered as a cause, not a description of sustained fibrillation. Thus, spiral reentry waves and 3D rotors remain as the spatial description of fibrillation. The picture of sustained fibrillation at present should be described in simple words as follows: the ventricular surface may be viewed as a sea of little reentry waves, usually also spirals, wandering on the ventricles; these waves arise from destabilization of one or a few greater spiral waves formed around an anatomical or dynamical singularity. Interestingly enough, if we reduce the singular region to a single cell or to a region comprising a few cells, the description of this singularity

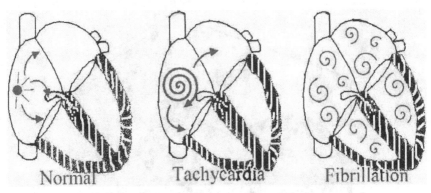

Fig. 7.10. Scheme of the transition to fibrillation. The normal cycle breaks in a tachycardia state characterized by one or a few great spiral waves. These waves rotate around a singular point and are preceded by a first duplication of period (alternans) and the spatial spread of such dynamical heterogeneity (spatial alternans). In a successive step, the mother spiral waves break in many smaller ones creating a state of chaotic excitation. These waves are scroll waves continuing deep in the ventricular tissue and organized around singularity filaments (for more details see R.H. Keldermann, Univ. of Utrecht, 3D Organization of Ventricular Fibrillation in a Heterogeneous Model of the Human Ventricles, 21-06-2006, slide presentation; http://bioinformatics.bio.uu.nl/rikkert/talks/CLS.pdf). With permission.

can be performed by using a low-dimensional model, as described in the previous section. The scheme of the transition to fibrillation, as seen on the ventricular surface, is illustrated in Fig. 7.10. The three-dimensional version of a scroll wave or rotor and transition to fibrillation were well depicted by Clayton *et al.* (2006), showing that the number of filaments increase substantially in the case of ventricular fibrillation. Moreover, filaments evolve in time; once generated, such one-dimensional singularities can move on the ventricle maintaining their dynamic features. The induced pathological dynamics can produce new singularities and also two singularities can merge and eventually annihilate or reduce to one. Thus, the evolution and spatial distribution of these singularities seem to be the key for the description of sustained ventricular fibrillation (Kirsten, 2007).

In order to understand sustained fibrillation and the therapy methods for stopping it, we need to resort to models of spatially extended systems of excitable cells. For modeling purposes, spatial structure represents a step further along the path of increasing complexity from simple systems, like a single forced auto-oscillator exhibiting only temporal complexity. However, we expect a "minimal qualitative model" description of sustained fibrillation; in fact, as the more recent simulations and experimental data show, also in the case of sustained fibrillation we have highly organized patterns of spatial complexity which are mainly represented by wandering reentry wavelets. By using statistical methods we can estimate the effective dimension of an unknown complex system (see following section). When applied to sustained fibrillation, these methods confirm that a great dimensionality reduction is attained, mainly due to the phenomena of dynamic auto-organization and mode slaving. Moreover, the property of qualitative universality may also be extended to these kinds of systems.

Thus, it is expected that the description of the relevant dynamics should be amenable to a drastic dimensionality reduction and that the main dynamical features should be described qualitatively in a universal manner, that is, not depending on the details of the system model. In fact, as described before, the B–Z reaction shows the same kind of behavior encountered in fibrillation and the associated precursor states, that is, spiral and concentric waves in two dimensions and rotors and singularity filaments in three dimensions. These are universal features exhibited by large classes of numerical and experimental systems. As an example, Fig. 7.11 shows another interesting biological system sharing similar qualitative dynamics (Cartwright *et al.*, 2009). That figure displays double spiralled concentric waves of mineralization (see also Fig. 7.8), which characterize the growth of nacre in bivalves.

As said before, for building a model we need to define the microscopic model of one constitutive element and the form of the coupling between such excitable elements. If for the microscopic excitable cell we choose a model of

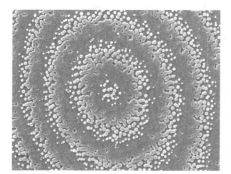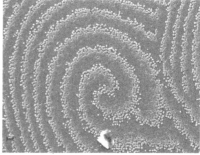

Fig. 7.11.   Concentric (left) and double spiral (right) waves in the growth of nacre in bivalve molluscs (after Cartwright *et al.*, 2009, with authors' permission). Nacre (or mother pearl) is an organic–inorganic composite material produced by some molluscs.

cardiac or neural excitable tissue, as for example the H–H equations or its simplified form, the BVDP-FHNs, we obtain an extended or spatial model of cardiac dynamics. Normally, these models are bidimensional in the form of an array of, say, $n$ by $n$ excitable elements, placed on a surface. However, the real heart tissue is three-dimensional and, thus, faithful models need also taking into account phenomena related to the tissue depth dimension. The consequences of this dimensional choice are also very important and are at the basis of our present knowledge about developed fibrillation. What is observed is that point singularities of the ventricular surface extend deeply in the tissue and produce a singularity filament. Rotor waves, which represent the extended versions of the planar spiral waves while maintaining and axial symmetry, are organized around these one-dimensional filaments.

The different models used to study rotor generation differ on the microscopic models utilized for describing a single excitable cell and on the mathematical form of the coupling terms between different cells. Microscopic models have evolved from the original FHN and H–H equations described in Sec. 3 to more sophisticated systems, which take into account the currents produced by other ions. Historically, the first modification of the H–H equation aimed at describing excitable heart cells was the Noble equations (1962). Such ODEs replicate very well the shape of the action potential and predicted new ionic currents that were later discovered. Mainly, the potassium current term was split into an instantaneous current and a slowly activating one (a consequence of the finding of two kinds of potassium channels in Purkinje fibers), and a current due to chloride anions was simultaneously introduced. Reuter (1967) basically demonstrated the existence of calcium channels. This feature together with the addition of further slow components in the potassium current led finally to the first model of a ventricular cell, the Beeler–Reuter model (1977). Successively, incorporation of sodium–calcium exchange led to the Di Francesco–Noble model (1985), and the same exchange during the action potential to the Hilgemann–Noble (1987) and Earn–Noble (1990) models. These models led in turn to the different versions of the Luo–Rudy model (1994a, 1994b) and became the starting point for recent models of excitation–contraction coupling. There exist actually more than 30 models of heart cells electrical activity (see, for example, *www.cellml.org*) and the historical review by Noble (2007). Of course, any of them can be used for building spatially extended 2D and 3D models of cardiac excitation by defining appropriate coupling between single cells. The common features they show are related to the comparison of rotors in 3D models, and spiral, and concentric waves in their analog 2D counterparts. For chemically mediated coupling, the coupling term is often of the diffusive type (the spatial diffusion of some chemical due to relative chemical gradients). We arrive in this way, i.e. coupling diffusively many spatially distributed excitable elements, at the so-called reaction–diffusion systems (see for example Ellner and Guckenheimer, 2006, Chap. 7: Spatial Patterns in Biology). As an example, we can build an extended model of the reaction–diffusion type based on the BVDP-FHN equations, say,

$$\dot{V} = V - \frac{V^3}{3} - W + I + \frac{\partial^2 V}{\partial x^2}$$
$$\dot{W} = \varepsilon(aV - bW + c). \tag{7.6}$$

Coupling is introduced here as a second partial derivative of the membrane potential $V$ with respect to the spatial variable $x$; the model describes a diffusive-like dynamics and is analytically tractable, easily allowing extraction of very useful information about its fundamental dynamic behavior.

The qualitative behavior of the extended, or reaction–diffusion BVDP-FHN equations, coincide with the general features described before, i.e. the comparison of concentric (spherical in 3D) waves, or mother giant spiral waves (rotor or scroll waves in 3D), the breaking of spiral waves in wandering wavelets, the development of singular points around spiral waves (spiral filaments and rotors in 3D) and others.

More complex extended models seem to give the same qualitative behavior related to spiral and rotor waves, either in two or in three dimensions. In this respect, the Luo–Rudy (1994a, 1994b) based model or also the simplified Kley and Bar one (Cao *et al.*, 2007), or a comparison (Zaritski *et al.*, 2005) between Pushchino, Barkley, Winfree, and two-component Oregonator model, a variant of the B-Z reaction, can be mentioned.

Thus, ventricular fibrillation seems to be a highly organized phenomenon and should be potentially modeled as such, i.e. by a deterministic non-linear dynamic model of reduced dimension, despite its spatially extended, higher dimensional character. This fact opens the door for having truly predictive models which can be used for preventive and therapeutic scopes. Moreover, increased model dimensionality by using more accurate microscopic models and/or more constitutive elements do not ensure more faithful dynamic description/prediction but increase the computational power needed for numerical integration and increase the complexity of the parameters to be explored, thus, rendering difficult the interpretation of related experimental results.

Simplified models of cardiac dynamics offer many opportunities beyond the purely academic interest: Understanding of the dynamic bifurcations that a generic system shows while attaining spatial complexity (fibrillation) should be the basis for developing methods directed to avoiding entering into such dangerous states (see, for example, Weiss *et al.*, 1999, and Karma, 2000, for drug fibrillation therapy and prevention). Moreover, the same approach can be used for attaining the difficult task of stopping developed fibrillation (see Weiss *et al.*, 2000, for 2D control, and Cao *et al.*, 2007, for 3D control, in which the inverse path from fibrillation to normal beating passing from scroll, and spherical waves, can be followed using the Barkley and Bar models).

## 7.5. Statistical Analysis

### 7.5.1. *To Begin With*

It is widely accepted that chaos and non-linear dynamical system theory provide a new paradigm for the analysis of time series. New tools and techniques are available to practitioners and the availability of computing power renders their application almost straightforward. Still, the adoption of rigorous statistical methods is strongly required in this field. In fact, it is not uncommon to have articles that propose new and interesting approaches that result somehow *ad hoc*, or heuristic. Also, the casual reader might find awkward that books that have the same title *"Non-linear time series analysis"* are, actually, very different (see e.g. Kantz and Schreiber, 2004; Fan and Yao, 2003). No doubt, putting together non-linear dynamicists and statisticians is well worth the effort.

Non-linear dynamics gives us many exploratory tools for the characterization of physiological signals. Combination of such tools together with rigorous statistical methods would allow inferring many peculiar features that, in first instance, answer to questions such as classifying and diagnosing pathological signals; secondly, they provide valuable information for building a model in a subsequent step. In the following, we review some of the most important issues when facing complex systems from a statistical point of view. Due to space constraints, many arguments are touched briefly, many others are missing. Besides the above-mentioned references, we refer to Abarbanel (1996), Chan and Tong (2001), Mees (2001), Small (2005), and Cutler and Kaplan (1997) as good starting points for the interested reader.

A first important issue deals with the reconstruction of the whole state space of the process when just one or few time series components are available. Let us introduce some notation. A dynamical system can be described by specifying $(i)$ a rule that governs the evolution of the process and $(ii)$ the space in which the process takes values. We will assume from now on that our state space is $M \subseteq \mathbb{R}^d$. Thus, we can describe the dynamics in two ways. If the time is a discrete variable, we have a $d$-dimensional map,

$$\mathbf{x}_{t+1} = F(\mathbf{x}_t), \quad t \in \mathbb{Z}^+. \tag{7.7}$$

In the case of continuous time, we have a system of $d$ ODEs:

$$\frac{d}{dt}\mathbf{x}(t) = F(\mathbf{x}(t)), \quad t \in \mathbb{Z}. \tag{7.8}$$

In both cases, $F : M \to M$ and $\mathbf{x} \in M$. In the following, we will adopt the map notation for convenience. In general, the states of the system are not observed directly but through an observation function $h : M \to \mathbb{R}$, a (non-linear) projection that defines the scalar time series we have in practice,

$$\mathbf{y}_t = h(\mathbf{x}_{t-1}) + s\eta_t \quad t \in \mathbb{Z}^+. \tag{7.9}$$

Here, $\eta_t$ is supposed to represent the measurement error and $s$ is a constant that determines the signal to noise ratio.

It is important to remark that the above-mentioned notation describes a context where a deterministic dynamical system is contaminated by *measurement noise* that does not interact with the dynamics. However, many physiological processes are better described by systems with *dynamic noise* for which the deterministic part and the stochastic part interact and give rise to many peculiar non-linear effects, such as the *stochastic resonance*. The task of assessing whether an observed system may be treated as (operationally) deterministic is still an open problem and a field of ongoing research (see, e.g. Small, 2005; Chan and Tong, 2001 and references therein). We will assume the measurement noise scenario even though the references provided also discuss the extension of some of the methods to the dynamic noise case.

Thus, we are given a univariate experimental time series $\mathbf{y} = \{y_1, \ldots, y_n\}$ of length $n$. Starting from $\mathbf{y}$ and according to Takens' *embedding theorem*, we can hope to reconstruct the state space dynamics of the system. Such theorem can be explained intuitively as follows: To describe the motion of a $d$-dimensional physical system one would need to know the relevant variable together with its derivatives of order up to $d$. In practice, one observes only **y**, but Takens' theorem states that, under appropriate conditions, lagged versions of **y** can be used as a proxy for such derivatives. Hence, the following *embedding vectors* can be built,

$$\mathbf{y}_t = (y_t, y_{t-\tau}, y_{t-2\tau} \cdots y_{t-(d_e-1)\tau}), \qquad (7.10)$$

provided that $d_e \leq 2d + 1$, the embedding of Eq. (7.4), contains the same information as the original system[a].

[a]More precisely, the theorem states that there exists a diffeomorphism between the true dynamics and the reconstructed one. A **diffeomorphism** is an isomorphism in the category of smooth or differentiable manifolds. It is an invertible function that maps one differentiable manifold into another, such that both the function and its inverse are smooth. Recall that informally, an isomorphism is a kind of mapping between objects, which shows a relationship between two properties or operations. A **manifold** is a mathematical space, for example, a line and a circle are one-dimensional manifolds, a plane and sphere are two-dimensional manifolds. The concept of manifolds is central to many parts of geometry and modern mathematical physics because it allows more complicated structures to be expressed in terms of properties of simpler spaces.

Clearly, the reconstruction process depends on two parameters: $d_e$, is the *embedding dimension*, that is, the dimension of the reconstructed space, and $\tau$, the *time delay* which gives the temporal distance between successive components of the embedding vector. Obtaining good estimates for $d_e$ and $\tau$ is not a trivial task. Even if many heuristic criteria have been proposed to this aim (Abarbanel, 1996; Kantz and Schreiber, 2004) different authors have pointed out that the estimation of such quantities is tantamount to a model selection procedure. In particular, in Chan and Tong (2001), the statistical approach to state space reconstruction is seen as a best subset selection problem within the non-parametric regression context. Within such framework, consistent estimators for the time delay and the embedding dimension are obtained.[b] Judd *et al.* (2001) and Small (2005) point out that, in analogy with modeling procedures, there is no unique reconstruction for a given time series; different embeddings may well capture different aspects of the dynamics. In the same references, further discussion on the reconstruction process including irregular embeddings and embeddings for stochastic dynamical systems are carried out. In conclusion, state space reconstruction is crucial and cannot be simply treated as an intermediate step to be carried out automatically.

[b]A consistent estimator converges with probability one to the true value of the parameter as the series' length approaches infinity. A sequence of estimators for a given parameter $\theta$ is said to be **consistent** if this sequence converges in probability to $\theta$. Intuitively, this means that estimators taken far enough in the sequence are more likely to be in the vicinity of the parameter being estimated, and in the limit they will be arbitrarily close to $\theta$ with probability one.

An example of a time series and its reconstruction is given in Fig. 7.12 (left), where we show time series of the monophasic action potential (MAP) of the toad *Bufo Arenarum* at fibrillation regime. This series is derived from an experiment described by Savino *et al.* (1989). The ventricles of such toads were externally driven by periodic pulses. By increasing the frequency of the stimulus, the authors observed a transition to the fibrillation regime similar to period-doubling transition to chaos. For further details see also Giannerini *et al.* (2007). The reconstructed attractor is shown in Fig. 7.12 (right) with a time delay $\hat{\tau} = 15$. (i.e. 30 ms) and an embedding dimension $\hat{d} = 4$.

Among the most important quantities motivated by chaos theory that can be used to characterize non-linear phenomena we should mention the so-called *dynamic invariants*. Such name derives from their property of

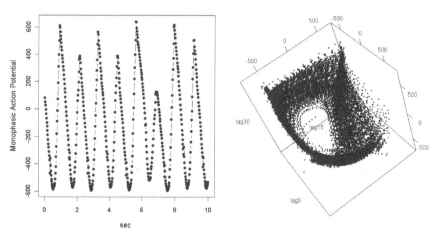

Fig. 7.12.   Time series of the monophasic action potential (MAP) at fibrillation regime (left). Phase space plot of three components of the reconstructed attractor, for $\tau = 15$, i.e. 30 ms, and $d_e = 4$ (right).

being invariant under smooth coordinate change. Hence, in theory, all of them should not depend on the reconstruction parameter used. In practice, the computation of the invariants for a range of parameters is advocated and can give useful information on the process under investigation. In the following sections, we will briefly describe some of the most important invariants.

### 7.5.2. *Lyapunov Exponents*

Lyapunov exponents (named after the Russian mathematician Aleksandr M. Lyapunov, 1857–1918) are important measures of stability and indicators of the presence of chaos. In particular, the maximum Lyapunov characteristic exponent (MLCE) measures the so-called *sensitivity to initial conditions* as it gives the rate of divergence of nearby starting trajectories on the attractor. Denote with $\mathbf{x}_0$ and $\mathbf{x}_0'$ two close initial conditions in the phase space and with $\mathbf{x}_n$ and $\mathbf{x}_n'$ their values after $n$ time steps, respectively. The MLCE may be then defined as,

$$\lambda_1 = \lim_{n\to\infty} \lim_{\mathbf{x}_0'\to\mathbf{x}_0} \frac{1}{n} \ln\left(\frac{\|\mathbf{x}_n - \mathbf{x}_n'\|}{\|\mathbf{x}_0 - \mathbf{x}_0'\|}\right). \tag{7.11}$$

This definition holds with probability one for almost all initial conditions. A positive MLCE is a necessary condition for the presence of chaos and indicates initial value sensitivity and short-term predictability.

Lyapunov exponents reflect the average rates of divergence over the whole attractor, for this reason, they are usually indicated as *global* exponents. However, a peculiar feature of a non-linear phenomenon is the strong non-uniformity in space with respect to many properties. For instance, a system with a positive MLCE might have an attractor with regions of enhanced predictability (Smith *et al.*, 1999; Bailey *et al.*, 1997; Chan and Tong, 2001). Hence, it is possible to work with *local* Lyapunov exponents (LLEs, also called *finite time Lyapunov exponents*), which provide valuable information on the heterogeneity of the system and allow the identification of regions with different dynamic structure. In brief, such exponents can be defined in terms of the distance between the unperturbed trajectory and the perturbed $k$-steps ahead in time,

$$\lambda_1(k, \mathbf{x}_0) = \frac{1}{k} \ln\left(\frac{\|\mathbf{x}_k - \mathbf{x}_k'\|}{\|\mathbf{x}_0 - \mathbf{x}_0'\|}\right). \tag{7.12}$$

Notice that there can be different versions of LLEs, depending on the kind of norm employed, the orientation of the perturbation, and the choice of which trajectory to follow (see Bailey *et al.*, 1997 and references therein for a discussion). As $k$ becomes large, the LLEs approach the corresponding global exponents. Estimating Lyapunov exponents from time series is a complex task that cannot be presented here. In the literature, several estimators have been proposed; the interested reader can refer to Giannerini and Rosa (2004) for a review. For an account of measures of initial value sensitivity in the stochastic case, see Chan and Tong (2001) and references therein.

### 7.5.3. *Dimensions and Entropies*

Other classes of dynamic invariants include dimensions and entropies. It is well known that chaotic phenomena are often associated with *strange attractors*, that is, objects with a fractional dimension. Such fact has motivated the study and the application of the different measures that can characterize fractal objects. One of the most used quantities is the *correlation dimension*, defined as follows:

$$D_2 = \lim_{\epsilon \to 0} \lim_{n \to \infty} \frac{d \ln C_2(\epsilon, n)}{d \ln \epsilon}, \qquad (7.13)$$

where $n$ is the length of the series and $C_2(\epsilon, n)$ is the *correlation integral*, namely, the fraction of phase space points that lie within a hypersphere of radius $\epsilon$. Interestingly, measures based on the correlation integral have attracted a great deal of attention and have been successfully applied in the analysis of the cardiovascular system. For instance, Small (2005) shows an application to categorize cardiac dynamics from observed ECG. Other applications are shown in Diks (1999). The reader can refer to Cutler (1993) for a review on recent developments on the theory of fractal dimension estimation.

Let us briefly discuss the class of dynamical invariants linked to Shannon's *entropy*. The entropy of a system is a measure of the uncertainty associated with a random variable, or it is a measure of how fast the system forgets about itself. Clearly, such measure of disorder is strictly related to both the kind and the strength of the dependence of a system. For this reason, many of the indexes motivated by the entropy are widely used in many applied fields and their theoretical properties have been investigated in detail. Shannon's entropy was introduced in the context of Information

Theory and is defined as follows,

$$H(X) = \int_{\mathbf{x} \in M} P(\mathbf{x}) \log(P(\mathbf{x})) dx, \qquad (7.14)$$

where $M$ is the domain of the system and $P(\mathbf{x})$ is the probability function. Hence, $H(X)$ measures the average uncertainty of a system and is of fundamental importance in communication engineering and coding theory. From its first appearance, many other entropy functionals were introduced and studied. Among the most widely used entropy measures in non-linear dynamics we mention the *Average Mutual Information* and the *Kolmogorov–Sinai* entropy. Interestingly, many of such functionals can be put in relation to each other. As we have remarked above, a peculiar feature of entropy measures is that they can characterize the dependence structure of a process. Hence, contrary to the Fourier analysis, they can be used for assessing the non-linear nature of an observed system.

Besides characterizing many peculiar features of non-linear phenomena, the *dynamic invariants* discussed in the previous sections can be used for building proper statistical tests. For instance, tests for chaos based on Lyapunov exponents are discussed in Bailey *et al.* (1997), Whang and Linton (1999), Giannerini and Rosa (2001), Shintani and Linton (2004), and Giannerini *et al.* (2007). Other tests for non-linearity that have captured the attention of the researchers in non-linear dynamics are the so-called *surrogate tests*.

Surrogate data methods can be regarded as a resampling approach for building tests for non-linearity when the distribution of the statistics employed in that field is unknown. The method can be summarized as follows: (*i*) select a null hypothesis regarding the process that has generated the observed series (DGP), for instance, $H_0$: the DGP is a linear stochastic process; (*ii*) by means of Monte Carlo methods generate a set of $B$ resampled series, called *surrogate series*, consistent with $H_0$; (*iii*) choose an appropriate test statistic having discriminatory power against $H_0$, compute it on the surrogates obtaining the distribution of the test statistic under the null hypothesis; and (*iv*) derive the significance level of the test by comparing such distribution with the value that the statistic takes on the original series.

After the introduction of the idea, several works that extend the method have been presented. In general, such extensions introduce either new test statistics or *ad hoc* algorithms for testing specific (not necessarily linear) hypotheses. For instance, Small *et al.* (2001) and Small (2005) study a class of such statistics based on the correlation integral. For interesting reviews on the topic see Schreiber and Schmitz (2000) and Kugiumtzis (2001). Note that, despite the fair amount of literature on surrogate data methods, to our knowledge, comprehensive studies on the theoretical properties of such tests are lacking. One notable exception is the contribution of Chan (1997).

## 7.6. Discussion

The physician, clinical engineer, paramedic, technician, or nurse should not be discouraged when looking at this chapter. They can skip it fully with no regrets. However, a quick glance led by sheer curiosity would not hurt, for daily medical practice even though often stands on previous medical experience (not totally discarding the common hearsay, the village healer methods or Old Mother Hutton's herbs), mostly relies and depends on well-trodden hard basic research and theories (including mathematical theories) that later were confirmed by animal experimentation and clinical trials. A suggested nice exercise is to search for the latter examples in medical history. Recall also essential and, in several respects, still valid contributions of Nicholas Rashevsky's School of Mathematical Biology developed over a long time span at the University of Chicago (Rashevsky, 1960).

The Hodgkin–Huxley equations, somewhat related or perhaps even inspired in Rashevsky's earlier concepts, gave us a good starting point to proceed thereafter with non-linear microscopic models of cardiac dynamics. Non-linearity appears as an intrinsic biological characteristic that, no matter how hard researchers try to circumvent by means of the linear counterpart, seems to defy the easier solutions offer by the latter. Thus, van der Pol, Bonhoeffer, FitzHugh and Nagumo were quickly visited to arrive at more recent authors as Winfree, Jalife, and others.

Non-linear dynamics and the onset of fibrillation was the subject dealt with next describing oscillation disappearance as caused by a topological characteristic, which manifests the existence of a vulnerable phase. More interesting than the vulnerable phase resetting is the possibility of having truly complex dynamic behavior associated with bifurcation routes to fibrillation. Moreover, we may expect the onset of fibrillation to be associated with destabilization at a lower-dimensional behavior, i.e. the breaking of a low-dimensional dynamic attractor. Several clinical studies were mentioned including examples such as the so-called electrical alternans, widely known in medical literature. The concept of cardiac dynamic disease is put forward pointing out to the importance of understanding dynamic instabilities for therapeutic purposes. Insight can be gained in the understanding of these complex phenomena through the use of appropriate models.

Extended models and connection with sustained fibrillation go back to the reentry idea introduced very early in this book. In fact, once spatial alternans have developed, there is an increased probability of VT as a state previous to fibrillation and several examples and experimental results are shown, as viewed from a bidimensional or tridimensional framework of nonlinear spiral waves and the possible appearance of new singularities. The section delves rather deeply in these aspects and uncovers a wide area to explore, both theoretically and experimentally.

The last section of this chapter tightly compresses the statistical approach to the problem, with ample backing up literature and not insignificant mathematical background concepts, from state spaces, Lyapunov exponents to dimensions and entropy. It is interesting here to point out the origin of the latter, how a communication engineer, Claude E. Shannon (no doubt a brilliant mathematical mind), based in the late 1940s in a purely technical environment, the Bell Telephone Laboratories, has projected over the years trespassing several lines and influencing the biomedical sciences (Shannon and Weaver, 1949). For sure, he never ever dreamt of such an interdisciplinary creative phenomenon.

Models are no doubt important for the understanding of complex systems. Their value depends on the model simplicity, which in terms of what was presented in the chapter is more or less equivalent to stating a dependence on the dimensionality; a good model shows low (or better, minimal) dimensionality but well describes the relevant aspects of the system dynamics. Such model helps, too, in the definition of the experimental protocols. The latter fact often occurs when modeling in other fields, as it is currently taking place in DNA research. Apparent trivial findings may bring up the question of how come we did not see it before, and the answer is simple: the search is motivated by a model and by an interpretation of facts, which, in turn, lead looking at facets of the experimental analysis that would have not be considered had we not had the model. It is not uncommon that the results do not confirm the model predictions, however, this should act as stimulus to reinterpret things in order to get a better model (remember: observe, think, and observe again). Last, but not least, models must predict as medicine needs to predict. Mere explanation is not enough if one aims at a heuristic and pragmatic value.

Good models are needed to understand why fibrillation is triggered and which are the pathologic and/or dynamic causes influencing cardiac dynamics. Such knowledge would improve prevention, that is, arrange for provisions (or measures) to anticipate how prone the individual is under given conditions of falling into it.

Another very significant and important situation refers to the high risk or borderline heart, one which is easily fibrillated due to, say, ischemia: How can fibrillation be avoided? How can it be efficiently defibrillated after fibrillation was established? Chaos control techniques in these respects might be surprisingly positive through different means, be they chemical, mechanical, or electrical. Paramount information here refers to how the effects are of dynamic parameters and variables to bring the whole system back to stable states that are not clinically dangerous.

The primary statistical information is in data analysis; from it, suggestions for dynamic models becomes possible, that is models that evolve with time, passing from one qualitative state to another. A complication is noise, present in any biological system. Statistical models can help in this respect to separate out the deterministic component from the statistical one. The so-called stochastic resonance can improve the signal-to-noise ratio, which has a deterministic origin. In a sense, stochastic resonance resembles noise insertion in an analog/digital converter to improve its precision, that is, paradoxically, noise addition improves the signal-to-noise ratio.

A good predictive model must take into account the high noise level of real data and, hence, must contain adequate statistical instruments to deal with the data and produce reliable results. In this context, all parameters need to be bounded by their respective typical deviations.

But nothing in science is easy and physicians usually are scared of mathematics and the math involved in the above-mentioned models is not easy either. Physicians, however, are not required to learn math, once a model is tested and proved useful, its application is mechanized as the operation of any machine is learned. Do the common computer users know computer intricacies? Does a driver know mechanics to drive a car? But they are aware of how powerful these machines are and how much better they accomplish by their use. Thus, diffusion and creation of sensitivity to the subject appears as a must, and this book, among its objectives, intends to make it known that models can be useful, or at least can spur the curiosity to know what they are about. As said before, when the model becomes part of a friendly software (in fact, an interface), the user forgets what is behind, at least partially, and in the end he or she sees only the benefits. Medical advances and development have demonstrated this many times already, as in ophthalmology or images, either in diagnostic or therapeutic systems. One calculated risk may not be enough a level of stability and predictivity of the model results to satisfy the requirements of medical practice.

## 7.7. Conclusions and Review Questions

Rather than trying to offer specific conclusions based on the hard theoretical issues, we are rather inclined to offer a brief general statement. Well after a century of tremendous advances in prevention of fibrillation and reversion of the arrhythmia, the subject still remains highly empirical and, whatever knowledge came from the approaches described here, it has not yet reached the medical profession and constitutes material restricted to the scientific circles. Nonetheless, such state of affairs should not be confused with failure, especially for the pragmatic mind, for history is plenty of cases showing how hard and long the way to full success can be.

**Multiple choice questions**

1. Qualitative or minimal modeling of complex systems is
    (A) a linear modeling technique
    (B) a bottom-up procedure
    (C) a top-down and non-linear approach

2. Why bottom-up faithful models of complex systems are not analytically solvable?
    (A) because of the high dimensionality of the model equations
    (B) because of the difficulty in constructing single element equations
    (C) because of the non-validity of the linear superposition principle

3. Qualitative or minimal modeling is based on
    (A) simplification of the model equations
    (B) dimensionality reduction, complexity, and universality of the underlying dynamics
    (C) linearization of the mathematical model

4. The BVDP-FHN equations are
    (A) a simplified model of the Hodgkin–Huxley equations

(B) a dynamical high dimensionality model equations

(C) a low dimensionality linear model equations

5. A relaxation oscillation corresponds to

   (A) the oscillation described by a linear harmonic oscillator

   (B) a non-linear oscillation described by a Poincaré limit cycle

   (C) none of the above

6. The phase space representation of the van der Pol oscillator is

   (A) the representation of the dynamics in a plane defined by its position and velocity

   (B) a statistical representation of the dynamics

   (C) both of the above

7. The vulnerable phase of a non-linear oscillator is

   (A) an undefined phase

   (B) a region of the phase space

   (C) a phase where an impulse of appropriate intensity can drive the oscillator to a singular point

8. The Feigenbaum scenario in the transition from periodicity to chaos consists of

   (A) the successive addition of incommensurate frequencies to the oscillator fundamental

   (B) a cascade of period-doubling bifurcations

   (C) an intermittent transition characterized by the generation of activity bursts

9. The Ruelle–Takens–Newhouse (RTN) theorem establishes that

   (A) dynamics with three incommensurate frequencies are unstable leading to complex or chaotic behavior

   (B) the number of Feigenbaum period-doubling bifurcations is finite

   (C) dynamics with more that three incommensurate frequencies are stable

10. Electric alternans are

    (A) a possible route to complex behavior

    (B) an experimental artifact

    (C) of no clinical significance

11. Established fibrillation is a phenomenon of

    (A) dynamical high dimensionality

(B) involving spatial dimensions

(C) both of the above

12. Universal behaviors of high-dimensional excitable systems are

(A) relaxation oscillations

(B) vulnerable phase and amplitude resetting

(C) spiral and scroll spatial waves

13. In established fibrillation we observe

(A) low-dimensional dynamics

(B) wandering wavelets

(C) periodic electrical oscillations

14. The embedding theorem allows to

(A) predict the onset of fibrillation

(B) reconstruct the phase space of the process from a scalar time series

(C) reconstruct the phase space of the process from a system of ODEs

15. The largest Lyapunov exponent of a dynamical system quantifies

(A) the sensitivity to initial conditions

(B) the dimensionality of the system

(C) the presence of bifurcations

# Chapter 8

# FINAL DISCUSSION, OVERALL CONCLUSIONS, AND LOOKING AHEAD

*Doubts may dangle out, or something was forgotten, or why not trying a little step further*

This last chapter attempts to round things out by looking back into what was said, tries to summarize the current situation of the subject by underlining those aspects that are still pending and, most difficult of all, wants to play the magician — the Nostradamus (Fig. 8.1) — by watching into the crystal ball to signal possible new avenues for research, development, and applications. During such endeavor, some references not given before will be brought up to better complete the list and partially compensate for ignorance and/or forgetfulness. No separate sections were considered necessary, rather following roughly the subject order of the chapters in a continuous easy discussion style.

We started the book (Introduction) by recalling the *Framingham Study*, as the best, longest and modern reference material, constantly being updated, which has become as some kind of aegis for cardiovascular disease at large and, more specifically, for the subject dealt with herein; after all, the primary concern is sudden death, and ventricular fibrillation usually stands out as standoffish lethal interloper. Observe in Table 8.1 that cardiovascular disease takes the first place only in the group over 65 years of age going down to the second cause of death in the 45–64 year old group. However, when looking at the 10 leading causes for the whole population irrespective of age, cardiac illness is first both in males and females with no significant difference between sexes and followed relatively close by cancer (Table 8.2). The third cause of death is cerebrovascular accident, but rather far behind the first two.

Not good reliable world data and per country for accidents (especially car and motorcycles) and violence, including wars and terrorism can be found, even though there are several websites. The subjective impression

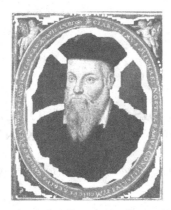

Fig. 8.1. Michel de Nostredame (14 Dec or 21 Dec 1503–2 July 1566). His name was latinized to **Nostradamus**. French apothecary and reputed foreseer. He published many prophecies. Portrait by his son Cesar. Downloaded from http://en.wikipedia.org/wiki/Nostradamus and modified.

when considering the daily public news regarding the latter causes would or could bring them to an unfortunate higher rank. What are the real numbers produced, say, in Corea, Vietnam, the former Yugoslavia, Afghanistan, Israel–Palestine, Iraq, Somalia, Kenya, and so many other places almost unknown or even forgotten, not to mention the two World Wars? An amazing website to visit is http://www.geocities.com/dtmcbride/hist/disasters-war.html.

Sticking to cars and motorcycles, in Argentina, for example, a total of 8,205 deaths due to accidents in highways or streets were reported during 2008, that is, 22/day or 683/month, on average (http://www.luchemos.org.ar/espa/mapa2008.htm). The ratio was close to 0.1, in 2003 (Fig. 8.2), of the former to cardiac causes, according to Sosa Liprandi *et al.* (2006). Other reports claim the figure is higher, something like 26 or even 27/day. Still, however, the heart is way ahead according to this information.

A total cardiovascular toll of about 21 million people in Latin America is anticipated during the first 10 years of the twenty-first century; such prediction was made in the World Congress of Cardiology, held in Buenos Aires, Argentina, in May 2008. Since the region currently holds about 560 million people, that would mean, in relative terms, slightly less than 4% (http://www.telam.com.ar/vernota.php?tipo=N&idPub=165268&id=228799&dis=1&sec=1). Now, taking into account an automotive overall park in the order of 85,000,000 units that led to almost 115,000 deaths in one year, Latin America yields a rate of slightly over 20 deaths/100,000

Table 8.1. Total deaths and leading cause of death by age group.

| | Calendar Year | | | | | | | |
|---|---|---|---|---|---|---|---|---|
| | 2003 | | 2004 | | 2005 | | 2006 | |
| | Number | Rank | Number | Rank | Number | Rank | Number | Rank |
| **Total under one year** | 447 | | 451 | | 420 | | 406 | |
| Congenital malformations | 116 | 1 | 120 | 1 | 113 | 1 | 120 | 1 |
| Sudden infant death syndrome | 48 | 3 | 53 | 2 | 42 | 2 | 53 | 2 |
| Short Gestation and low birth weight | 61 | 2 | 45 | 3 | 31 | 3 | 45 | 3 |
| Accidents | 15 | 6 | 15 | 5 | 21 | 4 | 15 | 5 |
| Maternal complications of pregnancy | 26 | 4 | 27 | 4 | 21 | 4 | 27 | 4 |
| Placenta and cord complications | 23 | 5 | 12 | 8 | 21 | 4 | *[1] | *[1] |
| **Total 1–14** | 218 | | 176 | | 180 | | 165 | |
| Accidents | 75 | 1 | 59 | 1 | 71 | 1 | 67 | 1 |
| Malignant neoplasms | 34 | 2 | 31 | 2 | 24 | 2 | 22 | 2 |
| Congenital anomalies | 17 | 3 | 12 | 4 | 15 | 3 | 13 | 3 |
| Homicide | 13 | 4 | 16 | 3 | 10 | 4 | 9 | 4 |
| Influenza and pneumonia | *[1] | *[1] | *[1] | *[1] | *[1] | *[1] | 6 | 5 |
| **Diseases of heart** | 11 | 5 | 6 | 5 | 6 | 5 | *[1] | *[1] |
| Suicide | 6 | 6 | *[1] | *[1] | *[1] | *[1] | *[1] | *[1] |
| **Total 15–24** | 564 | | 601 | | 599 | | 644 | |
| Accidents | 246 | 1 | 294 | 1 | 275 | 1 | 319 | 1 |
| Suicide | 100 | 2 | 102 | 2 | 99 | 2 | 115 | 2 |
| Homicide | 49 | 3 | 53 | 3 | 55 | 3 | 56 | 3 |
| Malignant neoplasms | 41 | 4 | 41 | 4 | 42 | 4 | 42 | 4 |

(Continued)

*Cardiac Fibrillation-Defibrillation*

Table 8.1.  (*Continued*)

| | 2003 | | 2004 | | 2005 | | 2006 | |
|---|---|---|---|---|---|---|---|---|
| | Number | Rank | Number | Rank | Number | Rank | Number | Rank |
| **Diseases of heart** | **18** | **5** | **14** | **5** | **20** | **5** | **13** | **5** |
| **Total 25–44** | 2,231 | | 2,161 | | 2,129 | | 2,089 | |
| Accidents | 574 | 1 | 564 | 1 | 620 | 1 | 603 | 1 |
| Malignant neoplasms | 339 | 2 | 338 | 2 | 303 | 2 | 334 | 3 |
| Suicide | 294 | 3 | 301 | 3 | 263 | 3 | 239 | 3 |
| **Diseases of heart** | **265** | **4** | **221** | **4** | **211** | **4** | **236** | **4** |
| Homicide | 89 | 5 | 88 | 5 | 98 | 5 | 92 | 5 |
| HIV | 89 | 5 | *[1] | *[1] | *[1] | *[1] | *[1] | *[1] |
| **Total 45–64** | 8,076 | | 8,207 | | 8,531 | | 8,708 | |
| Malignant neoplasms | 2,807 | 1 | 2,844 | 1 | 2,894 | 1 | 2,964 | 1 |
| **Diseases of heart** | **1,654** | **2** | **1,611** | **2** | **1,612** | **2** | **1,586** | **2** |
| Accidents | 560 | 3 | 640 | 3 | 704 | 3 | 779 | 3 |
| Chronic lower respiratory diseases | 335 | 4 | 343 | 4 | 352 | 4 | 343 | 4 |
| Diabetes mellitus | 334 | 5 | 343 | 4 | 337 | 5 | 341 | 5 |
| **Total 65 and over** | **34,269** | | **33,107** | | **34,156** | | **33,865** | |
| **Diseases of heart** | **9,199** | **1** | **8,765** | **1** | **9,063** | **1** | **8,713** | **1** |
| Malignant neoplasms | 7,820 | 2 | 7,723 | 2 | 7,744 | 2 | 7,638 | 2 |
| Cerebrovascular diseases | 3,203 | 3 | 2,896 | 3 | 2,578 | 3 | 2,395 | 4 |
| Chronic lower respiratory diseases | 2,296 | 5 | 2,177 | 5 | 2,318 | 4 | 2,290 | 5 |
| Alzheimer's disease | 2,360 | 4 | 2,206 | 4 | 2,283 | 5 | 2,434 | 3 |

Calendar Year

[1]These causes of death do not rank in the top five leading causes for these years.

*Note*: Based on criteria set by the National Center for Health Statistics.

*Source*: Department of Health (downloaded from http://www.ofm.wa.gov/databook/human/st10.asp) Last modified March 28, 2008; OFM Forecasting Division; E-mail: OFM.Forecasting@ofm.wa.gov

Table 8.2.   Ten leading causes of death in the USA — 2004. (downloaded from http://www.infoplease.com/ipa/A0005110.html)

Leading causes of death differ somewhat by age, sex, and race. In 2004, as in previous years, accidents were the leading cause of death for those under 34 years, while in older age groups, chronic diseases such as cancer and heart disease were the leading causes. The top two causes for males and females—heart disease and cancer—are exactly the same. However, suicide ranked eighth for males but was not ranked among the ten leading causes for females.

| Rank[1] | Causes of Death | All Persons | Causes of Death | Male | Causes of Death | Female |
|---|---|---|---|---|---|---|
|  | All causes | 2,397,615 | All causes | 1,181,668 | All causes | 1,215,947 |
| 1. | Diseases of heart | 652,486 | Diseases of heart | 321,973 | Diseases of heart | 330,513 |
| 2. | Malignant neoplasms (cancer) | 553,888 | Malignant neoplasms (cancer) | 286,830 | Malignant neoplasms (cancer) | 267,058 |
| 3. | Cerebrovascular diseases | 150,074 | Unintentional injuries | 72,050 | Cerebrovascular diseases | 91,274 |
| 4. | Chronic lower respiratory diseases | 121,987 | Cerebrovascular diseases | 58,800 | Chronic lower respiratory diseases | 63,341 |
| 5. | Unintentional injuries | 112,012 | Chronic lower respiratory diseases | 58,646 | Alzheimer's disease | 46,991 |
| 6. | Diabetes mellitus | 73,138 | Diabetes mellitus | 35,267 | Unintentional injuries | 39,962 |
| 7. | Alzheimer's disease | 65,965 | Influenza and pneumonia | 26,861 | Diabetes mellitus | 37,871 |
| 8. | Influenza and pneumonia | 59,664 | Suicide | 25,566 | Influenza and pneumonia | 32,803 |
| 9. | Nephritis, nephrotic syndrome, and nephrosis | 42,480 | Nephritis, nephrotic syndrome, and nephrosis | 20,370 | Nephritis, nephrotic syndrome, and nephrosis | 22,110 |
| 10. | Septicemia | 33,373 | Alzheimer's disease | 18,974 | Septicemia | 18,362 |

*Source:* U.S. National Center for Health Statistics, *Health, United States, 2007.*

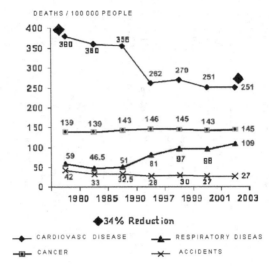

Fig. 8.2. Mortality rate per 100,000 inhabitants for: Cardiovascular Disease CVD (diamonds), showing 34% reduction from 1977 until 2003; Cancer (squares), kept constant; Respiratory Disease (triangles); Accidents (crosses). After Sosa Liprandi *et al.*, 2006, with kind permission.

inhabitants, while the World Health Organization reports 26 (http://www. clarin.com/diario/2009/05/10/sociedad/s-01915065.htm) and predicts, for 2030, the fifth position in accident-death-related causes instead of the ninth maintained nowadays (http://www.todotransito.cl/modules.php?name= News&file=article&sid=2201).

All over the world, road traffic accidents kill more than one million people a year, injuring another thirty-eight million (5 million of them seriously). The death toll on the world's roadways makes driving the **number one cause of death and injury for young people aged 15–44** (http:// www.crashtest.com/intro/). The question of how good these data are always dangles around without expecting satisfactory answers within a reasonable time, but we cannot prevent musing to ourselves, **so hard and slow to recover a cardiac patient and so easy and quick to lose a young healthy live.** No doubt, an interesting area to delve into and to think about, but it does belong neither to the cardiologist nor to the biomedical engineer, for sure, and predictions become a quicksand area in this particular subject, especially when one recalls the many times unexpected and crazy human behavior. The reader is left to his/her own conclusions.

Traditional concepts about fibrillation were brought up thereafter (Chap. 1) and, no doubt, anatomical and electrophysiological inhomogeneit-ies, even at the microstructure level, clearly showed up. The probabilistic nature of the arrhythmia so becomes its inherent characteristic, leading to the assertion, *the greater the inhomogeneity, the higher the probability of triggering the phenomenon.* Without discussion, then, the common and frequently seen myocardial ischemia, for example, introduces tissue differences that change cardiac topography, its properties and the normal pathways followed by the excitation waves; explanations and mechanisms of different kinds have been offered for fibrillation; however, in the end all converge to the closed circuit idea, as a dog persistently chasing and biting its own tail.

When the arrhythmia is looked at the atria, some relatively new aspects come up, as the possible association with an inflammatory process (Aviles *et al.*, 2003). The latter contribution has been widely cited. Drawing from these authors: "The presence of systemic inflammation determined by elevation in **C-reactive protein** (CRP) seems to be related to AF. Its measurement and cardiovascular assessment were performed at baseline in 5806 subjects enrolled in a cardiovascular study in which they were followed up for almost 8 years. AF was clinically and electrocardiographically identified. At baseline, 315 subjects (5%) had AF. Compared with subjects in the first CRP quartile (<0.97 mg/L), subjects in the fourth quartile (>3.41 mg/L) had more AF (7.4% vs 3.7%). Of 5491 subjects without AF at baseline, 897 (16%) developed AF during follow-up. Baseline CRP predicted higher risk for developing future AF." They concluded that CRP is not only associated with the presence of AF but may also predict patients at increased risk for future development of the arrhythmia. Other papers, as Ridker *et al.* (2000), reported CRP as another predictor of cardiovascular disease in women. It certainly gives a different reference framework to think about and work with.

Inflammation is the process by which the body responds to injury or infection. Evidence from clinical studies suggests that inflammation is important in atherosclerosis. CRP is one of the acute-phase proteins that increase during systemic inflammation (Taskinen *et al.*, 2002). It has been suggested that testing CRP levels in the blood may be an additional way to assess cardiovascular disease risk (such as atrial fibrillation). Even minimally oxidized, low-density lipoproteins (LDL) contain bioactive phospholipids capable of activating endothelial cells to induce secretion of monocyte chemoattractant protein-1 (MCP-1). Oxidized LDL and LDL lipolyzed with phospholipase contain lysophosphatidylcholine (lyso-PC), which, at low concentrations, has various proinflammatory effects on arterial cells and, at high concentrations, is cytotoxic. LDL modified by a protease and cholesterol esterase has been shown to be a potent inducer of adhesion and transmigration of monocytes and T cells through the endothelium. It also stimulates the secretion of

MCP-1 and interleukin-6 by macrophages and promotes smooth-muscle-cell proliferation and foam-cell formation. In short, proinflammatory mediators trigger the synthesis of **acute-phase reactants** in the liver, such as the CRP. **Acute-phase proteins** are a class of proteins whose plasma concentrations increase or decrease in response to inflammation.

As already stated before, ventricular fibrillation is rare in the pediatric population; when it does occur, ventricular fibrillation is usually a degeneration of other malignant arrhythmias, such as tachycardia. Perhaps, more oriented and controlled studies ought to be carried out while dividing the samples by age groups. Bibliography does not abound in this specific subject, most likely because it does not lend itself to experimentation while it relies only on relatively scarce clinical data. Pediatric cardiologists ought to place more attention to the eventual appearance of these kinds of cases.

Since nothing was said about *torsades de pointes* (French term that literally means "twisting of the points"), we should briefly refer to it as a rapid polymorphic ventricular tachycardia, prone to degenerate into fibrillation, with a characteristic twist of the QRS complex around the isoelectric baseline (Dessertenne, 1966; Hoshino *et al.*, 2006). It is also associated with a fall in arterial blood pressure, which can lead to fainting (Fig. 8.3). No doubt, it is a border line emergency and more studies to clearly explain its etiology are needed.

Disorder calls for order and the accepted and established method is an adequate electric shock although, even if so far not very practical chemicals show an alternative possible way out, in some specific circumstances

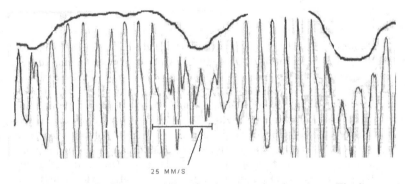

25 MM/S

Fig. 8.3. Printout of telemetry reading showing *torsades de pointes*. The line on top shows the characteristic "twist" around the isoelectric baseline. (anonymized ECG recording downloaded from http://en.wikipedia.org/wiki/File:Tosadesdepointes.jpg, freely available).

they might be recommendable (Chap. 2). In the latter respect, a quite attractive proposal indeed deserves mentioning (Kneller *et al.*, 2005) as complement of what was said before. These investigators discussed the mechanisms by which Na-channel blocking antiarrhythmic drugs terminate atrial fibrillation. By means of an ionically based mathematical model of vagotonic AF, these authors assessed the effects of applying pure Na-current ($I_{Na}$) inhibition during sustained arrhythmia. Under control conditions, AF was maintained by one or two dominant spiral waves, with fibrillatory propagation at critical levels of action potential duration (APD) dispersion. $I_{Na}$ inhibition terminated AF. During AF, $I_{Na}$ inhibition increased the size of primary rotors and reduced reentry rate (i.e. dominant frequency decreased by 33% at 60% $I_{Na}$ inhibition) while decreasing generation of secondary wavelets by wavebreak. Three mechanisms apparently contributed to $I_{Na}$ block-induced AF termination in the model, i.e. (1) enlargement of the center of rotation beyond the capacity of the computational substrate; (2) decreased anchoring to functional obstacles, increasing meander and extinction at boundaries; and (3) reduction in the number of secondary wavelets that could provide new primary rotors. Optical mapping in isolated sheep hearts confirmed that tetrodotoxin dose-dependently terminates AF while producing effects qualitatively like those of $I_{Na}$ inhibition in the mathematical model. The conclusion was that pure $I_{Na}$ inhibition terminates AF, producing activation changes consistent with clinical and experimental observations. These results provide insights into the mechanisms of Class I antiarrhythmic drug-induced AF termination.

Closely associated with defibrillation is the usual set of resuscitation maneuvers. There is news in this respect (Geddes *et al.*, 2007). This well known, and unfortunately not long ago gone researcher (Valentinuzzi, 2010) and his group, in Purdue University, introduced two new cardiopulmonary resuscitation (CPR) concepts: (1) the use of only rhythmic abdominal compression (OAC) to produce blood flow during CPR with ventricular fibrillation, and (2) a new way of describing coronary perfusion effectiveness, namely, the area between the aortic and right atrial pressure curves, summed over 1 min, the units being millimeters of mercury per second. They called this unit the coronary perfusion index (CPI). True mean coronary perfusion pressure is CPI/60. They also related CPI during CPR with ventricular fibrillation to the CPI for the normally beating heart in the same animal, obtained before each experiment. It was concluded that OAC-CPR produced 60% more coronary perfusion than standard chest-compression

CPR, with no damage to visceral organs. Other authors have not long ago reviewed this technique based mainly on Geddes' group previous reports (Adam *et al.*, 2009). The question they addressed was whether abdominal CPR could be used instead of external cardiac massage, either to protect a recent sternotomy or while chest compressions are not possible during a sternotomy.

Natalia Trayanova, who has been working in the area for many years, in an editorial note (Trayanova, 2008) underlined that many studies have been devoted to VF mechanisms in the short time period after VF onset (short-duration VF, lasting less than 1 min, as opposed to long-duration VF, over 5 min). Immediate defibrillation is prescribed if time from VF onset is less than 5 min, whereas giving CPR for up to 3 min in advance of the defibrillation shock is believed to improve outcome when VF persists for more than 5 min. There is evidence of the existence of intramural foci during VF, which seem to play a more important role than reentry mechanisms in the maintenance of the arrhythmia. Not all reentrant waves are equal in maintaining VF and raise the question regarding the universal nature of the mother rotor finding and its applicability to large hearts such as the human. Recall the difference made in Chap. 7 between triggering VF and maintenance of it.

In defibrillators, that is, the machines, there is a tendency to automatize the operation as much as possible trying also to reduce size and weight, envisioning even a miniature unit (http://www.implantchips.com/health/implantable-cardio-defibrillators/). No simple electrical descriptor provides a good measure of defibrillation efficacy and the waveform parameters that most directly influence defibrillation are voltage and duration. Voltage is a critical parameter for defibrillation because its spatial derivative defines the electrical field that interacts with the heart. Similarly, waveform duration is also critical because the shock interacts with the heart for the duration of the discharge. Shock energy is the most often cited metric of shock strength and an implantable cardioverter defibrillator (ICD's) capacity to defibrillate, but it is *not* a direct measure of effectiveness. Despite the physiological complexities of defibrillation, a simple approach in which the heart is modeled as passive resistor–capacitor (RC) network has proved useful for predicting efficient defibrillation waveforms. Kroll and Swerdlow (2007) proposed and discussed a model under two assumptions:

(1) the goal of both a monophasic shock and the first phase of a biphasic shock is to maximize the voltage change in the membrane at the end of the shock for a given stored energy; and

(2) the goal of the second phase of a biphasic shock is to discharge the membrane back to the zero potential, removing the charge deposited by the first phase.

Such model, continue Kroll and Swerdlow (2001), predicts that the optimal waveform rises in an exponential upward curve, but such an ascending waveform is difficult to generate efficiently. ICDs use electronically efficient capacitive-discharge waveforms, which require truncation for effective defibrillation. Even with optimal truncation, capacitive-discharge waveforms require more voltage and energy to achieve the same membrane voltage than do square waves and ascending waveforms. In ICDs, the value of the shock output capacitance is a key intermediary in establishing the relationship between stored energy and waveform voltage as a function of time, the key determinant of defibrillation efficacy. The RC model predicts that, for capacitive-discharge waveforms, stored energy is minimized when the **ICD's system time constant equals the cell membrane time constant**. Since the goal of phase two is to reverse the membrane charging effect of phase one, there is no advantage to additional waveform phases. The voltages and capacitances used in commercial ICDs vary widely, resulting in substantial disparities in waveform parameters. The development of present biphasic waveforms in the 1990s resulted in marked improvements in defibrillation efficacy. It is unlikely that substantial improvement in defibrillation efficacy will be achieved without radical changes in waveform design. In other words, these authors are strong supporters of the waveform concept. All said above regarding defibrillator apparatuses point out mostly to a technological endeavor where no basic new principles seem to be at sight. Materials, programming, and computer models appear as the main roads to follow.

Regarding DETECTION, ELECTRODES and PASTES, and EFFICACY and SAFETY, dealt with in Chaps. 4, 5 and 6, respectively, we think the subjects have been reasonably well covered so that, so far, there is nothing else to add except that, for sure, new algorithms and technologies, as for example the contribution by Park *et al.* (2009), will continue to show up, as is to be expected in the dynamic world we enjoy and sometimes suffer, too.

Theory, dealt with in Chap. 7, represents a well trodden and difficult avenue in this subject that, unfortunately, so far has not found the way to successful predictions and practical clinical applications, the latter being yet mostly empirical. Glass *et al.* (1991) edited a solid and thoughtful multi-author book devoted to non-linear dynamics of cardiac function. Three of its chapters delved, respectively, into ventricular fibrillation (by A.T. Winfree), ventricular defibrillation (by R.E. Ideker, A.S.L. Tang, D.W. Frazier, N. Shibata, P. Chen, and J.M. Wharton), and mechanically induced changes in electrophysiology and implications for arrhythmia (by M.J. Lab and A.V. Holden). The list of references is excellent and impressive, indeed; the conclusions of the book though are similar to what we say above. Still further work is awaited, more cross-talk between theoreticians and clinical people is needed and encouraged and outwardly and enthusiastically we claim it is full of bumps, but no doubt promising. Perhaps, it should be stated that the most difficult road is the best road.

Fibrillation and defibrillation are probabilistic events. We might try an appealing universal scaling, the *allometric law*, although in principle not directly related to the fibrillation–defibrillation overall phenomenon, it might find a place in it and at least deserves to be recalled bringing about a nice and well carried out paper by Noujaim, Lucca, Muñoz *et al.* (2004). The electrocardiographic PR interval measures the time taken by the electrical sinoatrial wave to propagate from atria to ventricles. From mouse to whale, this interval increases $10^1$ times whereas body mass BM augments $10^6$. Scaling of many biological processes (metabolic rate, life span, aortic diameter) can be described by the allometric equation $Y = Y_0.(BM)^b$, where $Y$ is the biological process and $b$ is the scaling exponent (where $b$ is an integer multiple of $1/4$). This paper assumed that the heart behaves as a set of "fractal-like" networks tending to minimize propagation time across the conducting system while ensuring a hemodynamically optimal atrioventricular activation sequence. The relationship $PR = BM^{1/4}$ was found and, subsequently, the authors collected previously published values of PR interval, heart rate, and BM of 541 mammals. The best fit for PR vs BM was described by the equation $PR = 53.BM^{0.24}$.

Inspired in the latter report, the following question seems pertinent: Would a relationship similar to the allometric equation be conceivable, say, between the probability of fibrillation and heart weight, or perhaps other parameter somehow related to the latter? Let us start with the basic allometric statement, that is, the relative rate of change of a given event $y$ is proportional to the relative rate of change of body mass or body weight $x$,

$$\frac{dy/dt}{y} = B\frac{dx/dt}{x}. \tag{8.1}$$

After integration and some easy algebraic manipulation, Eq. (8.1) becomes

$$\ln y = \ln A + B \ln x$$

or

$$y = A.x^B. \tag{8.2}$$

Originally, $y$ was the weight of an organ (heart, stomach, other) and $x$ was body weight or mass. The parameters A and B require numerical estimation by an appropriate procedure usually using empirical information.

By the same token, let us say that the probability of fibrillation $P_F$ follows a relationship with the number of ventricular diseased fibers $N_{DF}$ formally equal to Eq. (8.2), i.e.:

$$P_F = \alpha(N_{DF})^\beta. \tag{8.3}$$

Thus, $y$ in Eq. (8.2) is replaced by $P_F$ in Eq. (8.3), and $N_{DF}$ in the latter takes the place of $x$ in the former. After all, the number of diseased cardiac fibers (ischemic or infarcted or both) is part of the cardiac mass. Besides, since the electrocardiographic ST segment deviation is a traditional estimator of cardiac injury, why not stating that,

$$N_{DF} = \gamma.\Delta_{ST}, \tag{8.4}$$

or in words, the number of diseased ventricular fibers is proportional to the ST deviation ($\Delta$ indicating precisely "deviation"). Hence,

$$P_F = \alpha(\gamma.\Delta_{ST})^\beta. \tag{8.5}$$

After taking logarithms of both sides, the latter equation becomes:

$$\ln P_F = (\ln \alpha + \beta \ln \gamma) + \beta(\ln \Delta_{ST}),$$

which can be reduced to

$$Y = \delta + \beta(ST), \tag{8.6}$$

where $\delta = (\ln \alpha + \beta \ln \gamma)$ and $ST = \ln \Delta_{ST}$. The straight line (Eq. (8.6)) in log–log paper with the parameters $\alpha$ and $\beta$ would represent the probability of fibrillation as function of the ECG ST depression or elevation (Arini, Bonomini and Valentinuzzi 2010). Using published clinical data, these authors calculated the parameters of equation (8.6) above with which predictive probability values for VF could be anticipated when entering with a given ST-segment deviation. Validation, however, is still needed, but it looks as a promising avenue.

> *Allometry*, in general biology, measures the relative growth of a part in relation to the whole living organism. The term was first used by Snell in 1891 to express the mass of a mammal's brain as a function of the body mass BM. The term allometry describes the growth relation between two "components" of an organism (e.g. length vs volume of an organ): the specific growth velocity of a component $y$ is related to the specific growth velocity of another component (or the whole organism) $x$ in a constant way (Bertalanffy, 1957). The word *allometry* using the prefix *allos* derives from the Greek (else, different). To be considered in this respect as useful information, we recall from the preceding Chap. 7 Adler and Costabel (1975) who, based on the DNA content of 30 human hearts from different age groups and of different weight classes, determined the total number of heart muscle cells. The number of heart muscle cells is $2 \times 10^9$ in normal hearts of children and adults, and may rise to $4 \times 10^9$ in excessively hypertrophied hearts. Ventricular hypertrophy increases the probability of fibrillation; its fibrillatory threshold becomes lower as compared to the normal size heart.

To close this book, Webster Encyclopedia (2006) is recommended as good source material for several of the subjects treated herein. Another good source is the recent one by Josep Brugada and Luis Aguinaga (2010), produced by the Argentine Federation of Cardiology (FAC) and freely available in the WEB. Besides, the ethical issues often involved in defibrillation must be recalled and underlined. They encompass a complex and not easy to deal with set of aspects that project much beyond the scope of this book; however, as final remark, remember and keep always in mind the concept of **living and dying with dignity**.

# REFERENCES

Abarbanel HDI (1996) Analysis of observed chaotic data. Institute for Nonlinear Science. Springer Verlag, New York.

Adam Z, Adam S, Khan P, Dunning J (2009) Could we use abdominal compressions rather than chest compression in patients who arrest after cardiac surgery? *Interact Cardiovasc Thorac Surg* 8:148–151; doi:10.1510/icvts.2008.195974.

Addison PS, Watson JN, Clegg GR, Holzer M, Sterz F, Robertson CE (2000) Evaluating arrhythmias in ECG signals using Wavelet Transforms. *IEEE Eng Med Biol Mag* 19(5):104–109.

Adgey AA, Walsh SJ (2004) Theory and practice of defibrillation: Atrial fibrillation and DC conversion. *Heart* 90:1493–1498.

Adler CP, Costabel U (1975) Cell number in human heart in atrophy, hypertrophy, and under the influence of cytostatics. *Recent Adv Stud Cardiac Struct Metab* 6:343–355.

Afonso VX (1993) ECG QRS detection. In *Biomedical Digital Signal Processing*, ed Willis J. Tompkins, Prentice Hall, Englewood Cliffs, New Jersey, Chapter 12, pp. 236–264.

Afonso VX, Tompkins WJ (1995) Detecting ventricular fibrillation. *IEEE Eng Med Biol Mag* 14(2):152–159.

Akay M (1996) Wavelet representation of signals. Chapter 8 in Detection and estimation methods for biomedical signals. Academic Press, USA, pp. 157–241.

Akiyama T (1981) Intracellular recording of *in situ* ventricular cells during ventricular fibrillation. *Am J Physiol* 240:H465–H471.

Al Hatib F, Trendafilova E Daskalov I (2000) Transthoracic electrical impedance during external defibrillation: Comparison of measured and modelled waveforms. *Physiol Meas* 21:145–153; doi:10.1088/0967-3334/21/1/318.

Alatawi F, Gurevitz O, White R (2005) Prospective, randomized comparison of two biphasic waveforms for the efficacy and safety of transthoracic biphasic cardioversion of atrial fibrillation. *Heart Rhythm* 2:382–387.

Alexander S, Kleiger R, Lown B (1961) Use of external electric countershock in the treatment of ventricular tachycardia. *J Am Med Assoc* 177:916.

Alizadeh A, Haghjoo M, Arya A, Fazelifar AF, Alasti M, Bagherzadeh AA, Sadr-Ameli MA (2006) Inappropriate ICD discharge due to *T*-wave over-sensing in a patient with Brugada syndrome. *J Interv Card Electrophysiol* 15(1) January.

Amann A, Tratnig R, Unterkofler K (2005) Reliability of old and new ventricular fibrillation detection algorithms for automated external defibrillators. *Biomed Eng Online* 4:60. Published online Oct 27; doi:10.1186/1475-925X-4-60.

243

Amann A, Tratnig R, Unterkofler K (2007) Detecting ventricular fibrillation by time-delay methods. IEEE Trans Biomed Eng 54(1):174–177.

American Society for Hospital Engineering of the American Hospital Association (1994) Electromagnetic interference: Causes and concerns in the health care environment. Healthcare Facilities Management Series, Chicago, IL, AHA, August.

ANSI/AAMI PC69 (2000) Active implantable medical devices. Electromagnetic compatibility. EMC test protocols for implantable cardiac pacemakers and implantable cardioverter defibrillators. *American National Standards Institute.*

Armayor MR, Savino GV, Valentinuzzi ME, Clavin OE, Monzón JE, Arredondo MT (1978) Ventricular defibrillation thresholds with capacitor discharge. *Int Symp and Workshop on Biomed Eng* (New Delhi, India), Febr, pp. 146–147. Full paper in Trends in Biomedical Engineering, 1978, editor SK Guha, CBME Publications, New Delhi, India, pp. 231–250. Also in *Med Biol Eng Comput* 1979, 17(4):435–442.

Arredondo MT, Armayor MR, Clavin OE, Valentinuzzi ME, Scidá EE (1980) Effect of body hypothermia on transventricular simple capacitor discharge defibrillation thresholds. *Am J Physiol 238 (Heart Circ Physiol 7)*:H675–H685.

Arredondo MT, Armayor MR, Valentinuzzi ME (1982) Electrical defibrillation thresholds with transventricular simple-capacitor discharge under conditions of ischemia by acute coronary occlusion. *Med Prog Technol* 8:175–181.

Arredondo MT, Armayor MR, Valentinuzzi ME, Ruiz E (1984) Transventricular simple capacitor discharge defibrillation thresholds after coronary ligation and body hypothermia. *J Biomed Eng* 6(4):284–288.

Arnsdorf and Bradley (2008) Patient information: Implantable cardioverter-defibrillators. *UpToDate for Patients*, Samuel Levy MD, Section Editor, http://www.uptodate.com/patients/content/topic.do?topicKey=~vYXPq 0f2CRDHW.

Atkins DL, Sirna S, Kieso R, Charbonnier F, Kerber RE (1988) Pediatric defibrillation: Importance of paddle size in determining transthoracic impedance. *Pediatrics* 82(6):914–918.

Aupetit JF, Timour Q, Chevrel G, Loufoua-Moundanga J, Omar S, Faucon G (1993) Attenuation of the ischaemia-induced fall of electrical ventricular fibrillation threshold by a calcium antagonist, diltiazem. *Naunyn Schmiedebergs Arch Pharmacol* 348(5):509–514 (Nov).

Aviles RJ, Martin DO, Apperson-Hansen C, Houghtaling PL, Rautaharju P, Kronmal RA, Tracy RP, Van Wagoner DR, Psaty BM, Lauer MS, Chung MK (2003) Inflammation as a risk factor for atrial fibrillation. *Circulation* 108:3006–3010; Published online before print November 17, 2003, doi:10.1161/01.CIR.0000103131.70301.4F.

Aylward PE, Kieso R, Hite P, Charbonnier F, Kerber RE (1985) Defibrillator electrode-chest wall coupling agents: Influence on transthoracic impedance and shock success. *J Am Coll Cardiol* 6:682–686.

Babbs CF, Tacker WA, van Vleet JF, Bourland JD, Geddes LA (1980) Therapeutic indices for transchest defibrillation shocks: Effective, damaging and lethal doses. *Am Heart J* 99(6):734–738.

Babbs CF, Whistler SJ, Yim GKW, Tacker WA, Geddes LA (1980) Dependence of defibrillation threshold upon extracellular/intracellular $K^+$ concentrations. *J Electrocardiol* 13(1):73–78.

Bailey B, Ellner S, Nychka DW (1997) Chaos with confidence: Asymptotic and applications of local Lyapunov exponents. *In Cutler and Kaplan*, pp. 115–133.

Barbaro V, Bartolini P, Bellocci F, Caruso F, Donato A, Gabrielli D, Militello C, Montenero AS, Zecchi P (1999) Electromagnetic interference of digital and analog cellular telephones with implantable cardioverter defibrillators: *In vitro* and *in vivo* studies. *Pacing Clin Electrophysiol* (PACE) 22(4):626–634; doi:10.1111/j.1540-8159.1999.tb00504.x.

Bardy, G, Gliner, B, Kudenchuk, P (1995) Truncated biphasic pulses for transthoracic defibrillation. *Circulation* 91:1768–1774.

Bardy GH, Lee KL, Mark DB, Pool JE, Packer DL, Boineau R, Domanski M, Troutman C, Anderson J, Johnson G, McNulty SE, Clapp-Channing N, Davidson-Ray LD, Fraulo ES, Fishbein DP, Luceri RM (2005) Amiodarone or an implantable cardioverter-defibrillator for congestive heart failure. *New Engl J Med* 352(3):225–237. Erratum in *New Engl J Med* 2005 May 19; 352(20):2146.

Bardy G, Marchlinski F, Sharma A (1996) Multicenter comparison of truncated biphasic shocks and standard damped sine wave monophasic shocks for transthoracic ventricular defibrillation. *Circulation* 94:2507–2514.

Bardy GH, Zaghi H, Gartman D, Poole JE, Kudenchuk PK, Dolack GL, Johnson G, Troutman C (1994) A prospective randomized comparison of defibrillation efficacy of truncated pulses and damped sine wave pulses in humans. *J Cardiovasc Electrophysiol* 5(9):725–730, doi:10.1111/j.1540-8167.1994.tb01195.x.

Bassen H (2008) Low frequency magnetic emissions and resulting induced voltages in a pacemaker by iPod portable music players. *Biomed Eng OnLine* 7:7; doi:10.1186/1475-925X-7-7; http://www.biomedical-engineering-online.com/content/7/1/7.

Baumert J, Schmitt C, Ladwig KH (2006) Psychophysiologic and affective parameters associated with pain intensity of cardiac cardioverter defibrillator shock discharges. *Psychosom Med* 68:591–597.

Bayés de Luna AJ (1999) Características del electrocardiograma normal (Characteristics of the normal ECG). In *Electrocardiografía Clínica* (Clinical Electrocardiography), Ediciones Espaxs, Barcelona, Spain. Chap 2, pp. 31–45. In Spanish.

Beck CS, Pritchard WH, Feil HS (1947) Ventricular fibrillation of long duration abolished by electric shock. *J Am Med Assoc* (JAMA) 135:985–986.

Beeler GW, Reuter H (1977) Reconstruction of the action potential of ventricular myocardial fibres. *J Physiol* 268:177–210.

Belousov B P (1959) A periodic reaction and its mechanism (in Russian). *Compilation of Abstracts on Radiation Medicine* 147:145.

Bennet M, Dennett D, Hacker P, Searle J, Robinson D (2007) Neuroscience & Philosophy. Columbia University Press, New York, USA, 215 pp.

Bernstein T (1973) A grand success: The first legal electrocution was fraught with controversy which flared between Edison and Westinghouse. *IEEE Spectrum* Febr, pp. 54–58.

Bertalanffy L von (1957) Quantitative laws in metabolism and growth. *Q Rev Biol* 32(3):217–231.

Blair HA (1935) On the quantity of electricity and the energy in electrical stimulation. *J Gen Physiol* (London): 951–964; downloaded from www.jgp.org, February 23, 2008.

Bonhoeffer KF (1948) Activation of passive iron as a model for the excitation of nerve. *J Gen Physiol* 32:69–91.

Bonhoeffer KF (1953) Modelle der Nervenerregung. *Naturwissenschaften* 40:301–311; doi:10.1007/BF00632438. Bostrom U (1991) Interference from mobile telephones: A challenge for Clinical Engineers. *Clin Eng Update* 10, Nov.

Bostrum U (1991) Interference from mobile telephones: A challenge for Clinical Engineers. *Clin Eng Update* 10, Nov.

Brugada P, Brugada J (1992) Right bundle branch block, persistent ST segment elevation and sudden cardiac death: A distinct clinical and electrocardiographic syndrome. A multicenter report. *J Am Coll Cardiol* 20(6):1391–1396.

Brugada J, Aguinaga L (editors) (2010) Ablación por Catéter de Arritmias Cardíacas (In Spanish, Catheter Ablation of Cardiac Arrhythmias). Federación Argentina de Cardiología (FAC). Available at http://www.fac.org.ar/1/publicaciones/libros/ablacion/.

Boyer M, Koplan BA (2005) Atrial flutter. *Circulation* 112:e334–e336.

BMJ editorial (2003) Risk factor scoring for coronary heart disease. Prediction algorithms need regular updating. *Br Med J* 327:1238–1239 (29 Nov).

Bradley JR, Salil GP (2003) Effects of elevated extracellular potassium ion concentration on anodal excitation of cardiac tissue. *J Cardiovasc Electrophysiol* 14(12):1351–1355. doi:10.1046/j.1540-8167.2003.03167.x.

Bristow M, Saxon L, Boehmer J, Krueger S, Kass D, De Marco T, Carson P, DiCarlo L, DeMets D, White B, DeVries D, Feldman A (2004). Cardiac-resynchronization therapy with or without an implantable defibrillator in advanced chronic heart failure. *N Engl J Med* 350(21):2140–2150.

Brooks L, Zhang Y, Dendi R, Anderson RH, Zimmerman B, Kerber RE (2009) Selecting the transthoracic defibrillation shock directional vector based on VF amplitude improves shock success. *J Cardiovasc Physiol* May 4; abstract freely available at http://www.ncbi.nlm.nih.gov/pubmed/19460079.

Burrus CS, Gopinath RA, Guo H (1998) Generalizations of the basic multi-resolution wavelet system. In Introduction to wavelets and wavelet transforms. A primer. Burrus CS, Gopinath RA and Guo, eds, Prentice Hall, New Jersey, USA. Chapter 7, pp. 98–147.

Butter C, Meisel E, Tebbenjohanns J, Engelmann L, Fleck E, Schubert B, Hahn S, Pfeiffer D (2001) Transvenous biventricular defibrillation halves energy requirements in patients. *Circulation* 104:2533.

Cammilli L, Grassi G (1998) Implantable electric heart defibrillation system with attenuation of the pain resulting from the electric shock. United States Patent #6167305; Application #09/057206; Publication Date 12/26/2000; Filing Date 04/08/1998.

Cammilli L, Mugelli A, Grassi G, Alcidi L, Melissano G, Menegazzo G, Silvestri V (1991) Implantable pharmacological defibrillator (AIPhD): Preliminary investigations in animals. *Pacing and Clinical Electrophysiology* (PACE) 14(2):381–6; doi:10.1111/j.1540-8159.1991.tb05126.x.

Cancelas JA, Koevoet WLM, de Koning AE, Mayen AEM, Rombouts EJC, Ploemacher RE (2000) Connexin-43 gap junctions are involved in multiconnexin-expressing stromal support of hemopoietic progenitors and stem cells. *Blood* 96(2):498–505.

Cao Z, Li P, Zhang H, Xie F, and Hu G (2007) Turbulence control with local pacing and its implication in cardiac defibrillation. *Chaos* 17:015107.

Carlsson E, Olsson BS, Hertervig E (2002) The role of the nurse in enhancing quality of life in patients with an implantable cardioverter-defibrillator: The Swedish Experience. *Prog Cardiovasc Nur* 17(1):18–25.

Cartwright J, Gonzalez DL, and Piro O (1999a) Universality in three-frequency resonances. *Phys Rev E* 59(3):2902–2906.

Cartwright J, Gonzalez DL, Piro O, and Zanna M, (1999b) Teoria dei sistemi dinamici: Una base matematica per i fenomeni non-lineari in biologia. *Sistema Naturae* 2:215–254.

Cartwright J, Checa AG, Escribano B, Sainz-Díaz I (2009) Spiral and target patterns in bivalve nacre manifest a natural excitable medium from layer growth of a biological liquid crystal. *Proc Natl Acad Sci* (PNAS) 106(26):10499–10504.

CAST (Cardiac Arrhythmia Suppression Trial) (1989) Effect of encainide and flecainide on mortality in a randomized trial of arrhythmia suppression after myocardial infarction. *N Engl J Med* 321:406–412.

Cechi GA, González DL, Magnasco MO, Mindlin GB, Piro O, Santillán AJ (1993) Periodically kicked hard oscillators. *Chaos* 3:51–62.

Chan KS (1997) *On the validity of the method of surrogate data*. In Cutler and Kaplan, pp. 77–97.

Chan KS, Tong H (2001) *Chaos: A statistical perspective*. Springer Verlag, New York.

Chapman PD, Vetter JW, Souza JJ, Troup PJ Wetherbee JN, Hoffmann RG (1988) Comparative efficacy of monophasic and biphasic truncated exponential shocks for nonthoracotomy internal defibrillation in dogs. *J Am Coll Cardiol* 12:739–745.

Chen PS, Shibata N, Dixon EG, Martin RO, Ideker RE (1986) Comparison of the defibrillation threshold and the upper limit of ventricular vulnerability. *Circulation* 73:1022–1028.

Chen PS, Wolf PD, Ideker RE (1991): Mechanism of cardiac defibrillation: A different point of view. *Circulation* 84: 913–919.

Cheng Y, Zhuang S, Nikolski, V, Efimov, IR, Wallick, DW (2002) Virtual electrode-induced phase singularity in a rabbit model of chronic myocardial infarction. *Eng Medicine Biology 24th Ann Conf and Annual Fall Meeting*

*Biomed Eng Soc*, EMBS/BMES Second Joint Conf Proc 2:1430-1; doi:10.1109/IEMBS.2002.1106465.

Chorro FJ, Blasco E, Trapero I, Cánoves J, Ferrero A, Mainar L, Such-Miquel L, Sanchis J, Bodí V, Cerdá JM (2007) Selective myocardial isolation and ventricular fibrillation. *Pacing Clin Electrophysiol* (PACE) 30(3):359.

Chorro FJ, Guerrero J, Ferrero A, Tormos A, Mainar L, Mollet J, Cánoves J, Porres JC, Sanchos J, López-Merino V, Duch L (2002) Effects of acute reduction of temperature on ventricular fibrillation activation patterns. *Am J Physiol Heart Circ Physiol* 283(6):H2331–H2340.

Chung-Wah Siu, Hung-Fat Tse, Chu-Pak Lau (2005) Inappropriate implantable cardioverter defibrillator shock from a transcutaneous muscle stimulation device therapy. *J Interv Cardiac Electrophysiol* 13(1):73–75; doi:10.1007/s10840-005-0357-3.

Clayton RH, Murray A (1998) Comparison of techniques for time-frequency analysis of the ECG during human ventricular fibrillation. *IEE Proc Sci Meas Technol* 45(6):301–306.

Clayton RH, Murray A, Campbell RWF (1994) Recognition of ventricular fibrillation using neural networks. *Med Biol Eng Comput* 32:217–220.

Clayton RH, Murray A, Campbell RWF (1995) Frequency analysis of ventricular fibrillation. *IEE Colloquium Signal Processing in Cardiography* 3:1–4.

Clayton RH, Zhuchkovab EA, and Panfilov AV (2006) Phase singularities and filaments: Simplifying complexity in computational models of ventricular fibrillation. *Prog Biophys Mol Biol* 90:378–398.

Cleland J, Daubert J, Erdmann E, Freemantle N, Gras D, Kappenberger L, Tavazzi L (2005) The effect of cardiac resynchronization on morbidity and mortality in heart failure. *N Engl J Med* 352(15):1539–1549.

Connell PN, Ewy GA, Dahl CF, Ewy MD (1973) Transthoracic impedance to defibrillator discharge. Effect of electrode size and electrode-chest wall interface. *J Electrocardiol* 6(4):313-M.

Coronel R, Wilms-Schopman FJG, de Groot JR (2002) Origin of ischemia-induced phase 1b ventricular arrhythmias in pig hearts. *J Am Coll Cardiol* 39:166–176.

Crampton R (1980) Accepted, controversial and speculative aspects of ventricular defibrillation. *Prog Cardiovasc Dis* 23(3):167–186.

Croisier H, Guevara MR, Dauby PC (2009) Bifurcation analysis of a periodically forced relaxation oscillator: Differential model versus phase-resetting map. *Phys Rev E* 79: 016209.

Cummins RO, Chesemore K, White RD (1990) Defibrillator failures. Causes of problems and recommendations for improvement. Defibrillator Working Group. *J Am Med Assoc* (JAMA) 264(8), August 22.

Cutler CD (1993) A review of the theory and estimation of fractal dimension.In C.D. Cutler, ed, Dimension estimation and models, volume 1 of Nonlinear Time Series Chaos, pp. 1–107, World Scientific Publishers, Singapore.

Cutler CD, Kaplan DT (eds) (1997) *Nonlinear dynamics and time series: Building a bridge between the natural and statistical sciences*, volume 11 of *Fields Institute Communications*. American Mathematical Society, Providence, RI.

Dahl CF, Ewy GA, Ewy MD, Thomas ED (1976) Transthoracic impedance to direct current discharge: Effect of repeated countershocks. *Med Instrum* 10(3):151–154.

Damani SB, Topol EJ (2009) Molecular genetics of atrial fibrillation. *Genome Medicine* 1:54; doi:10.1186/gm54; http://blogs.openaccesscentral.com/blogs/bmcblog/entry/.

Darbar D, Olgin JE, Mille JM, Friedman PA (2001) Localization of the origin of arrhythmias for ablation: From electrocardiography to advanced endocardial mapping systems. *J Cardiovasc Electrophysiol* 12:1309–1325.

Defares JG, Sneddon IN (1961) The Mathematics of Medicine and Biology. Year Book Medical Publishers, Chicago (see Chapter X, pp. 593–597).

de Jongh AL, Entcheva EG, Replogle JA, Booker RS, Kenknight BH, Claydon FJ (1999) Defibrillation efficacy of different electrode placements in a human thorax model. *Pacing Clin Electrophysiol* (PACE) 22(1 Pt 2):152–157.

de Paola AA, Figueiredo E, Sesso R, Veloso HH, Nascimento LO (2003) Effectiveness and costs of chemical versus electrical cardioversion of atrial fibrillation. *Int J Cardiol* 88(2–3):157–66.

Dessertenne F (1966). La tachycardie ventriculaire a deux foyers opposés variables (in French). Ventricular tachycardia with two variable opposing foci. *Arch Mal Cœur Vaiss* 59(2):263–272.

Di Francesco D, Noble D (1985) A model of cardiac electrical activity incorporating ionic pumps and concentration changes. *Philos Trans R Soc Lond B Biol Sci* 240:61–81.

Diks C (1999) Nonlinear time series analysis, volume 4 of *Nonlinear Time Series and Chaos*. World Scientific Publishing, Singapore.

Diodato MD, Shah NR, Prasad SM, Gaynor SL, Lawton JS, Damiano RJ (2004) Donor heart preservation with pinacidil: The role of the mitochondrial $K_{ATP}$ channel. *Ann Thorac Surg* 78:620–627.

DeSilva RA, Lown B (1978) Energy requirement for defibrillation of a markedly overweight patient. *Circulation* 57(4):827–830.

Dosdall DJ, Ideker RE (2007) Intracardiac atrial defibrillation. *Heart Rhythm* Mar; 4(3 Suppl):S51–6. Epub 2006 Dec 28.

Dyro JF (2004) The Clinical Engineering Handbook. Association for the Advancement of Medical Instrumentation, USA, 696 pp. ISBN: 9780122265709.

Earn YE, Noble D (1990) A model of the single atrial cell: Relation between calcium current and calcium release. *Proc R Soc Lond B Sci* 240:83–96.

Edwards KE, Wenstone R (2000) Successful resuscitation from recurrent ventricular fibrillation secondary to butane inhalation. *Br J Anaesth* 84(6):803–805.

Echt DS, Cato EL, DR Coxe DR (1989) pH-dependent effects of lidocaine on defibrillation energy requirements in dogs. Circulation 80:1003–1009.

Efimov IR, Fedorov VV (2005) Chessboard of atrial fibrillation: reentry or focus? Single or multiple source(s)? Neurogenic or myogenic? *Am J Physiol Heart Circ Physiol* 289:H977–H979; doi:10.1152/ajpheart.00456.

Efimov IR, Kroll MW, Tchou PJ (eds) (2008) Cardiac Bioelectric Therapy: Mechanisms and Practical Implications. Springer, New York, 704 pp.

250           *Cardiac Fibrillation-Defibrillation*

Einthoven W (1903) Ein neues Galvanometer (in German, A new galvanometer). *Ann Phys* 4 (Suppl):1059–1071.

Eisenberg M (2006) The resuscitation greats. Bernard Lown and defibrillation. *Resuscitation* 69(2):171–173.

Elabbady TZ, Chapman FW, Sullivan JL, Nova RC, Borschowa LA (1999) Defibrillator method and apparatus. US Patent No. 5999852, December.

Ellner SP, Guckenheimer J (2006) *Dynamic Models in Biology*, Princeton University Press, 329 pp.

Ewy GA (1992) Optimal technique for electrical cardioversion of atrial fibrillation. *Circulation* 86:1645–1647 (see also http://circ.ahajournals.org/).

Ewy GA, Ewy MD, Nuttall AJ, Nuttall AW (1972) Canine transthoracic resistance. *J Appl Physiol* 32(1):91–94.

Ewy GA, Horan WJ, Ewy MD (1977) Disposable defibrillator electrodes. *Heart Lung* 6(1):127–130.

Fado S (2003) Biphasic and monophasic shocks for transthoracic defibrillation: A meta analysis of randomised controlled trials. *Resuscitation* 58(1):9.

Fan J and Yao Q (2003) *Nonlinear time series. Nonparametric and parametric methods*. Springer Series in Statistics, Springer-Verlag, New York.

Fatema, K, Barnes ME, Bailey KR, Abhayaratna WP, Cha S, Seward JB, Tsang TSM (2008) Minimum vs maximum left atrial volume for prediction of first atrial fibrillation or flutter in an elderly cohort: A prospective study. *Eur J Echocardiogr*, online on September 11; doi:10.1093/ejechocard/jen235.

Feigenbaum MJ (1978) Quantitative universality for a class of non-linear transformations. *J Stat Phys* 19:25–52.

Feigenbaum MJ (1980) Universal behaviour in non-linear systems. *Los Alamos Sci* 1:4–27.

Feingold M, González DL, Piro, Viturro H (1988) Phase locking, period doubling, and chaotic phenomena in externally driven excitable systems. *Phys Rev A, Gen Phys, 3rd Series* 37:4060–4063.

Feldman CL, Amazeen PG, Klein MD, Lown B (1970) Computer detection of ventricular ectopic beats. *Comput Biomed Res* 3(6):666–674.

Fish RM, Geddes LA (2003) Medical and Bioengineering Aspects of Electrical Injuries. Lawyers & Judges Publishers, Tucson, AZ, 498 pp.

FitzHugh R (1961) Impulses and physiological states in theoretical models of nerve membrane. *Biophys J* 1:445–466.

Fogarty TJ, Howell TA (1995) Implantable defibrillator electrodes. US Patent Issued on November 7 of said year.

Freysz M, Timour Q, Bertrix L, Loufoua J, Aupetit JF, Faucon G (1995) Bupivacaine hastens the ischemia-induced decrease of the electrical ventricular fibrillation threshold. *Anesth Analg* 80(4):657–663.

Garfinkel A, Young-Hoon K, Voroshilovsky O, Qu Z, Kil JR, Moon-Hyoung L, Karagueuzian HS, Weiss JN, Peng-Sheng C (2000) Preventing ventricular fibrillation by flattening cardiac restitution. *Proc Natl Acad Sci* 97(11):6061–6066.

Garrey WE (1914) The nature of fibrillary contraction of the heart: Its relations to tissue mass and form. *Am J Physiol* 33:397–414.

Geddes LA (1976) Electrical ventricular defibrillation. Chapter 3 in IEE Medical Electronics, Monographs 18–22, eds D. W. Hill and B.W. Watson, Peter Peregrinus Ltd, pp. 42–72, London, England.

Geddes LA (1984) A short history of the electrical stimulation of excitable tissues, including electrotherapeutic applications. *Physiologist* (supplement) 27(1):S1–S47.

Geddes LA (1987) Cardiac Fibrillation and Defibrillation (*Fibrilación-Defibrilación Cardíaca*), Book Review, *MEBC News*, N° 1, January, p. N7.

Geddes L A 1994 Electrodes for transchest and ICD defibrillation and multi-functional electrodes. In Defibrillation of the Heart: ICDs, AEDs and Manual, ed. W A Tacker Jr, Saint Louis, MO, Mosby-Year Book, pp. 82–118.

Geddes LA (1997) Historical evolution of circuit models for the electrode-electrolyte interface. *Ann Biomed Eng* 25:1–14.

Geddes LA, Baker LE (1989) Principles of Applied Biomedical Instrumentation. Third Edition, John Wiley & Sons, New York, USA, 961 pp.

Geddes LA, Bakken EE (2007) Who first performed cardiac pacing: Why, when, and where? *IEEE/EMB Magazine* 26(3):77–79.

Geddes LA, Roeder RA (1995) Handbook of Electrical Hazards and Accidents. Lawyers & Judges Publishers, Tuczon, AZ, 726 pp.

Geddes LA, Roeder R. (2001) Measurement of the direct-current (faradic) resistance of the electrode-electrolyte interface for commonly used electrode materials. *Ann Biomed Eng* 29(2):181–186.

Geddes LA, Rundell A, Lottes A, Kemeny A, Otlewski M (2007) A new cardiopulmonary resuscitation method using only rhythmic abdominal compression: A preliminary report. *Am J Emerg Med* 25:786–790.

Geddes LA, Tacker WA, Cabler P, Gothard R, Kidder H (1975) The decrease in transthoracic impedance during successive ventricular defibrillation trials. *Med Instrum* 9:179–180.

Geddes LA, Tacker WA, Schoenlein BS, Minton M, Grubbs S, Wilcox P (1976) The prediction of the impedance of the thorax to defibrillating current. *Med Instrum* 10:159–62.

Giannerini S and Rosa R (2001) New resampling method to assess the accuracy of the maximal Lyapunov exponent estimation. *Physica D*, 155:101–111.

Giannerini S and Rosa R (2004) Assessing chaos in time series: Statistical aspects and perspectives. *Stud Nonlinear Dynam Econometrics*, 8 (2, Article 11).

Giannerini S, Rosa R, González DL (2007) Testing chaotic dynamics in systems with two positive Lyapunov exponents: A bootstrap solution. *Int J Bifurcat Chaos* 17(1):169–182.

Gillberg J (2007) Detection of cardiac tachyarrhythmias in implantable devices. *J Electrocardiol* 40:S123–S128.

Glass L, Perez R (1982) Fine structure of phase locking. *Phys Rev Lett* 48:1772–1775.

Glass L, Guevara MR, Bélair J, Shrier A (1984) Global bifurcations of a periodically forced biological oscillator. *Phys Rev A* 29:148–157.

Glass L, Hunter P, McCulloch A (editors) (1991) *Theory of Heart*. Springer-Verlag, New York, 611 pp.

Glass L, Nagai Y, Hall K, Talajic M, Nattel S (2002) Predicting the entrainment of reentrant cardiac waves using phase resetting curves. *Phys Rev E* 65:021908.

Gliner, BE, Jorgenson, DB, Poole, JE (1998) Treatment of out-of-hospital cardiac arrest with a low-energy impedance-compensating biphasic waveform automatic external defibrillator. *Biomed Instrum Technol* 32,631–644.

Gold MR, Higgins S, Klein R, Gilliam FR, Kopelman H, Hessen S, Payne J, Strickberger SA, Breiter D, Hahn S (2002) Efficacy and temporal stability of reduced safety margins for ventricular defibrillation. Primary Results from the Low Energy Safety Study (LESS). *Circulation* 105:2043.

Gold M, Olsovsky M, Pelini M (1998) Comparison of single- and dual-coil active pectoral defibrillation systems. *J Am Coll Cardiol* 31:1391–1394.

Gonzalez, DL (1987) Sincronización y caos en osciladores no-lineales, PhD Dissertation, *Universidad Nacional de La Plata, Physics Department*, 393 pp.

Gonzalez DL, Piro O, (1984) One dimensional Poincaré map for a non-linear driven oscillator, analytical derivation and geometrical properties *Phys Lett A* 101(9):455–458.

Gonzalez, DL, Rosso, O (1997) Qualitative modeling of complex biological systems. In *Proc Second Italian-Latin-American Meeting Applied Math*, Rome, pp. 132–135.

Goyal R, Harvey M, Horwood L, Bogun F, Castellani M, Chan KK, Daoud E, Niebauer M, Ching Man K, Morady F, Strickberger SA (1996) Incidence of lead system malfunction detected during implantable defibrillator generator replacement. *Pacing Clin Electrophysiol* (PACE) 19(8):1143–1146; doi:10.1111/j.1540-8159.1996.tb04183.x.

Guan D, Powell C, Malkin R (2000) Defibrillation impedance: Including an inductive element. *Comput Cardiol* 27:549–552.

Guevara MR, Glass L, Shrier A (1981) Phase locking, period doubling bifurcations and irregular dynamics in periodically stimulated cardiac cells. *Science* 214:1350.

Gunn HM (1989) Heart weight and running ability. *J Anat* 167: 225–233.

Gurvich NL, Yuniev GS (1946) Restoration of regular rhythm in the mammalian fibrillating heart. *Am Rev Soviet Med* 3:236–239.

Gurvich NL, Yuniev GS (1947) Restoration of heart rhythm during fibrillation by a condenser discharge. *Amer Rev Soviet Med* 4:252.

Gutstein DE, Danik SB, Lewitton S, France D, Liu F, Chen FL, Zhang J, Ghodsi N, Morley GE, Fishman GI (2005) Focal gap junction uncoupling and spontaneous ventricular ectopy. *Am J Physiol Heart Circ Physiol* 289:H1091–H1098. First published May 13, 2005; doi: 10.1152/ajpheart.00095.2005, 0363-6135/05.

Guttman R, Feldman L, Jakobsson EJ (1980) Frequency entrainment of squid axon membrane. *J Membr Biol* 56(1):9–18.

Györke I, Hester N, Jones LR, Györke S (2004) The role of calsequestrin, triadin, and junction in conferring cardiac ryanodine receptor responsiveness to luminal calcium. *Biophys J* 86:2121–2128.

Hanada E, Antoku Y, Tani S, Kimura M, Hasegawa A, Urano S, Ohe K, Yamaki M, Nose Y (2000). Electromagnetic interference on medical equipment by low-power mobile telecommunication systems. *IEEE Trans Electromag Compatibility* 42(4):470–476; doi:10.1109/15.902316.

Hilborn RC (2001) Chaos and Nonlinear Dynamics: An Introduction for Scientists and Engineers. USA: Oxford University Press, 2nd ed.

Hilgemann DW, Noble D (1987) Excitation-contraction coupling and extracellular calcium transients in rabbit atrium: Reconstruction of basic cellular mechanisms. *Proc Royal Soc Lond B Biol Sci* 230:163–205.

Hille B (2001) Ionic Channels of Excitable Membranes, 2nd ed, Sinauer Associates, Sunderland, MA 01375, 722 pp.

Hillman H (1983) A unnatural way to die. *New Scientist* Oct 27, pp. 276–278.

Himel HD, Dumas JH, Kiser AC, Knisley SB (2007) Translesion stimulus-excitation delay indicates quality of linear lesions produced by radiofrequency ablation in rabbit hearts. *Physiol Meas* 28:611–623; doi:10.1088/0967-3334/28/6/001.

Hodgkin AL, Huxley AF (1952) A quantitative description of membrane current and its application to conduction and excitation in nerve. *J Physiol* (London) 117:500–544.

Hoff HE, Geddes LA, McGrady JD (1966) The contribution of the horse to knowledge of the heart and circulation. III. James Mackenzie, Thomas Lewis and the nature of atrial fibrillation. *Connecticut Medicine* 30(1):43–48. This is the 3rd of a series of four outstanding articles dealing with studies made with the horse as experimental animal.

Hoffa M, Ludwig C (1850) Einige neue Versuche über Herzbewegung (in German, A new investigation about cardiac movement). *Zeitschrift für rat Medizin* (Journal for Counselling Medicine) 9:107–144.

Hoffman BF, Cranefield PF (1960) Electrophysiology of the Heart. McGraw-Hill Book Co., New York, 323 pp. (see p. 261).

Hooker DR (1930) Chemical factors in ventricular fibrillation. *Am J Physiol* 92(3):639–647.

Hoshino K, Ogawa K, Hishitani T, Isobe T, Etoh Y (2006) Successful uses of magnesium sulfate for torsades de pointes in children with long QT syndrome. *Pediatrics Int* 48(2):112–117; doi:10.1111/j.1442-200X.2006.02177.x.

Hulting J, Nygards ME (1976) Evaluation of a computer-based system for detecting ventricular arrhythmias. Acta Med Scan 199 (2):53–60.

Ideker RE, Chen P-S, Shibata N, Colavita PG, Wharton JM (1987) Current concepts of the mechanisms of ventricular defibrillation. In Nonpharmacological Theory of Tachyarrhythmias, eds G Breithardt, M Borggrefe, DP Zipes, pp. 449–464, Futura Pub Co, Mount Kisco, New York.

Ideker RE, Fine MJ, Baker R G, Calfee RV (1987) Implantable defibrillation electrodes. United States Patent 4827932, published on 05/09/1989.

International Organization for Standardization (ISO) 14708-1 (2000) Implants for surgery. Active implantable medical devices – Part 1: General requirements for safety, marking and for information to be provided by the manufacturer. *Geneva, Switzerland.*

Irnich W (1990) The fundamental law of electrostimulation and its application to defibrillation. *Pacing Clin Electrophysiol* (PACE) 13:1433–1447.

Irnich W (2002) Georges Weiss' fundamental law of electrostimulation is 100 Years old. *Pacing Clin Electrophysiol (PACE)* 25:245–248; doi:10.1046/j.1460-9592.2002.00245.x.

Jalife J (2000) Ventricular fibrillation: Mechanisms of initiation and maintenance. *Annual Rev Physiol* 62:25–50 March; (doi:10.1146/annurev.physiol.62.1.25).

Jalife J, Berenfeld (2004) Molecular mechanisms and global dynamics of fibrillation: An integrative approach to the underlying basis of vortex-like reentry. *J Theor Biol* 230:475–487.

Jané R, Rix H, Caminal P, Laguna P (1991) Alignment methods for averaging of high-resolution cardiac signals: A comparative study of performance. *IEEE Trans Biomed Eng* 38(6):571–579.

Jenkins JM, Caswell SA (1996) Detection algorithms in implantable defibrillators. *Proc IEEE* 84:428–445.

Johansson BW (1984) Cardiac responses in relation to heart size. *Cryobiology* 21:627–636.

Jones JL, Jones RE, Balasky G (1987) Improved cardiac cell excitation with symmetrical biphasic defibrillator waveforms. *Am J Physiol* 253:H1418–H1424.

Judd K, Small M, Mees AI (2001) Achieving good nonlinear models: Keep it simple, vary the embedding, and get the dynamics right. In Mees AI, editor, *Nonlinear Dynamics and Statistics*, pp. 65–80.

Jalife J, Antzelevich C (1979) Phase resetting and annihilation of pacemaker activity in cardiac tissue. *Science* 206:695.

Kalter HH, Schwartz ML (1948) Electrical alternans. *NY State J Med* 1:1164–1166.

Kantz H, Schreiber T (2004) *Nonlinear time series analysis.* Cambridge University Press, Cambridge, second edition.

Karma A (2000) New paradigm for drug therapies of cardiac fibrillation. *PNAS* 97(11):5687–5689.

Karma A, Gilmour RF (2007) Nonlinear dynamics of heart rhythm disorders. *Phys Today* 60:51–57.

Keener JP, Lewis TJ (1999) The biphasic mystery: why a biphasic shock is more effective than a monophasic shock for defibrillation. *J Theor Biol* 200:1–17.

KenKnight B, Walker R, Ideker R (2000) Marked reduction of ventricular defibrillation threshold by application of an auxiliary shock to a catheter electrode in the left posterior coronary vein of dogs. *J Cardiovasc Electrophysiol* 11: 900–906.

Kerber RE, Kouba C, Martins J, Kelly K, Low R, Hoyt R, Ferguson D, Bailey L, Bennett P, Charbonnier F (1984) Advance prediction of transthoracic impedance in human defibrillation and cardioversion: Importance of impedance in determining the success of low-energy shocks. *Circulation* 70(2):303–308.

Kerber RE, Martins JB, Kienzle MG, Constantin L, Olshansky B, Hopsond R and Charbonnier F (1988) Energy, current, and success in defibrillation and cardioversion: Clinical studies using an automated impedance-based method of energy adjustment *Circulation* 77:1038–1046.

Kerber RE, Pandian NG, Hoyt R, Jensen SR, Koyanagi S, Grayzel J, Kieso R (1983) Effect of ischemia, hypertrophy, hypoxia, acidosis, and alkalosis on canine defibrillation. *Heart Circulatory Physiol* 244(6):H825–H831.

Kerber RE, Sarnat W (1979) Factors influencing the success of ventricular defibrillation in man. *Circulation* 60(2):226–230.

Kerber RE, Vance S, Schomer SJ, Mariano DJ, Charbonnier F (1992) Transthoracic defibrillation: Effect of sternotomy on chest impedance. *J Am Coll Cardiol* 20:94–97.

Khedun SM, Leary WP, Lockett CJ, Maharaj B (1991) Changes in myocardial electrolytes and ventricular fibrillation threshold induced by alcohol feeding in laboratory rats. *Japn Heart J* 32(3):373–379.

Kirsten HWJ, Tusscher T, Hren R, Panfilov AV (2007) Organization of ventricular fibrillation in the human heart. *Circ Res* 100:e87.

Kneller J, Kalifa J, Zou R, Zaitsev AV, Warren M, Berenfeld O, Vigmond EJ, Leon LJ, Nattel S, Jalife J (2005) Mechanisms of atrial fibrillation termination by pure sodium channel blockade in an ionically-realistic mathematical model. *Circ Res* 96:e35–e47.

Koning G, Schneider H, Hoelen AJ, Reneman RS (1975) Amplitude-duration relation for direct ventricular defibrillation with rectangular current pulses. *Med Biol Eng* 13(3):388–395.

Kontos MC, Ellenbogen KA, Wood MA, Damiano RJ, Akosah KO, Nixon JV, Stambler BS (1997) Factors associated with elevated impedance with a non-thoracotomy defibrillation lead system. *Am J Cardiol* 79(1):48–52.

Koster RW, Dorian P, Chapman FW, Schmitt PW, O'Grady SG, Walker RG (2004) A randomized trial comparing monophasic and biphasic waveform shocks for external cardioversion of atrial fibrillation. *Am Heart J* 147:e20.

Kouwenhoven WB, Hooker RD (1933) Resuscitation by counter-shock. *Elec Eng* 52:475–477.

Kouwenhoven WB, Milnor WR, Knickerbocker GG, Chesnut WR (1957) Closed chest defibrillation of the heart. *Surgery* 42:550–561.

Köhler BU, Hennig C, Orglmeister R (2002) The principles of software QRS detection. *IEEE Eng Med Biol Mag* 21(1):42–57.

Krauthamer V, Smith TC (2004) Acute effects of adrenergic agents on post-defibrillation arrest time in a cultured heart model. *Cell Mol Life Sci* (CMLS) 61(24):3093–3099; doi:10.1007/s00018-004-4372-9.

Kroll, MW, Dahl, RW, Sundquist, SK, Nelson, RS (1995) One piece disposable threshold test can electrode for use with an implantable cardioverter defibrillator system. US Patent #5662696; Application #08/535666; Publication Date 09/02/1997; Filing Date 09/28/1995.

Kroll MW, Swerdlow CD (2001) Optimizing defibrillation waveforms for ICDs *J Interv Cardiac Electrophysiol* 18(3):247–263.

Kugiumtzis D (2001) On the reliability of the surrogate data test for nonlinearity in the analysis of noisy time series. *Int J Bifurcat Chaos* 11(7):1881–1896.

Kuo, S, Dillman, R. (1978) Computer detection of ventricular fibrillation. *Comput Cardiol* 347–349.

Laciar E, Jané R, Brooks DH (2003) Improved alignment method for noisy high-resolution ECG and Holter records using multiscale cross-correlation. *IEEE Trans Biomed Eng* 50(3):344–353.

Laguna P, Simón B, Sörnmo L (1997) Improvement in high-resolution ECG analysis by interpolation before time alignment. *Comput Cardiol* 24:617–620.

Lang DJ, Bach SM (1990) Algorithms for fibrillation and tachyarrhythmia detection. *J Electrocardiol* 23 (Suppl):46–50.

Lapicque L (1909) Definition experimentale de l'excitation. *CR Acad Sci* 67(2):280–283.

Larson L, Blanchard E, Herman L, Léger MM, McNellis R, Quigley T, Toth S (2003) Current status of implantable cardioverter defibrillators. *JAPA* 2:11–17.

Lateef F, Swee, HL, Anantharaman V, Lim CS (2000) Changes in chest electrode impedance. *Am J Emerg Med* 18(4):381–384.

Lerman BB, Engelstein ED (1995) Increased defibrillation threshold due to ventricular fibrillation duration: Potential mechanisms. *J Electrocardiol* 28 Suppl:21–24.

Lerman BB, Halperin HR, Tsitlik JE, Brin K, Clark C, Wand Deal OC (1987) Relationship between canine transthoracic impedance and defibrillation threshold. *J Clin Invest* 80:797–803.

Levy D, Brink S (2005) A Change of Heart: How the People of Framingham, Massachusetts, Helped Unravel the Mysteries of Cardiovascular Disease. Knopf, ISBN: 0-375-41275-1.

Lewis T (1910) Notes upon alternation of the heart. *Q J Med* 4:141–144.

Lewis T (1925) The Mechanism and Graphic Registration of the Heart Beat, 3rd ed, Shaw, London, pp. 319–374.

Li C, Zheng C, Tai C (1995) Detection of ECG characteristic points using wavelet transforms. *IEEE Trans Biomed Eng* 42:21–28.

Lin D, Jenkins JM, Wiesmeyer MD, Jadvar H, Di Carlo LA (1986) Analysis of time and frequency domain patterns of endocardial electrograms to distinguish ventricular tachycardia from sinus rhythm. *Comput Cardiol* 13: 171–174.

Lopin, ML, Ayati S (1998) Electrotherapy circuit having controlled peak current. US Patent #5 800 462, issued on Sept 1st.

Lown B (1967a) Electrical reversion of cardiac arrhythmias. *Heart* 29:469–489. Freely downloaded from www.heart.bmj.com on 20 March 2008.

Lown B (1967b) Electrical reversion of cardiac arrhythmias. *Br Heart J* 29(4):469–489.

Lown B (2002) Defibrillation and cardioversion. *Cardiovasc Res* 55(2):220–224.

Lown B, Neuman J, Amarasingham R, Berkovits BV (1962) Comparison of alternating current with direct current electroshock across the closed chest. *Amer J Cardiol* 10:223.

Luo C, Rudy Y (1994a) A dynamical model of the cardiac ventricular action potential I: Simulation of ionic currents and concentration changes. *Circ Res* 74:1071–1097.

Luo C, Rudy Y (1994b) A dynamic model of the cardiac ventricular action potential: After-depolarizations, trigger activities, and potentiation. *Circ Res* 74:1097–1113.

MacDonald CF (1892) The infliction of the death penalty by means of electricity: Being a report of seven cases. *Trans Medical Society New York*, pp. 400–427.

Machin W (1978) Thoracic impedance of human subjects. *Med Biol Eng Comput* 16:169–178.

Malkin RA, Guan D, Wikswo JP (2006) Experimental evidence of improved transthoracic defibrillation with electroporation-enhancing pulses. *IEEE Trans Biomed Eng* 53(19):1901–1910.

MacWilliam JA (1887) Fibrillar contraction of the heart. *J Physiol* 8:296–310.

Mallat S (1989) Multifrequency channel decomposition of images and wavelet models. *IEEE Trans Acoust Speed Signal Process* 37:2091–2110.

Mallat S, Zhong S (1992) Characterization of signals from multiscale edges. *IEEE Trans Pattern Anal Machine Intell* 14:710–32.

Malmivuo J, Plonsey R (1995) Bioelectromagnetism: Principles and Applications of Bioelectric and Biomagnetic Fields. Oxford University Press, New York, 482 pp.

Mandel J (1964) The Statistical Analysis of Experimental Data. Interscience Publishers, New York, 410 pp.

Martínez JP, Almeida R, Olmos S, Rocha AP, Laguna P (2004) A wavelet-based ECG delineator: Evaluation on standard databases. *IEEE Trans Biomed Eng* 51(4):570–581

Massé S, Downar E, Chauhan V, Sevaptsidis E, Nanthakumar K (2007) Ventricular fibrillation in myopathic human hearts: Mechanistic insights from *in vivo* global endocardial and epicardial mapping. *Am J Physiol Heart Circ Physiol* 292:H2589–H2597. First published January 26, 2007; doi:10.1152/ajpheart.01336.2006 0363-6135/07.

Mazur A, Wang L, Anderson ME, Yee R, Theres H, Pearson A, Olson W, Wathen M (2001) Functional similarity between electrograms recorded from an implantable cardioverter defibrillator emulator and the surface electrocardiogram. *Pacing Clin Electrophysiol* (PACE) 24(1):34–40.

Mayer S, Geddes LA, Bourland JD, Ogborn L (1992) Faradic resistance of the electrode/electrolyte interface. *Med Biol Eng Comput* 30(5):538–542.

McAdams ET, Lackermeier A, McLaughlin JA, Macken D, Jossinet J (1995) The linear and non-linear electrical properties of the electrode-electrolyte interface. *Biosens Bioelectron* 10:67–74.

Mees AI (editor) (2001) *Nonlinear Dynamics and Statistics*. Birkhäuser, Boston.

Merillat JC, Lakatta EG, Hano O, Guarnieri T (1990) Role of calcium and the calcium channel in the initiation and maintenance of ventricular fibrillation. *Circ Res* 67:1115–23.

Millet-Roig J, Rieta-Ibáñez JJ, Vilanova E, Mocholi A, Chorro FJ (1999) Time-frequency analysis of a single ECG to discriminate between ventricular tachycardia and ventricular fibrillation. *Comput Cardiol* 26:711–714.

Mines GR (1913) On dynamics equilibrium in the heart. *J Physiol* (Lond) 46:349–382.

Mines GR (1914) On circulating excitations in heart muscle and their possible relation to tachycardia and fibrillation. *Trans R Soc Can* 8:43–52.

Mirowski M (1971) Standby defibrillator and method of operation, US Patent 3,614,955.

Mirowski M, Mower MM, Langer A, Heilman MS, Schreibman J (1978) A chronically implanted system for automatic defibrillation in active conscious dogs. Experimental model for treatment of sudden death from ventricular fibrillation. *Circulation* 58(1):90–94.

Mirowski M, Mower MM, Reid PR (1980a) The automatic implantable defibrillator. *Am Heart J* 100(6):1089–1092.

Mirowski M, Reid PR, Mower MM, Watkins L, Gott VL, Schaube JF, Langer A, Heilman MS, Kolenik SA, Fischell RE, Weisfeldt ML (1980b) Termination of malignant ventricular arrhythmias with an implanted automatic defibrillator in human beings. *New Engl J Med* 303:322–324.

Mirowski M, Reid PR, Watkins L, Weisfeldt ML, Mower MM (1981) Clinical treatment of life-threatening ventricular tachyarrhythmias with the automatic implantable defibrillator. *Am Heart J* 102(2):265–270.

Mittal S, Ayati S, Stein KM, Schwartzman D, Cavlovich D, Tchou PJ, Markowitz SM, Slotwiner DJ, Scheiner MA, Lerman BB (2000) Transthoracic cardioversion of atrial fibrillation: Comparison of rectilinear biphasic versus damped sine wave monophasic shocks. *Circulation* 101:1282–1287.

Moe GK, Abildskov JA (1959) Atrial fibrillation as a self-sustaining arrhythmia independent of focal discharge. *Am Heart J* 58:59–70.

Monzón JE, Guillén SG (1985) New instrument of programmed current for research and clinical use. *IEEE Trans BME* 32(11):928–935.

Monzón JE, Valentinuzzi ME (1982) Transventricular defibrillation thresholds using quarter and half sinusoidal pulses. *Med Biol Eng Comput* 20:756–760.

Moore TW, DiMeo FN, Dubin SF (1977) The half-cycle sinusoid as an alternative defibrillating waveform in low-energy applications. *Ann Biomed Eng* 5(2):157–163.

Moreno J, Zaitsev AV, Warren M, Berenfeld O, Kalifa J, Lucca E, Mironov S, Guha P, Jalife J (2005) Effect of remodelling, stretch and ischaemia on ventricular fibrillation frequency and dynamics in a heart failure model. *Cardiovascular Research* 65:158–166.

Moss AJ (2003) History of atrial fibrillation. *Ann Noninvasive Electrocardiol* 8(1):90 (January).

Mower MM (1993) Mortality and implantable cardioverter-defibrillators. *Circulation* 88(1):332–334.

Mower MM (1995) Implantable cardioverter defibrillator therapy: 15 years experience and future expectations. In the beginning: From dogs to humans. *Pacing Clin Electrophysiol* (PACE) 18(3 Pt 2):506–511.

Mower MM, Hause RG (1993) Developmental history, early use, and implementation of the automatic implantable cardioverter defibrillator. *Prog Cardiovasc Dis* 36(2):89–96.

Munhoz Da Fontoura Tavares N, Araújo De Oliveira, Miguel R, Atié J (2004) Recurrent ventricular fibrillation secondary to aortic valve tumor. *Heart Rhythm* 1(3):348–351; doi:10.1016/j.hrthm.2004.04.023.

Nagumo J, Arimoto S, Yoshizawa S (1962) An active pulse transmission line simulating nerve axon. *Proc IRE* 50:2061–2070.

Newhouse S, Ruelle D, Takens F (1978) Occurrence of strange axiom — A attractors near quasi-periodic flows of $T^m$, $m \geq$ 3. *Commun Math Phys* 64:35–40.

Nielsen JC, Kottkamp H, Zabel M, Aliot E, Kreutzer U, Bauer A, Schuchert A, Neuser H, Schumacher B, Schmidinger H, Stix G, Clémenty J, Danilovic D, Hindricks G (2008) Automatic home monitoring of implantable cardioverter defibrillators. *Europace*, published online April 22, 2008; doi:10.1093/europace/eun099.

Noble D (1962) A modification of the Hodgkin-Huxley equations applicable to Purkinje fibre action and pacemaker potential. *J Physiol* 160:317–352.

Noble D (2007) From the Hodgkin-Huxley axon to the virtual heart. *J Physiol* 580(1):15–22.

Nolasco JB, Dahlen RW (1968) A graphic method for the study of alternation in cardiac action potentials. *J Appl Physiol* 25:191–196.

Noujaim SF, Lucca E, Muñoz V, Persaud D, Berenfeld O, Meijler FL, Jalife (2004) From mouse to whale. A universal scaling relation for the PR interval of the electrocardiogram of mammals. *Circulation* 110:2802–2808.

Obeid AI, Verrier RL, Lown B (1978) Influence of glucose, insulin, and potassium on vulnerability to ventricular fibrillation in the canine heart. *Circ Res* 43(4):601–608.

Olivera JM, Ruiz E, De Majo R (1991) Defibrilador de corriente controlada (in Spanish, Constant current defibrillator). *Mundo Electrónico* (Barcelona, Spain) 219:49–53.

Pan J, Tompkins WJ (1985) A real-time QRS detection algorithm. *IEEE Trans Biomed Eng* 32:230–236.

Panfilov A (2006) Is heart size a factor in ventricular fibrillation? Or how close are rabbit and human hearts? *Heart Rhythm* 3(7):862–864.

Pannizzo F, Mercando AD, Fisher JD, Furman S (1988) Automatic methods for detection of tachyarrhythmias by antitachycardia devices. *Pacing Clin Electrophysiol* (PACE) 11:308–316.

Park J, Lee S, Jeon M, Jeon M (2009) Atrial fibrillation detection by heart rate variability in Poincare plot. *Bio Med Eng Online* 8:38 (11 December 2).

Pedrote A, Morales FJ, García-Riesco L, Errazquin F (2006) Documented exercise-induced cardiac arrest in a paediatric patient with hypertrophic cardiomyopathy. *Europace* 8(6):430–433; doi:10.1093/europace/eul044.

Pichel RH, Valentinuzzi ME (2001) An honorable death? *PACE* 24(7):1152–1153. See also Cardiovascular Failure: Pathophysiological Bases and Management, eds EIC Cabrera Fischer, AI Christian and JC Trainoni, Fundación Universitaria René G. Favaloro, Buenos Aires, pp. IX–X.

Pines JM, Pollack CV, Diercks DB, Chang AM, Shofer FS, Hollander JE (2009) The association between emergency department crowding and adverse cardiovascular outcomes in patients with chest pain. *Acad Emerg Med* 16:617–625.

Pomeau Y, Manneville P (1980) Intermittent transitions to turbulence in dissipative dynamical systems. *Commun Math Phys* 74:189.

Poole, JE, White, RD, Kanz, K-G (1997) Low-energy impedance-compensating biphasic waveforms terminate ventricular fibrillation at high rates in victims of out-of-hospital cardiac arrest. *J Cardiovasc Electrophysiol* 8:1373–1385.

Prevost JL, Batelli F (1899a) La mort par la décharges électriques. *CR Acad Sci Paris D* 128:651–654.

Prevost JL, Batelli F (1899b) La mort par la décharges électriques. *CR Acad Sci Paris D* 128:668–670.

Prevost JL, Batelli F (1899c) Sur quelques effets des décharges électriques sur le coeur des mamifères. *CR Acad Sci Paris D* 129:1267–1268.

Prevost JL, Batelli F (1899d) La mort par la courant électrique: Courant alternatif à bas voltage. *J Physiol Pathol Gen* (Paris) 1:399–412.

Prevost JL, Batelli F (1900) Influence du nombre des périodes sur les effets mortels des courant alternatifs. *J Physiol Pathol Gen* (Paris) 2:755–766.

Puglisi JL, Savino GV, Valentinuzzi ME (1989) Defibrillation thresholds with multiple pulses and angular leads. *Rev Bras Eng Caderno Eng Bioméd* 6(2):569–576.

Ragheb T, Geddes LA. (1991) The polarization impedance of common electrode metals operated at low current density. *Ann Biomed Eng* 19(2):151–163.

Rashba EJ, Shorofsky SR, Peters RW, Gold MR (2004) Optimization of atrial defibrillation with a dual-coil active pectoral lead system. *J Cardiovasc Electrophysiol* 15:790–4.

Rashevsky N (1960) Mathematical Biophysics. Dover Publications, 3rd ed, New York, two volumes, 488 pp and 462 pp, respectively (see Chapter XXXI, pp. 379–388).

Rattes MF, Jones DL, Sharma AD, Klein GJ (1987) Defibrillation threshold: A simple and quantitative estimate of the ability to defibrillate. *Pacing Clin Electrophysiol* (PACE) 10(1):70–77; doi:10.1111/j.1540-8159.1987.tb05926.x.

Reuter H (1967) The dependence of slow inward currents in Purkinje fibres on the extracellular calcium concentration. *J Physiol* 192:479–492.

Reyes-Juárez JL, Juárez-Rubí R, Rodríguez G, Zarain-Herzberg A (2007) Transcriptional analysis of the human cardiac calsequestrin gene in cardiac and skeletal myocytes. *J Biol Chem* 282 (49):35554–35563.

Rials SJ, Wu Y, Ford N, Pauletto FJ, Abramson SV, Rubin AM, Marinchak RA, Kowey PR (1995) Effect of left ventricular hypertrophy and its regression on ventricular electrophysiology and vulnerability to inducible arrhythmia in the feline heart. *Circulation* 91:426–430.

Rials SJ, Wu Y, Xiaoping X, Filart RA, Marinchak RA, Kowey PR (1997) Regression of left ventricular hypertrophy with captopril restores normal ventricular action potential duration, dispersion of refractoriness, and vulnerability to inducible ventricular fibrillation. *Circulation* 96: 1330–1336.

Ridker PM, Hennekens ChH, Buring JE, Rifai N (2000) C-reactive protein and other markers of inflammation in the prediction of cardiovascular disease in women. *New Engl J Med* 342(12):836–843.

Robicsek F (1984) Biochemical termination of sustained fibrillation occurring after artificially induced ischemic arrest. *J Thorac Cardiovasc Surg* 87(1):143–145.

Robinovitch LG (1907) Resuscitation of electrocuted animals: Choice of the electric current and method used and application to human beings; experimental study of the respiration and blood pressure during electrocution and resuscitation. *J Mental Pathol* 8(2):74–81.

Robinovitch LG (1909) Induction coil specifically constructed according to our indication for purposes of resuscitation of subjects in a condition of apparent death caused by chloroform, morphine, electrocution, etc. *J Mental Pathology* 8(3):129–145.

Rogers JM, Ideker RE (2000) Editorial. Fibrillating myocardium: Rabbit Warren or Beehive? *Circ Res* 86:369.

Ruiz de Gauna S, Lazkano A, Ruiz J, Aramendi E (2004) Discrimination between ventricular tachycardia and ventricular fibrillation using the continuous Wavelet Transform. *Comput Cardiol* 31:21–24.

Ruiz E, Arredondo MT, Valentinuzzi ME, Peres da Costa C (1987) Ventricular fibrillation threshold: Influence of the type of electrical stimulus. *J Clin Eng* 12(3):233–237, May–June.

Ruiz GA, Felice CJ, Valentinuzzi ME (2005) Non-linear response of electrode-electrolyte interface at high current density. *Chaos Solitons Fractals* 25(3):649–654. Available on-line on March 2, 2005.

Ruiz E, Valentinuzzi ME (1994) Heart weight affects spontaneous defibrillation but not ventricular fibrillation threshold. *Pacing Clin Electrophysiol* (PACE) 17(12, Part I):2255–2262.

Santel DJ, Kallok MJ, Tacker WA (1985) Implantable defibrillator electrode systems: A brief review. *Pacing Clin Electrophysiol* (PACE) 8(1):123–131.

Savino G, Romanelli L, Gonzalez DL, Piro O, Valentinuzzi M (1989) Evidence for chaotic behavior in driven ventricles. *Biophys J* 56:273–280.

Savino GV, Ruiz E, Valentinuzzi ME (1983) Transventricular impedance during fibrillation. *IEEE Trans BME* 30(6):364–367.

Savino GV, Tirado MC, Valentinuzzi ME (1986) Decrease in transventricular impedance during successive defibrillation shocks. *Innov Technol Biol Med* 7(4):482–490.

Savino GV, Valentinuzzi ME (1988) Ventricular fibrillation-defibrillation in the toad *Bufo paracnemis. Int J Cardiol* 19(1):19–25.

Schreiber T and Schmitz A (2000) Surrogate time series. *Physica D*, 142(3–4):346–382.

Schwan HP (1968) Polarization impedance and measurements in biological materials. *Trans NY Acad Sci* 148:191–209.

Schechter DC (1971) Early experience with resuscitation by means of electricity. *Surgery* 69(3):360–372.

Schechter DC (1983) Exploring the Origins of Electrical Cardiac Stimulation. Medtronic, Inc., Minneapolis, MN, 181 pp. It can be found in The Bakken Museum.

Schuckers SA (2006) Automated arrhythmia analysis. In *Encyclopedia of Medical Devices*, ed John G. Webster, vol 1, pp. 69–84, John Wiley, Hoboken, New Jersey.

Shannon CE, Weaver W (1949) *The Mathematical Theory of Communication*, University of Illinois Press, Urbana, IL, 117 pp.

Shintani M, Linton O (2004) Nonparametric neural network estimation of Lyapunov exponents and a direct test for chaos. *J Econometrics* 120(1):1–33.

Silberberg J (1993) Performance degradation of electronic medical devices due to electromagnetic interference. *Compliance Eng* 10(5), Fall. An updated version was published in *Compliance Engineering's European Edition's 1995 Annual Reference Guide* with the title "Electronic medical devices and EMI" (pp. F-10–F-15); http://www.ce-mag.com.

Small M (2005) Applied Nonlinear Time Series Analysis. World Scientific Publishers, Singapore, Applications in Physics, Physiology and Finance.

Small M, Judd K, and Mees AI (2001) Testing time series for nonlinearity. *Statistics Comput* 11:257–268.

Small M, Yu DJ, Harrison RG, Robertson C, Clegg G, Holzer M, Sterz F (1999) Characterizing nonlinearity in ventricular fibrillation. *Comput Cardiol* 26:17–20.

Smith LA, Ziehmann C, Fraedrich K (1999) Uncertainty dynamics and predictability in chaotic systems. *Q J Research Meteorol Soc* 125:2855–2886.

Smith WT, Fleet WF, Johnson TA, Engle CL, Cascio WE (1995) The Ib phase of ventricular arrhythmias in ischemic *in situ* porcine heart is related to changes in cell-to-cell electrical coupling. *Circulation* 92:3051–3060.

Sosa Liprandi, María I., Harwicz, Paola S. y Sosa Liprandi Álvaro (2006) Causas de muerte en la mujer y su tendencia en los últimos 23 años en la Argentina. (In Spanish, Women death causes in Argentina and its tendency during the last 23 years). *Revista Argentina de Cardiología* July/August 74(4):297–303; http://www.scielo.org.ar/scielo.php?pid=S1850-37482006000500007&script=sci_arttext.

Steinhaus DM, Cardinal DS, Mongeon L, Musley SK, Foley L, Corrigan S (2002) Internal defibrillation: Pain perception of low energy shocks. *Pacing Clin Electrophysiol* (PACE) 25:1090–1093; doi:10.1046/j.1460-9592.2002.01090.x.

Strickberger SA, Man K, Souza J, Zivin A, Weiss R, Knight BP, Goyal R, Daoud EG, Morady F (2007) A prospective evaluation of two defibrillation safety margin techniques in patients with low defibrillation energy requirements. *J Cardiovasc Electrophysiol* 9(1):41–46.

Strohmenger HU, Hemmer W, Lindner KL, Schickling J, Brown, CG (1997) Median fibrillation frequency in cardiac surgery: Influence of temperature and guide to countershock therapy. *Chest* 111:1560–1564; http://chestjournals.org/cgi/content/abstract/111/6/1560.

Strohmenger HU, Eftestol T, Sunde K, Wenzel V, Mair M, Ulmer H, Lindner KH, Steen PA (2001) The predictive value of ventricular fibrillation: Electrocardiogram signal frequency and amplitude variables in patients with out-of-hospital cardiac arrest. *Anaesth Analg* 93:1428–1433.

Suárez JE, Bravo AI (2006) Conexinas y sistema cardiovascular (in Spanish, Connexins and the cardiovascular system). *Revista Argentina Cardiología* (Buenos Aires) 74(2):March/April.

Swerdlow C, Shehata M, Belk P, Cao J, Kremers MS, Saba S (2007) Automatic determination of the upper limit of vulnerability using ICD electrograms. *Circulation* 116:II-535.

SWORD (1996) Effect of d-sotalol on mortality in patients with left ventricular dysfunction after recent and remote myocardial infarction. *Lancet* 348: 7–12.

Tacker WA, Geddes LA (1980) Electrical Defibrillation. CRC Press, Boca Raton, FL, USA, 192 pp.

Tang AS, Yabe S, Wharton JM, Dolker M, Smith WM, Ideker RE (1989) Ventricular defibrillation using biphasic waveforms: The importance of phasic duration. *J Am Coll Cardiol* 13:207–214.

Tang W, Weil MH, Sun S, Povoas HP, Klouche K, Kamohara T, Bisera J (2001) A comparison of biphasic and monophasic waveform defibrillation after prolonged ventricular fibrillation. *Chest* 120:948–954.

Taskinen S, Kovanen PT, Jarva H, Meri S, Pentikainen MO (2002) Binding of C-reactive protein to modified low-density-lipoprotein particles: Identification of cholesterol as a novel ligand for C-reactive protein. *Biochem J* 367:403–412.

Thakor NV (1984) From Holter monitors to automatic defibrillators: Developments in ambulatory arrhythmia monitoring. *IEEE Trans Biomed Eng* 31 (12):770–778.

Thakor N, Zhu Y, Pan K (1990) Ventricular tachycardia and fibrillation detection by a sequential hypothesis testing algorithm. *IEEE Trans Biomed Eng* 37:837–843.

Thomas ED, Ewy GA, Dahl CF, Ewy MD (1977) Effectiveness of direct current defibrillation: role of paddle electrode size. *Am Heart J* 93(4):463–467.

Throne RD, Jenkins JM, DiCarlo LA (1991) A comparison of four new time-domain techniques for discriminating monomorphic ventricular tachycardia from sinus rhythm using ventricular waveform morphology. *IEEE Trans Biomed Eng* 38 (6):561–570.

Todd MM (1983) Atrial fibrillation induced by the right atrial injection of cold fluids during thermodilution cardiac output determination: A case report. *Anesthesiology* 59(3):253–255.

Toivonen L, Viitasalo M, Jarvinen A (1992) The performance of the probability density function in differentiating supraventricular from ventricular rhythms. *Pacing Clin Electrophysiol* (PACE) 15:726–730.

Toyomi S, Noriyuki T, Takio S (1959) Directional difference of conduction velocity in the cardiac ventricular syncytium studied by microelectrodes. *Circ Res* 7:262.

Trayanova N (2008) The long and the short of long and short duration ventricular fibrillation. *Circ Res* 102:1151.

Traube L (1872) Ein Fall von Pulsus bigeminus nebst Bemerkungen über die Leberschwellungen bei Klappenfehlern und über akute Leberatrophie (A case of bigeminal pulse together with remarks about liver swelling due to valvular insufficiency and about acute hepatic atrophy). *Berl Klin Wochenschr* 9:185–188.

Troup P (1990) Early development of defibrillation devices. *IEEE Eng Med Biol Magazine* 9(2):19–24; ISSN: 0739-5175, doi:10.1109/51.57861.

Tyson JJ, Glass L (2004) Arthur T. Winfree (1942–2002), Editorial. *J Theor Biology* 230:433–439.

Ujhelyi M, Hoyt RH, Burns K, Fishman RS, Musley S, Silverman MH (2004) Nitrous oxide sedation reduces discomfort caused by atrial defibrillation shocks. *Pacing Clin Electrophysiol* (PACE) 27(4):485–491; doi:10.1111/j.1540-8159.2004.00468.x.

Ujhelyi MR, Sims JJ, Dubin SA, Vender J, Winecoff Miller A (2001) Defibrillation energy requirements and electrical heterogeneity during total body hypothermia. *Cri Care Med* 29(5):1006–1011.

Upile T, Jerjes W, Maaytah M, Singh S, Hopper C, Mahil J (2006) Reversible atrial fibrillation secondary to a mega-oesophagus. *BMC Ear Nose Throat Disord.* 6:15; doi:10.1186/1472-6815-6-15. Electronic version at www.biomedcentral.com/1472-6815/6/15.

Vaidya D, Morley GE, Samie FH, Jalife J (1999) Reentry and fibrillation in the mouse heart: A challenge to the critical mass hypothesis. *Circ Res* 85:174–181. On line version at http://circres.ahajournals.org/cgi/content/full/85/2/174.

Valencia Martín J, Climent Payá VE, Marín Ortuño F, Monmeneu Menadas JV, Martínez Martínez JG, García Martínez M, Criado A, García de Burgos Rico F, Sogorb Garri F (2002) The efficacy of scheduled cardioversion in atrial fibrillation. Comparison of two schemes of treatment: Electrical versus pharmacological cardioversion. *Revista Española Cardiol* 55(2):113–120 (in Spanish).

Valentinuzzi ME (1995) Defibrillation energy (Letter to the Editor) PACE, 18:1465–1466.

Valentinuzzi ME (2004) A new beginning for human health. *IEEE/EMB Magazine,* July–August, 23(4):67–72.

Valentinuzzi ME (2004) Understanding the Human Machine: A Primer for Bioengineering. World Scientific Publisher, New Jersey & Singapore, 396 pp, 8 chapters. Series on Bioengineering & Biomedical Engineering, volume. 4, ISBN: 981-238-930-X & ISBN: 981-256-043-2 (pbk); see the section on Essentials of Electrophysiology.

Valentinuzzi ME (2008) Honor Thy Profesión. Chapter 62 in *Career Development in Bioengineering and Biotechnology,* eds Guruprasad Madhavan, Barbara Oakley & Luis Kun, Springer Verlag.

Valentinuzzi ME (2010) Leslie A. Geddes . . . Farewell. *Biomed Eng On Line* 9:1 Jan 5.

Valentinuzzi ME, Arredondo MT, Monzón JE, Armayor MR, Clavin OE, Guillén SG, Ruiz E, Savino GV, Valdez E, Chialvo DR, Spinelli JC (1986) Fibrilación-Defibrilación Cardíaca: Revisión Crítica (Cardiac Fibrillation-Defibrillation: Critical Review). Intermédica, Buenos Aires, (xvii + 129) pp.(in Spanish).

Valentinuzzi ME, Baker LE, Powell T (1974) Heart rate response to the Valsalva maneuver. *Med Biol Eng* 12(6):817–822.

Valentinuzzi ME, Hoff HE (1970) Catheterization in the snake: Correlation of cardiac events. *Cardiovasc Res Center Bull* (Houston, TX)8(3):102–118.

Valentinuzzi ME, Hoff HE (1972) The sinus venosus-atrial Wenckebach-Luciani phenomenon. *J Electrocardiol* 5:1–14.

Valentinuzzi ME, Hoff HE, Geddes LA (1973) A two compartment model for the release and action of acetylcholine in the heart. *Circ Res* 33(5):532–538.

Valentinuzzi ME, Ruiz E, Peres da Costa C (1984) Ventricular fibrillation thresholds in the three-toed sloth (*Bradypus tridactylus*). *Acta Physiol Pharmacol Latinoam* 34:313–322.

van der Pol B, van der Mark J (1928) The heartbeat considered as a relaxation oscillation and an electrical model of the heart. *Phil Mag* (Suppl) 6, 763–775. Also in *Arch Neerdl de Physiol de l'Homme et des Animaux* 1929, 14:418–443.

Veltri EP, Mower MM, Mirowski M (1988) Ambulatory monitoring of the automatic implantable cardioverter-defibrillator: A practical guide. *Pacing Clin Electrophysiol* (PACE) 11(3):315–25.

Verrier RL, Brooks WW, Lown B (1978) Protective zone and the determination of vulnerability to ventricular fibrillation threshold. *Am J Physiol* 234(5):H592–H596.

Verrier RL, Lown B (1982) Prevention of ventricular fibrillation by use of low-intensity electrical stimuli. *Ann N Y Acad Sci* 382:355–370.

Verrier RL, Calvert A, Lown B (1975) Effect of posterior hypothalamic stimulation on ventricular fibrillation threshold. *Am J Physiol* 228(3): 923–927.

Vulpian EFA (1874) Note sur les effets de la faradisation directe des ventricules du coeur du chien. *Arch Physiol* i:975.

Wang TJ, Massaro JM, Levy D, Vasan RS, Wolf PA, D'Agostino RB, Larson MG, Kannel WB, Benjamin EJ (2003) A risk score for predicting stroke or death for individuals with new-onset atrial fibrillation in the community: The Framingham Heart Study. *J Am Med Assoc* (JAMA) 290:1049–1056.

Ware DL, Atkinson JB, Brooks MJ, Echt DS (1993) Ventricular defibrillation in canines with chronic infarction, and effects of lidocaine and procainamide. *Pacing Clin Electrophysiol* (PACE) 16(2):337–346.

Webster JG (ed.) (2006) *Encyclopedia of Medical Devices and Instrumentation.* Wiley-Interscience, ISBN: 978-0471263586.

Weiss G (1901) Sur la possibilité de render comparables entre eux les appareils servant a l'excitation électrique. *Arch Italian Biol* 35:413–447.

Weiss JN, Chen P-S, Qu Z, Karagueuzian HS, and Garfinkel A (2000) How do we stop the waves from breaking? *Circ Res* 87:1103–1107.

Weiss JN, Garfinkel A, Karagueuzian HS, Qu Z, Chen PS (1999) Chaos and the transition to ventricular fibrillation: A new approach to antiarrhythmic drug evaluation. *Circulation* 99(21):2819–2826.

Westrum BL (1993) Adaptive-Rate Pacing. Perspectives in Cardiac Rhythm Management. Cardiac Pacemakers, Inc., Saint, MN, 114 pp.

Whang Y-J, Linton O (1999) The asymptotic distribution of nonparametric estimates of the Lyapunov exponent for stochastic time series. *J Econometrics* 91(1):1–42.

White, RD (1997) Early out-of-hospital experience with an impedance compensating low-energy biphasic waveform automatic external defibrillator. *J Intervent Cardiac Electrophysiol* 1:203–208.

Wiggers C, Wegria R (1940) Ventricular fibrillation due to single localized induction and condenser shocks applied during the vulnerable phase of ventricular systole. *Am J Physiol* 128:500–505.

Wilson CM, Bailey A, Allen JD, Anderson J, Adgey AAJ (1989) Cardiac injury with damped sine and trapezoidal defibrillator waveforms. *Eur Heart J* 10(7):628–636.

Winfree (1970) Integrated view of the resetting of a circadian clock. *J Theor Biol* 28:327–374.

Winfree AT (1972) Spiral waves of chemical activity. *Science* 175:634–636.

Winfree AT (1973) Scroll shaped waves of chemical activity in three-dimensions. *Science* 181:634–636.

Winfree AT (1983) Sudden cardiac death: A problem in topology? *Scientific American* 248(5):144–161.

Winfree AT (1994) Electrical turbulence in three-dimensional heart muscle. *Science* 266:1003–1006.

Winecoff, AP, Sims JJ, Markel, ML, Ujhelyi MR (1997) Pinacidil's effects on defibrillation outcomes: Role of increased potassium conductance via the KATP channel. *J Cardiovasc Pharmacol Ther* 2(3):171–180; doi:10.1177/107424849700200304.

Witkowski FX, Penkoske PA, Plonsey R (1990) Mechanism of cardiac defibrillation in open-chest dogs with unipolar dc-coupled simultaneous activation and shock potential recordings. *Circulation* 82(1):244–260.

Wu T-J, Yashima M, Doshi R, Kim YH, Athill CA, Ong JJ, Czer L, Trento A, Blanche C, Kass RM, Garfinkel A, Weiss JN, Fishbein MC, Karagueuzian HS, Chen PS (1999) Relation between cellular repolarization characteristics and critical mass for human ventricular fibrillation. *J Cardiovasc Electrophysiol* 10:1077–1086.

Yuan Q, Fan GC, Dong M, Altschafl B, Diwan A, Ren X, Hahn HH, Zhao W, Waggoner JR, Jones LR, Jones WK, Bers DM, Dorn GW, Wang HS, Valdivia HH, Chu G, Kranias EG (2007) Sarcoplasmic reticulum calcium overloading in junctin deficiency enhances cardiac contractility but increases ventricular automaticity. *Circulation* Published online Jan 15; doi:10.1161/CIRCULATIONAHA.106.654699.

Zaritski RM, Ju J, Ashkenazi, (2005) Spontaneous formation of multiarmed spiral waves in various simple excitable media. *Intern J Bifurc Chaos* 15(12):4087–4094.

Zhabotinsky AM (1964) Periodic processes of malonic acid oxidation in a liquid phase (in Russian)*Biofizika* 9:306–311.

Zhang Y R, Ramabadran S, Boddicker KA, Bawaney I, Davies LR, Zimmerman MB, Wuthrich S, Jones JL, Kerber RE (2003) Triphasic waveforms are superior to biphasic waveforms for transthoracic defibrillation. *J Am Coll Cardiol* 42:568–575, doi:10.1016/S0735-1097(03)00656-9.

Zhang X, Zhu Y, Thakor N, Wang Z (1999) Detecting ventricular tachycardia and fibrillation by complexity measure. *IEEE Trans Biomed Eng* 46:548–555.

Zimmerman D, Farkhani F, Wesley RC (1994) Automated precision current delivery: An alternative method for cardiac defibrillation. *Pacing Clin Electrophysiol* (PACE) 17:595–602.

Zipes DP (1975) Electrophysiological mechanisms involved in ventricular fibrillation. *Circulation* 41–52(Suppl III):120–130.

Zipes DP, Fisher J, King RM, Nicoll A, Jolly WW (1975) Termination of ventricular fibrillation in dogs by depolarizing a critical amount of myocardium. *Am J Cardiol* 36:37–44.

Zoll PM, Linenthal AJ, Gibson W (1956) Termination of ventricular fibrillation in man by externally applied electric counter-shock. *New Engl J Med* 254:727–732.

# ABOUT THE AUTHORS

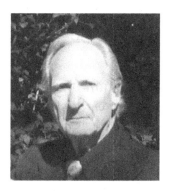

Max E. Valentinuzzi
Professor and Career Investigator
*Universidad de Buenos Aires* (UBA)
and
*Consejo Nacional de Investigaciones
Científicas y Técnicas* (CONICET)
Argentina
maxvalentinuzzi@arnet.com.ar

**Max E. Valentinuzzi**, native of Buenos Aires City, graduated as Telecommunications Engineer at the University of Buenos Aires and earned a PhD in Physiology and Biophysics from Baylor College of Medicine (Houston, Texas, USA). For several years, he developed his activities in the latter moving, thereafter, back to Argentina to the National University of Tucumán. Currently, he is Honorary Professor with the Institute of Biomedical Engineering at the University of Buenos Aires and Honorary Fellow Investigator of the National Research Council of Argentina (CONICET). Recognized with several awards, he produced more than 100 papers in the fields of bioimpedance, cardiovascular system, numerical deconvolution and education (http://www.ieeeghn.org/wiki/index.php/Max_Valentinuzzi_Oral_History). Textbook by the same author: *Understanding the Human Machine. A Primer for Bioengineering*, WSPC, Singapore, 2004.

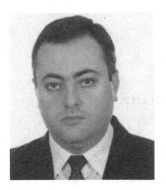

Eric Laciar Leber
Professor and Career Investigator
*Universidad Nacional de San Juan* (UNSJ)
and
*Consejo Nacional de Investigaciones
Científicas y Técnicas* (CONICET)
Argentina

**Eric Laciar Leber** was born in San Juan, Argentina, in 1970. He received his Electronics Engineering degree (with honours) from *Universidad Nacional de San Juan* (UNSJ), San Juan (Argentina), in 1997, and PhD degree in Biomedical Engineering from *Universitat Politècnica de Catalunya*, Barcelona (Spain), in 2004. Currently, he is a Professor in the *Departamento de Electrónica y Automática* of the UNSJ and a Career Investigator of *Consejo Nacional de Investigaciones Científicas y Técnicas* (CONICET). His research areas include digital processing and analysis of biomedical signals in cardiorespiratory and brain diseases.

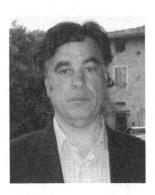

Diego González
Investigator
*Consiglio Nazionale delle Ricerche* (CNR)
and
*Università di Bologna*
Italy

**Diego L. Gonzalez** was born in Buenos Aires, Argentina, in 1951. He qualified as a pianoforte Professor in 1971. He received his degree in Physics from the University of La Plata in Argentina in 1981 and the PhD on Theoretical Physics from the same University in 1987. His PhD focused on synchronisation and chaos in non-linear oscillators. He worked from 1988 for the Italian CNR at LAMEL Institute in the field of microelectronics and from 1999 to 2008, he collaborated with the Acoustical Laboratory of the St. George School Foundation and the CNR at Venice. Presently, he is with the CNR Institute for Microsystems and Microelectronics and Associate Researcher of the Statistical Department of Bologna University. His main research interests are the theory of non-linear dynamics and chaos and their application to the modelling of complex dynamical systems, with particular emphasis on biological systems. In this last field, Dr. Gonzalez has developed an original theory about the pitch perception of complex sounds based on qualitative non-linear modelling, and is at present developing a new mathematical theory of the genetic code. Dr. Gonzalez has published more than 70 works in the field of non-linear dynamics and its applications to the modelling of biological and physical systems.

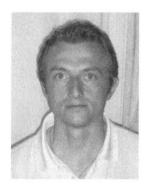

Simone Giannerini
Professor and Investigator
Department of Statistics
*Università di Bologna*
Italy

**Simone Giannerini** was born in 1970 in Castiglione dei Pepoli (Bologna). He received his degree in Statistics and a PhD in Statistics from Bologna University. He also obtained a MSc in Statistics from the London School of Economics. Since 2005 he has been Assistant Professor at the Statistics Department, Bologna University. His research interests include time series analysis, the connections between chaos theory and statistics with applications in biology, physics and econometrics.

# INDEX